NURSE POCKET DRUG GUIDE 2006

P9-ECR-563

EDITOR

Judith A. Barberio, PhD, APRN, BC-ANP, GNP, FNP
Assistant Professor
Rutgers, The State University of New Jersey
College of Nursing
Newark, New Jersey

CONSULTING EDITOR

Leonard G. Gomella, MD, FACS
The Bernard W. Godwin, Jr., Professor
Chairman, Department of Urology
Jefferson Medical College
Thomas Jefferson University
Philadelphia, Pennsylvania

McGraw-Hill
MEDICAL PUBLISHING DIVISION
New York Chicago San Francisco Lisbon London Madrid Mexico City Milan
New Delhi San Juan Seoul Singapore Sydney Toronto

The McGraw·Hill Companies

Nurse's Pocket Drug Guide 2006

Copyright © 2006 by Judith A. Barberio. Based on *Clinician's Pocket Drug Reference 2005*. Copyright © 2005 by Leonard G. Gomella. Published by The McGraw-Hill Companies, Inc. All rights reserved. Printed in Canada. Except as permitted under the United States Copyright Act of 1976, no part of this publication may be reproduced or distributed in any form or by any means, or stored in a data base or retrieval system, without the prior written permission of the publisher.

1 2 3 4 5 6 7 8 9 0   WBCWBC   0 9 8 7 6 5 4

ISBN: 0-07-145731-3
ISSN: 1550-2554

Notice

Medicine is an ever-changing science. As new research and clinical experience broaden our knowledge, changes in treatment and drug therapy are required. The authors and the publisher of this work have checked with sources believed to be reliable in their efforts to provide information that is complete and generally in accord with the standards accepted at the time of publication. However, in view of the possibility of human error or changes in medical sciences, neither the authors nor the publisher nor any other party who has been involved in the preparation or publication of this work warrants that the information contained herein is in every respect accurate or complete, and they disclaim all responsibility for any errors or omissions or for the results obtained from use of the information contained in this work. Readers are encouraged to confirm the information contained herein with other sources. For example and in particular, readers are advised to check the product information sheet included in the package of each drug they plan to administer to be certain that the information contained in this work is accurate and that changes have not been made in the recommended dose or in the contraindications for administration. This recommendation is of particular importance in connection with new or infrequently used drugs.

This book was set in Times Roman by Pine Tree Composition, Inc.
The editors were Janet Foltin and Harriet Lebowitz.
The production supervisor was Sherri Souffrance.
Project management was provided by Pine Tree Composition, Inc.
The cover designer was Mary McKeon.
The text designer was Marsha Cohen/Parallelogram Graphics.
The index was prepared by Ann Salinger
Webcom Limited was printer and binder.

This book is printed on acid-free paper.

CONTENTS

ASSOCIATE EDITORS

Aimee Gelhot Adams, PharmD
Director, Primary Care Pharmacy
  Practice Residency
University of Kentucky Medical
  Center
Assistant Professor
College of Pharmacy and Depart-
  ment of Medicine
University of Kentucky
Lexington, Kentucky

Steven A. Haist, MD, MS, FACP
Professor of Medicine
Division of General Medicine
Department of Internal Medicine
University of Kentucky Medical
  Center
Lexington, Kentucky

Kelly M. Smith, PharmD
Associate Professor
Division of Pharmacy Practice and
  Science
University of Kentucky College of
  Pharmacy
Director, Drug Information Center
University of Kentucky Medical
  Center
Lexington, Kentucky

PREFACE

On behalf of the entire editorial board, we are pleased to present the second edition of the *Nurse's Pocket Drug Guide*. This book is based on the basic drug presentation style used since 1983 in the *Clinician's Pocket Reference*.

Our goal is to identify the most frequently used and clinically important medications and herbs based on input from our readers and editorial board. The book includes over 1000 generic medications and herbs and is designed to represent a cross section of those used in health care practices across the country.

The style of drug presentation includes key "must know" facts of commonly used medications and herbs, which represents the essential information for both the student and practicing nurse, and health care provider. A unique feature is the inclusion of common uses of medications and herbs rather than just the official labeled indications. These recommendations are based on the actual uses of the medication and herbs supported by publications and community standards of care. All uses have been reviewed by our editorial board. New in this edition is the inclusion of antimicrobial spectrum for the majority of antibiotics, useful for accurate prescribing practices.

It is essential that students, registered nurses, and advanced-practice nurses learn more than the name and dose of the medications they prescribe and administer. Certain common side effects and significant contraindications are associated with most prescription medications. Although nurses and other health care practitioners should ideally be completely familiar with the entire package insert of any medication prescribed, such a requirement is unreasonable. References such as the *Physician's Desk Reference* and in many cases the drug manufacturer's Web site make package inserts readily available for many medications, but may not provide key data for generic drugs and those available over the counter. The limitations of difficult-to-read package inserts were acknowledged by the Food and Drug Administration in early 2001, when it noted that health care providers do not have time to read the many pages of small print in the typical package insert. In the future, package inserts will likely be redesigned to ensure that important drug interactions, contraindications, and common side effects are highlighted for easier practitioner reference. We have made this key prescribing information available to you now in this pocket-sized book. Information in this book is meant for use by health care professionals who are familiar with these commonly prescribed medications.

We are pleased about the popularity of the first edition. The previous edition has been completely reviewed and updated by our editorial board. Over three dozen key new medications and thirty herbs have been added, with changes in indications and available forms of other drugs updated based on new FDA approvals.

We express special thanks to our families for their support of this book and the entire project. The contributions of the members of the editorial board are deeply appreciated. Janet Foltin, Linda Davoli, and the team at McGraw-Hill have been supportive in our goal of creating a pocket reference for nursing professionals.

Your comments and suggestions are always welcome and encouraged because improvements to this book would be impossible without the interest and feedback of our readers. We hope this book will help you learn some of the key elements in prescribing medications and allow you to care for your patients in the best way possible.

Judith A. Barberio, PhD, APRN, BC-ANP, GNP, FNP
Newark, NJ
JABPHD83@aol.com

Leonard G. Gomella, MD, FACS
Philadelphia, PA
Leonard.Gomella@jefferson.edu

MEDICATION KEY

Medications are listed by prescribing class, and the individual medications are then listed in alphabetical order by generic name. Some of the more commonly recognized trade names are listed for each medication (in parentheses after the generic name).

> **Generic Drug Name (Selected Common Brand Names [Controlled Substance])** WARNING: Summary of the "Black Box" precautions that are deemed necessary by the FDA. These are significant precautions and contraindications concerning the individual medication. **Uses:** This includes both FDA labeled indications bracketed by * and other "off label" uses of the medication. Because many medications are used to treat various conditions based on the medical literature and not listed in their package insert, we list common uses of the medication rather than the official "labeled indications" (FDA approved) based on input from our editorial board **Action:** How the drug works. This information is helpful in comparing classes of drugs and understanding side effects and contraindications. *Spectrum:* Included for most antibiotics **Dose:** *Adults.* Where no specific pediatric dose is given, the implication is that this drug is not commonly used or indicated in that age group. At the end of the dosing line, important dosing modifications may be noted (ie, take with food, avoid antacids, etc) **Caution:** [pregnancy/fetal risk categories, breast-feeding] cautions concerning the use of the drug in specific settings **Contra:** Contraindications **Supplied: Common dosing forms** SE: Common or significant side effects **Notes:** Other key information about the drug. **Interactions:** Common drug—drug, drug—herb, and drug—food interactions that may change the drug response **Labs:** Common laboratory test results that are changed by the drug or significant lab monitoring requirements **NIPE:** Nursing Indications and/or Patient Education) Significant information that the nurse must be aware of with administration of the drug or information that should be given to any patient taking the drug.

CONTROLLED SUBSTANCE CLASSIFICATION

Medications under the control of the US Drug Enforcement Agency (Schedule I–V controlled substances) are indicated by the symbol [C]. Most medications are "uncontrolled" and do not require a DEA prescriber number on the prescription. The following is a general description for the schedules of DEA controlled substances:

Schedule (C-I) I: All nonresearch use forbidden (eg, heroin, LSD, mescaline, etc).

Schedule (C-II) II: High addictive potential; medical use accepted. No telephone call-in prescriptions; no refills. Some states require special prescription form (eg, cocaine, morphine, methadone).

Schedule (C-III) III: Low to moderate risk of physical dependence, high risk of psychologic dependence; prescription must be rewritten after 6 months or five refills (eg, acetaminophen plus codeine).

Schedule (C-IV) IV: Limited potential for dependence; prescription rules same as for schedule III (eg, benzodiazepines, propoxyphene).

Schedule (C-V) V: Very limited abuse potential; prescribing regulations often same as for uncontrolled medications; some states have additional restrictions.

FDA FETAL RISK CATEGORIES

Category A: Adequate studies in pregnant women have not demonstrated a risk to the fetus in the first trimester of pregnancy; there is no evidence of risk in the last two trimesters.

Category B: Animal studies have not demonstrated a risk to the fetus, but no adequate studies have been done in pregnant women.

or

Animal studies have shown an adverse effect, but adequate studies in pregnant women have not demonstrated a risk to the fetus during the first trimester of pregnancy and there is no evidence of risk in the last two trimesters.

Category C: Animal studies have shown an adverse effect on the fetus, but no adequate studies have been done in humans. The benefits from the use of the drug in pregnant women may be acceptable despite its potential risks.

or

No animal reproduction studies and no adequate studies in humans have been done.

Category D: There is evidence of human fetal risk, but the potential benefits from the use of the drug in pregnant women may be acceptable despite its potential risks.

Category X: Studies in animals or humans or adverse reaction reports, or both, have demonstrated fetal abnormalities. The risk of use in pregnant women clearly outweighs any possible benefit.

Category ?: No data available (not a formal FDA classification; included to provide complete data set).

BREAST-FEEDING

No formally recognized classification exists for drugs and breast-feeding. This shorthand was developed for the *Clinician's Pocket Drug Reference*.

+   Compatible with breast-feeding
M   Monitor patient or use with caution
+/–   Excreted, or likely excreted, with unknown effects or at unknown concentrations
?/–   Unknown excretion, but effects likely to be of concern
–   Contraindicated in breast-feeding
?   No data available

ABBREVIATIONS

ac: before meals (*ante cibum*)
ABMT: autologous bone marrow transplantation
ACE: angiotensin-converting enzyme
ACEI: angiotensin-converting enzyme inhibitor
ACLS: advanced cardiac life support
ACS: acute coronary syndrome
ADH: antidiuretic hormone
ADHD: attention-deficit hyperactivity disorder
AF: atrial fibrillation
Al: aluminum
ALL: acute lymphocytic leukemia
ALT: alanine aminotransferase
AMI: acute myocardial infarction
AML: acute myelogenous leukemia
amp: ampule
ANC: absolute neutrophil count
aPTT: activated partial thromboplastin time
APAP: acetaminophen [*N*-acetyl-*p*-aminophenol]
ARB: angiotensin II receptor blocker
ARDS: adult respiratory distress syndrome
ASA: aspirin (acetylsalicylic acid)
AUC: area under the curve
AV: atrioventricular
AVM: arteriovenous malformation
BB: beta-blocker
BCL: B-cell lymphoma

BMT: bone marrow transplantation
BSA: body surface area
BUN: blood urea nitrogen
Ca: calcium
CA: cancer
CAD: coronary artery disease
cap: capsule
CAP: cancer of prostate
CBC: complete blood count
CCB: calcium channel blocker
CF: cystic fibrosis
CHF: congestive heart failure
CLL: chronic lymphocytic leukemia
CML: chronic myelogenous leukemia
CMV: cytomegalovirus
CNS: central nervous system
Contra: contraindicated
COPD: chronic obstructive pulmonary disease
CP: chest pain
CPP: central precocious puberty
CR: controlled release
CrCl: creatinine clearance
CRF: chronic renal failure
CV: cardiovascular
CVA: cerebrovascular accident
CVH: common variable hypergammaglobulinemia
D_5LR: 5% dextrose in lactated Ringer's solution
D_5NS: 5% dextrose in normal saline
D_5W: 5% dextrose in water

DC: discontinue

DI: diabetes insipidus

DKA: diabetic ketoacidosis

dL: deciliter

DN: diabetic nephropathy

DVT: deep venous thrombosis

Dz: disease

EC: enteric-coated

ECC: emergency cardiac care

ECG: electrocardiogram

ELISA: enzyme-linked immunosorbent assay

EPS: extrapyramidal symptoms

ESRD: end-stage renal disease

ET: endotracheal

EtOH: ethanol

ext: extract

Fe: iron

FSH: follicle-stimulating hormone

5-FU: fluorouracil

Fxn: function

g: gram

GABA: gamma-aminobutyric acid

G-CSF: granulocyte colony-stimulating factor

GERD: gastroesophageal reflux disease

GFR: glomerular filtration rate

GH: growth hormone

GI: gastrointestinal

GIST: gastrointestinal stromal tumor

GM-CSF: granulocyte-macrophage colony-stimulating factor

GnRH: gonadotropin-releasing hormone

gt, gtt: drop, drops (*gutta*)

HA: headache

HCL: hairy cell leukemia

Hct: hematocrit

HCTZ: hydrochlorothiazide

HF: heart failure

Hgb: hemoglobin

HIT: heparin-induced thrombocytopenia

HIV: human immunodeficiency virus

HMG-CoA: hydroxymethylglutaryl coenzyme A

hs: at bedtime (*hora somni*)

HSV: herpes simplex virus

5-HT: 5-hydroxytryptamine

HTN: hypertension

Hx: history

I: iodine

IBD: irritable bowel disease

IBS: irritable bowel syndrome

ICP: intracranial pressure

Ig: immunoglobulin

IM: intramuscular

inf: infusion

INH: isoniazid

inj: injection

INR: international normalized ratio

I&O: intake and output

ISA: intrinsic sympathomimetic activity

IT: intrathecal

ITP: idiopathic thrombocytopenic purpura

IV: intravenous

K: potassium

L/d: liters per day

LDL: low-density lipoprotein

LFT: liver function test

LH: luteinizing hormone

LHRH: luteinizing hormone-releasing hormone

Li: lithium

liq: liquid

LMW: low molecular weight

LVD: left ventricular dysfunction

LVEF: left ventricular ejection fraction

MAC: *Mycobacterium avium* complex

MAO/MAOI: monoamine oxidase/in-hibitor

mEq: milliequivalent

Mg: magnesium

MI: myocardial infarction, mitral in-sufficiency

mL: milliliter

MRSA: methicillin-resistant *Staphylococcus aureus*

MS: multiple sclerosis

MSSA: methicillin-sensitive *Staphylococcus aureus*

MTT: monotetrazolium

MTX: methotrexate

MyG: myasthenia gravis

Na: sodium

ng: nanogram

NG: nasogastric

NHL: non-Hodgkin's lymphoma

NIDDM: non-insulin-dependent dia-betes mellitus

NPO: nothing by mouth (*nil per os*)

NS: normal saline

NSAID: nonsteroidal antiinflamma-tory drug

N/V: nausea and vomiting

N/V/D: nausea, vomiting, diarrhea

OCP: oral contraceptive pill

OD: overdose

OTC: over the counter

P: phosphorus

PAT: paroxysmal atrial tachycardia

pc: after eating (*post cibum*)

PCP: *Pneumocystis jiroveci* pneumo-nia

PCWP: pulmonary capillary wedge pressure

PDGF: platelet-derived growth factor

PE: pulmonary embolus, physical ex-amination, pleural effusion

PFT: pulmonary function test

pg: picogram

PID: pelvic inflammatory disease

plt: platelet

PMDD: premenstrual dysphoric dis-order

PO: by mouth (*per os*)

PPD: purified protein derivative

PR: by rectum

prep: preparation

PRG: pregnancy

PRN: as often as needed (*pro re nata*)

PSA: prostate-specific antigen

PSVT: paroxysmal supraventricular tachycardia

Pt: patient

PT: prothrombin time

PTCA: percutaneous transluminal coronary angioplasty

PTH: parathyroid hormone

PTT: partial thromboplastin time

PUD: peptic ulcer disease

PVC: premature ventricular contrac-tion

PVD: peripheral vascular disease

PWP: pulmonary wedge pressure

q: every (*quaque*)

q_h: every _ hours

qd: every day

qh: every hour

qhs: every hour of sleep (before bed-time)

qid: four times a day (*quater in die*)

qod: every other day

RA: rheumatoid arthritis

RCC: renal cell carcinoma

RDA: recommended dietary al-lowance

RDS: respiratory distress syndrome

RSV: respiratory syncytial virus

RT: reverse transcriptase

RTA: renal tubular acidosis

Rx: treatment

Rxn: reaction

SCr: serum creatinine

SIADH: syndrome of inappropriate antidiuretic hormone

SL: sublingual

SLE: systemic lupus erythematosus

soln: solution

SPAG: small particle aerosol generator

SQ: subcutaneous

SSRI: selective serotonin reuptake inhibitor

SSS: sick sinus syndrome

S/Sxs: signs and symptoms

stat: immediately (*statim*)

suppl: supplement

supp: suppository

SVT: supraventricular tachycardia

Sx: symptom

Sz: seizure

tab/tabs: tablet/tablets

TB: tuberculosis

TCA: tricyclic antidepressant

TFT: thyroid function test

TIA: transient ischemic attack

tid: three times a day (*ter in die*)

tinc: tincture

TMP: trimethoprim

TMP–SMX: trimethoprim–sulfamethoxazole

TPA: tissue plasminogen activator

tri: trimester

tsp: teaspoon

TTP: thrombotic thrombocytopenic purpura

ULN: upper limits of normal

URI: upper respiratory infection

UTI: urinary tract infection

VF: ventricular fibrillation

VT: ventricular tachycardia

w/: with

WHI: Women's Health Initiative

w/in: within

wk: week

WNL: within normal limits

w/o: without

WPW: Wolff–Parkinson–White syndrome

wt: weight

ZE: Zollinger–Ellison (syndrome)

<: less than, younger than

>: greater than, older than

↑: increase

↓: decrease

⊘: not recommended, do not take

CLASSIFICATION (Generic and common brand names)

ALLERGY

Antihistamines

Azelastine (Astelin, Optivar)
Cetirizine (Zyrtec)
Chlorpheniramine (Chlor-Trimeton)
Clemastine Fumarate (Tavist)

Cyproheptadine (Periactin)
Desloratadine (Clarinex)
Diphenhydramine (Benadryl)

Fexofenadine (Allegra)
Hydroxyzine (Atarax, Vistaril)
Loratadine (Claritin, Alavert)

Miscellaneous Antiallergic Agents

Budesonide (Rhinocort, Pulmicort)

Cromolyn Sodium (Intal, NasalCrom, Opticrom)

Montelukast (Singulair)

ANTIDOTES

Acetylcysteine (Mucomyst)
Amifostine (Ethyol)
Charcoal (Superchar, Actidose, Liqui-Char Activated)

Dexrazoxane (Zinecard)
Digoxin Immune Fab (Digibind)
Flumazenil (Romazicon)
Ipecac Syrup (OTC Syrup)

Mesna (Mesnex)
Naloxone (Narcan)
Physostigmine (Antilirium)
Succimer (Chemet)

ANTIMICROBIAL AGENTS

Antibiotics

AMINOGLYCOSIDES
Amikacin (Amikin)
Gentamicin (Garamycin, G-Mycitin)

Neomycin
Streptomycin

Tobramycin (Nebcin)

CARBAPENEMS
Ertapenem (Invanz)

Imipenem–Cilastatin (Primaxin)

Meropenem (Merrem)

CEPHALOSPORINS, FIRST GENERATION

Cefadroxil (Duricef, Ultracef)

Cefazolin (Ancef, Kefzol)

Cephalexin (Keflex, Keftab)

Cephradine (Velosef)

CEPHALOSPORINS, SECOND GENERATION

Cefaclor (Ceclor)

Cefmetazole (Zefazone)

Cefonicid (Monocid)

Cefotetan (Cefotan)

Cefoxitin (Mefoxin)

Cefprozil (Cefzil)

Cefuroxime (Ceftin [oral], Zinacef [parenteral])

Loracarbef (Lorabid)

CEPHALOSPORINS, THIRD GENERATION

Cefdinir (Omnicef)

Cefditoren (Spectracef)

Cefixime (Suprax)

Cefoperazone (Cefobid)

Cefotaxime (Claforan)

Cefpodoxime (Vantin)

Ceftazidime (Fortaz, Ceptaz, Tazidime, Tazicef)

Ceftibuten (Cedax)

Ceftizoxime (Cefizox)

Ceftriaxone (Rocephin)

CEPHALOSPORINS, FOURTH GENERATION

Cefepime (Maxipime)

FLUOROQUINOLONES

Ciprofloxacin (Cipro)

Gatifloxacin (Tequin)

Levofloxacin (Levaquin, Quixin Ophthalmic)

Lomefloxacin (Maxaquin)

Moxifloxacin (Avelox)

Norfloxacin (Noroxin)

Ofloxacin (Floxin, Ocuflox Ophthalmic)

Sparfloxacin (Zagam)

Trovafloxacin (Trovan)

MACROLIDES

Azithromycin (Zithromax)

Clarithromycin (Biaxin)

Dirithromycin (Dynabac)

Erythromycin (E-Mycin, E.E.S., Ery-Tab)

Erythromycin and Sulfisoxazole (Eryzole, Pediazole)

KETOLIDE

Telithromycin (Ketek)

PENICILLINS

Amoxicillin (Amoxil, Polymox)

Amoxicillin and Clavulanic Acid (Augmentin)

Ampicillin (Amcill, Omnipen)

Ampicillin–Sulbactam (Unasyn)

Dicloxacillin (Dynapen, Dycill)

Mezlocillin (Mezlin)

Nafcillin (Nallpen)

Oxacillin (Bactocill, Prostaphlin)

Penicillin G, Aqueous (Potassium or Sodium) (Pfizerpen, Pentids)

Penicillin G Benzathine
  (Bicillin)
Penicillin G Procaine
  (Wycillin)

Penicillin V (Pen-Vee K,
  Veetids)
Piperacillin (Pipracil)
Piperacillin–Tazobactam
  (Zosyn)

Ticarcillin (Ticar)
Ticarcillin/Potassium
  Clavulanate
  (Timentin)

TETRACYCLINES

Doxycycline
  (Vibramycin)

Tetracycline
  (Achromycin V,
  Sumycin)

MISCELLANEOUS ANTIBACTERIAL AGENTS

Aztreonam (Azactam)
Clindamycin (Cleocin,
  Cleocin-T)
Fosfomycin (Monurol)
Linezolid (Zyvox)
Metronidazole (Flagyl,
  MetroGel)

Quinupristin–Dalfo-
  pristin (Synercid)
Trimethoprim–
  Sulfamethoxazole
  [Co-Trimoxazole]
  (Bactrim, Septra)

Vancomycin (Vancocin,
  Vancoled)

Antifungals

Amphotericin B
  (Fungizone)
Amphotericin B Choles-
  teryl (Amphotec)
Amphotericin B Lipid
  Complex (Abelcet)
Amphotericin B Liposo-
  mal (AmBisome)
Caspofungin (Cancidas)

Clotrimazole (Lotrimin,
  Mycelex)
Clotrimazole and
  Betamethasone
  (Lotrisone)
Econazole (Spectazole)
Fluconazole (Diflucan)
Itraconazole (Sporanox)
Ketoconazole (Nizoral)

Miconazole (Monistat)
Nystatin (Mycostatin)
Oxiconazole (Oxistat)
Sertaconazole (Ertaczo)
Terbinafine (Lamisil)
Triamcinolone and
  Nystatin (Mycolog-II)
Voriconazole (VFEND)

Antimycobacterials

Clofazimine (Lamprene)
Dapsone (Avlosulfon)
Ethambutol (Myambutol)

Isoniazid (INH)
Pyrazinamide
Rifabutin (Mycobutin)

Rifampin (Rifadin)
Rifapentine (Priftin)
Streptomycin

Antiprotozoals

Nitazoxanide (Alinia)

Antiretrovirals

Abacavir (Ziagen)
Amprenavir (Agenerase)

Delavirdine (Rescriptor)
Didanosine [ddI] (Videx)

Efavirenz (Sustiva)
Fosamprenavir (Lexiva)

Indinavir (Crixivan)
Lamivudine (Epivir, Epivir-HBV)
Lopinavir/Ritonavir (Kaletra)

Nelfinavir (Viracept)
Nevirapine (Viramune)
Ritonavir (Norvir)
Saquinavir (Fortovase)
Stavudine (Zerit)

Tenofovir (Viread)
Zalcitabine (Hivid)
Zidovudine (Retrovir)
Zidovudine and Lamivudine (Combivir)

Antivirals

Acyclovir (Zovirax)
Adefovir (Hepsera)
Amantadine (Symmetrel)
Atazanavir (Reyataz)
Cidofovir (Vistide)
Emtricitabine (Emtriva)
Enfuvirtide (Fuzeon)
Famciclovir (Famvir)

Foscarnet (Foscavir)
Ganciclovir (Cytovene, Vitrasert)
Interferon Alfa-2b and Ribavirin Combination (Rebetron)
Oseltamivir (Tamiflu)
Palivizumab (Synagis)

Peg Interferon Alfa 2a (Pegasys)
Penciclovir (Denavir)
Ribavirin (Virazole)
Rimantadine (Flumadine)
Valacyclovir (Valtrex)
Valganciclovir (Valcyte)
Zanamivir (Relenza)

Miscellaneous Antimicrobial Agents

Atovaquone (Mepron)
Atovaquone/Proguanil (Malarone)

Pentamidine (Pentam 300, NebuPent)

Trimetrexate (Neutrexin)

ANTINEOPLASTIC AGENTS

Alkylating Agents

Altretamine (Hexalen)
Busulfan (Myleran, Busulfex)

Carboplatin (Paraplatin)
Cisplatin (Platinol)
Procarbazine (Matulane)

Triethylenetriphosphamide (Thio-Tepa, Tespa, TSPA)

NITROGEN MUSTARDS

Chlorambucil (Leukeran)
Cyclophosphamide (Cytoxan, Neosar)

Ifosfamide (Ifex, Holoxan)
Mechlorethamine (Mustargen)

Melphalan [L-PAM] (Alkeran)

NITROSOUREAS

Carmustine [BCNU] (BiCNU, Gliadel)

Streptozocin (Zanosar)

Antibiotics

Bleomycin Sulfate (Blenoxane)

Dactinomycin (Cosmegen)

Daunorubicin (Daunomycin, Cerubidine)

Doxorubicin
  (Adriamycin, Rubex)

Epirubicin (Ellence)
Idarubicin (Idamycin)

Mitomycin (Mutamycin)

Antimetabolites

Cytarabine [ARA-C]
  (Cytosar-U)
Cytarabine Liposome
  (DepoCyt)
Floxuridine (FUDR)
Fludarabine Phosphate
  (Flamp, Fludara)

Fluorouracil [5-FU]
  (Adrucil)
Gemcitabine (Gemzar)
Mercaptopurine [6-MP]
  (Purinethol)
Methotrexate (MRX,
  Folex, Rheumatrex)

6-Thioguanine [6-TG]
  (Tabloid)

Hormones

Abarelix (Plenaxis)
Anastrozole (Arimidex)
Bicalutamide
  (Casodex)
Estramustine Phosphate
  (Estracyt, Emcyt)
Exemestane (Aromasin)

Fluoxymesterone
  (Halotestin)
Flutamide (Eulexin)
Fulvestrant (Faslodex)
Goserelin (Zoladex)
Leuprolide (Lupron,
  Viadur, Eligard)

Levamisole (Ergamisol)
Megestrol Acetate
  (Megace)
Nilutamide (Nilandron)
Tamoxifen (Nolvadex)
Triptorelin (Trelstar
  Depot, Trelstar LA)

Mitotic Inhibitors

Etoposide [VP-16]
  (VePesid)
Vinblastine (Velban,
  Velbe)

Vincristine (Oncovin,
  Vincasar PFS)

Vinorelbine (Navelbine)

Miscellaneous Antineoplastic Agents

Aldesleukin [Interleukin-
  2, IL-2] (Proleukin)
Aminoglutethimide
  (Cytadren)
L-Asparaginase (Elspar,
  Oncaspar)
BCG [Bacillus Calmette-
  Guérin] (TheraCys,
  Tice BCG)
Bevacizumab (Avastin)
Bortezomib (Velcade)
Cladribine (Leustatin)

Dacarbazine (DTIC)
Docetaxel (Taxotere)
Gefitinib (Iressa)
Gemtuzumab Ozogam-
  icin (Mylotarg)
Hydroxyurea (Hydrea,
  Droxia)
Imatinib (Gleevec)
Irinotecan (Camptosar)
Letrozole (Femara)
Leucovorin (Wellcovorin)
Mitotane (Lysodren)

Mitoxantrone
  (Novantrone)
Paclitaxel (Taxol)
Pemetrexed (Alimta)
Rasburicase (Elitek)
Thalidomide (Thalomid)
Topotecan (Hycamtin)
Trastuzumab (Herceptin)
Tretinoin, Topical
  [Retinoic Acid]
  (Retin-A, Avita,
  Renova)

CARDIOVASCULAR AGENTS

Aldosterone Antagonist

Eplerenone (Inspra)

Alpha$_1$-Adrenergic Blockers

Doxazosin (Cardura)   Prazosin (Minipress)   Terazosin (Hytrin)

Angiotensin-Converting Enzyme Inhibitors

Benazepril (Lotensin)   Lisinopril (Prinivil,   Quinapril (Accupril)
Captopril (Capoten)   Zestril)   Ramipril (Altace)
Enalapril (Vasotec)   Moexipril (Univasc)   Trandolapril (Mavik)
Fosinopril (Monopril)   Perindopril Erbumine
                               (Aceon)

Angiotensin II Receptor Antagonists

Candesartan (Atacand)   Irbesartan (Avapro)   Telmisartan (Micardis)
Eprosartan (Teveten)   Losartan (Cozaar)   Valsartan (Diovan)

Antiarrhythmic Agents

Adenosine (Adenocard)   Dofetilide (Tikosyn)   Procainamide (Pronestyl,
Amiodarone (Cordarone,   Esmolol (Brevibloc)   Procan)
  Pacerone)   Flecainide (Tambocor)   Propafenone (Rythmol)
Atropine   Ibutilide (Corvert)   Quinidine (Quinidex,
Digoxin (Lanoxin,   Lidocaine (Anestacon   Quinaglute)
  Lanoxicaps)   Topical, Xylocaine)   Sotalol (Betapace,
Disopyramide (Norpace,   Mexiletine (Mexitil)   Betapace AF)
  NAPamide)

Beta-Adrenergic Blockers

Acebutolol (Sectral)   Carvedilol (Coreg)   Pindolol (Visken)
Atenolol (Tenormin)   Labetalol (Trandate,   Propranolol (Inderal)
Atenolol and Chlorthali-   Normodyne)   Timolol (Blocadren)
  done (Tenoretic)   Metoprolol (Lopressor,
Betaxolol (Kerlone)   Toprol XL)
Bisoprolol (Zebeta)   Nadolol (Corgard)
Carteolol (Cartrol,   Penbutolol (Levatol)
  Ocupress Ophthalmic)

Calcium Channel Antagonists

Amlodipine (Norvasc)
Bepridil (Vascor)
Diltiazem (Cardizem,
    Cartia XT, Dilacor,
    Diltia XT, Tiamate,
    Tiazac)

Felodipine (Plendil)
Isradipine (DynaCirc)
Nicardipine (Cardene)
Nifedipine (Procardia,
    Procardia XL, Adalat,
    Adalat CC)

Nimodipine (Nimotop)
Nisoldipine (Sular)
Verapamil (Calan,
    Isoptin)

Centrally Acting Antihypertensive Agents

Clonidine (Catapres)

Methyldopa (Aldomet)

Diuretics

Acetazolamide (Diamox)
Amiloride (Midamor)
Bumetanide (Bumex)
Chlorothiazide (Diuril)
Chlorthalidone
    (Hygroton)
Furosemide (Lasix)
Hydrochlorothiazide (Hy-
    droDIURIL, Esidrix)

Hydrochlorothiazide and
    Amiloride
    (Moduretic)
Hydrochlorothiazide and
    Spironolactone
    (Aldactazide)
Hydrochlorothiazide and
    Triamterene (Dyazide,
    Maxzide)

Indapamide (Lozol)
Mannitol
Metolazone (Mykrox,
    Zaroxolyn)
Spironolactone
    (Aldactone)
Torsemide (Demadex)
Triamterene (Dyrenium)

Inotropic/Pressor Agents

Digoxin (Lanoxin,
    Lanoxicaps)
Dobutamine (Dobutrex)
Dopamine (Intropin)
Epinephrine (Adrenalin,
    Sus-Phrine, EpiPen)

Inamrinone (Inocor)
Isoproterenol (Isuprel)
Milrinone (Primacor)
Nesiritide (Natrecor)
Norepinephrine
    (Levophed)

Phenylephrine
    (Neo-Synephrine)

Lipid-Lowering Agents

Atorvastatin (Lipitor)
Cholestyramine
    (Questran,
    LoCHOLEST)
Colesevelam (Welchol)
Colestipol (Colestid)

Ezetimibe (Zetia)
Fenofibrate (Tricor)
Fluvastatin (Lescol)
Gemfibrozil (Lopid)
Lovastatin (Mevacor,
    Altocor)

Niacin (Niaspan)
Pravastatin (Pravachol)
Rosuvastatin (Crestor)
Simvastatin (Zocor)

Lipid-Lowering/Antihypertensive Combinations

Amlodipine/Atorvastatin
(Caduet)

Vasodilators

Alprostadil
[Prostaglandin E$_1$]
(Prostin VR)
Epoprostenol (Flolan)
Fenoldopam (Corlopam)
Hydralazine (Apresoline)
Isosorbide Dinitrate
(Isordil, Sorbitrate,
Dilatrate-SR)

Isosorbide Mononitrate
(Ismo, Imdur)
Minoxidil (Loniten,
Rogaine)
Nitroglycerin (Nitrostat,
Nitrolingual, Nitro-
Bid Ointment, Nitro-
Bid IV, Nitrodisc,
Transderm-Nitro)

Nitroprusside (Nipride,
Nitropress)
Tolazoline (Priscoline)
Treprostinil Sodium
(Remodulin)

CENTRAL NERVOUS SYSTEM AGENTS

Antianxiety Agents

Alprazolam (Xanax)
Buspirone (BuSpar)
Chlordiazepoxide (Lib-
rium, Mitran, Libritabs)
Clorazepate (Tranxene)

Diazepam (Valium)
Doxepin (Sinequan,
Adapin)
Hydroxyzine (Atarax,
Vistaril)

Lorazepam (Ativan)
Meprobamate (Equanil,
Miltown)
Oxazepam (Serax)

Anticonvulsants

Carbamazepine (Tegretol)
Clonazepam (Klonopin)
Diazepam (Valium)
Ethosuximide (Zarontin)
Fosphenytoin (Cerebyx)
Gabapentin (Neurontin)

Lamotrigine (Lamictal)
Levetiracetam (Keppra)
Lorazepam (Ativan)
Oxcarbazepine (Trileptal)
Pentobarbital (Nembutal)
Phenobarbital

Phenytoin (Dilantin)
Tiagabine (Gabitril)
Topiramate (Topamax)
Valproic Acid (Depak-
ene, Depakote)
Zonisamide (Zonegran)

Antidepressants

Amitriptyline (Elavil)
Bupropion (Wellbutrin,
Zyban)
Citalopram (Celexa)
Desipramine (Norpramin)
Doxepin (Sinequan,
Adapin)

Escitalopram (Lexapro)
Fluoxetine (Prozac,
Sarafem)
Fluvoxamine (Luvox)
Imipramine (Tofranil)
Mirtazapine (Remeron)
Nefazodone (Serzone)

Nortriptyline (Aventyl,
Pamelor)
Paroxetine (Paxil)
Phenelzine (Nardil)
Sertraline (Zoloft)
Trazodone (Desyrel)
Venlafaxine (Effexor)

Antiparkinson Agents

Amantadine (Symmetrel)
Apomorphine (Apokyn)
Benztropine (Cogentin)
Bromocriptine (Parlodel)

Carbidopa/Levodopa (Sinemet)
Entacapone (Comtan)
Pergolide (Permax)
Pramipexole (Mirapex)

Ropinirole (Requip)
Selegiline (Eldepryl)
Tolcapone (Tasmar)
Trihexyphenidyl (Artane)

Antipsychotics

Aripiprazole (Abilify)
Chlorpromazine (Thorazine)
Clozapine (Clozaril)
Fluphenazine (Prolixin, Permitil)
Haloperidol (Haldol)
Lithium Carbonate (Eskalith, Lithobid)

Mesoridazine (Serentil)
Molindone (Moban)
Olanzapine (Zyprexa)
Perphenazine (Trilafon)
Prochlorperazine (Compazine)
Quetiapine (Seroquel)
Risperidone (Risperdal)

Thioridazine (Mellaril)
Thiothixene (Navane)
Trifluoperazine (Stelazine)
Ziprasidone (Geodon)

Sedative Hypnotics

Chloral Hydrate (Aquachloral, Supprettes)
Diphenhydramine (Benadryl)
Estazolam (ProSom)
Flurazepam (Dalmane)

Hydroxyzine (Atarax, Vistaril)
Midazolam (Versed)
Pentobarbital (Nembutal)
Phenobarbital
Propofol (Diprivan)

Quazepam (Doral)
Secobarbital (Seconal)
Temazepam (Restoril)
Triazolam (Halcion)
Zaleplon (Sonata)
Zolpidem (Ambien)

Miscellaneous CNS Agents

Atomoxetine (Strattera)
Galantamine (Reminyl)
Memantine (Namenda)

Nimodipine (Nimotop)
Rivastigmine (Exelon)

Sodium Oxybate (Xyrem)
Tacrine (Cognex)

DERMATOLOGIC AGENTS

Acitretin (Soriatane)
Acyclovir (Zovirax)
Alefacept (Amevive)
Anthralin (Anthra-Derm)
Amphotericin B (Fungizone)

Bacitracin, Topical (Baciguent)
Bacitracin and Polymyxin B, Topical (Polysporin)
Bacitracin, Neomycin, and Polymyxin B,

Topical (Neosporin Ointment)
Bacitracin, Neomycin, Polymyxin B, and Hydrocortisone, Topical (Cortisporin)

Bacitracin, Neomycin, Polymyxin B, and Lidocaine, Topical (Clomycin)

Calcipotriene (Dovonex)

Capsaicin (Capsin, Zostrix)

Ciclopirox (Loprox)

Ciprofloxacin (Cipro)

Clindamycin (Cleocin)

Clotrimazole and Betamethasone (Lotrisone)

Dibucaine (Nupercainal)

Doxepin, Topical (Zonalon)

Econazole (Spectazole)

Efalizumab (Raptiva)

Erythromycin, Topical (A/T/S, Eryderm, Erycette, T-Stat)

Finasteride (Proscar, Propecia)

Gentamicin, Topical (Garamycin, G-Mycitin)

Haloprogin (Halotex)

Imiquimod Cream, 5% (Aldara)

Isotretinoin [13-*cis* Retinoic acid] (Accutane, Amnesteem, Claravis, Sotret)

Ketoconazole (Nizoral)

Lactic Acid and Ammonium Hydroxide [Ammonium Lactate] (Lac-Hydrin)

Lindane (Kwell)

Metronidazole (Flagy, MetroGel)

Miconazole (Monistat)

Minoxidil (Loniten, Rogaine)

Mupirocin (Bactroban)

Naftifine (Naftin)

Neomycin Sulfate (Myciguent)

Nystatin (Mycostatin)

Oxiconazole (Oxistat)

Penciclovir (Denavir)

Permethrin (Nix, Elimite)

Pimecrolimus (Elidel)

Podophyllin (Podocon-25, Condylox Gel 0.5%, Condylox)

Pramoxine (Anusol Ointment, Proctofoam-NS)

Pramoxine and Hydrocortisone (Enzone, Proctofoam-HC)

Selenium Sulfide (Exsel Shampoo, Selsun Blue Shampoo, Selsun Shampoo)

Silver Sulfadiazine (Silvadene)

Steroids, Topical (Table 5, page 272)

Tacrolimus (Prograf, Protopic)

Tazarotene (Tazorac)

Terbinafine (Lamisil)

Tolnaftate (Tinactin)

Tretinoin, Topical [Retinoic Acid] (Retin-A, Avita, Renova)

DIETARY SUPPLEMENTS

Calcium Acetate (Calphron, Phos-Ex, PhosLo)

Calcium Glubionate (Neo-Calglucon)

Calcium Salts [Chloride, Gluconate, Gluceptate]

Cholecalciferol [Vitamin D_3] (Delta D)

Cyanocobalamin [Vitamin B_{12}]

Ferric Gluconate Complex (Ferrlecit)

Ferrous Gluconate (Fergon)

Ferrous Sulfate

Folic Acid

Iron Dextran (DexFerrum, InFeD)

Iron Sucrose (Venofer)

Magnesium Oxide (Mag-Ox 400)

Magnesium Sulfate

Phytonadione [Vitamin K] (AquaMEPHYTON)

Potassium Supplements (Kaon, Kaochlor, K-Lor, Slow-K, Micro-K, Klorvess)

Pyridoxine [Vitamin B_6]

Sodium Bicarbonate [$NaHCO_3$]

Thiamine [Vitamin B_1]

EAR (OTIC) AGENTS

Acetic Acid and Aluminum Acetate (Otic Domeboro)

Benzocaine and Antipyrine (Auralgan)

Ciprofloxacin, Otic (Cipro HC Otic)

Neomycin, Colistin, and Hydrocortisone (Cortisporin-TC Otic Drops)

Neomycin, Colistin, Hydrocortisone, and Thonzonium (Cortisporin-TC Otic Suspension)

Neomycin, Polymyxin, and Hydrocortisone (Cortisporin Ophthalmic and Otic)

Polymyxin B and Hydrocortisone (Otobiotic Otic)

Sulfacetamide and Prednisolone (Blephamide)

Triethanolamine (Cerumenex)

ENDOCRINE SYSTEM AGENTS

Antidiabetic Agents

Acarbose (Precose)

Chlorpropamide (Diabinese)

Glimepiride (Amaryl)

Glipizide (Glucotrol)

Glyburide (DiaBeta, Micronase, Glynase)

Glyburide/Metformin (Glucovance)

Insulins (Table 6, page 275)

Metformin (Glucophage)

Miglitol (Glyset)

Nateglinide (Starlix)

Pioglitazone (Actos)

Repaglinide (Prandin)

Rosiglitazone (Avandia)

Tolazamide (Tolinase)

Tolbutamide (Orinase)

Hormone and Synthetic Substitutes

Calcitonin (Cibacalcin, Miacalcin)

Calcitriol (Rocaltrol)

Cortisone Systemic, Topical

Desmopressin (DDAVP, Stimate)

Dexamethasone (Decadron)

Fludrocortisone Acetate (Florinef)

Glucagon

Hydrocortisone Topical & Systemic (Cortef, Solu-Cortef)

Methylprednisolone (Solu-Medrol)

Prednisolone

Prednisone

Testosterone (AndroGel, Androderm, Striant, Testim, Testoderm)

Vasopressin [Antidiuretic Hormone, ADH] (Pitressin)

Hypercalcemia Agents

Etidronate Disodium (Didronel)

Gallium Nitrate (Ganite)

Pamidronate (Aredia)

Zoledronic acid (Zometa)

Obesity

Sibutramine (Meridia)

Osteoporosis Agents

Alendronate (Fosamax)   Risedronate (Actonel)   Zoledronic Acid
Raloxifene (Evista)   Teriparatide (Forteo)   (Zometa)

Thyroid/Antithyroid

Levothyroxine   Potassium iodide   Propylthiouracil [PTU]
   (Synthroid, Levoxyl)   [Lugol's solution]
Liothyronine (Cytomel)   (SSKI, Thyro-Block)
Methimazole (Tapazole)

Miscellaneous Endocrine Agents

Cinacalcet (Sensipar)   Demeclocycline   Diazoxide (Hyperstat,
                           (Declomycin)   Proglycem)

EYE (OPHTHALMIC) AGENTS

Glaucoma Agents

Acetazolamide (Diamox)   Dipivefrin (Propine)   Levobunolol (A-K Beta,
Apraclonidine (Iopidine) Dorzolamide (Trusopt)   Betagan)
Betaxolol, Ophthalmic   Dorzolamide and   Levocabastine (Livostin)
   (Betoptic)   Timolol (Cosopt)   Lodoxamide (Alomide)
Brimonidine (Alphagan)   Echothiophate Iodine   Rimexolone (Vexol
Brinzolamide (Azopt)   (Phospholine   Ophthalmic)
Carteolol (Cartrol,   Ophthalmic)   Timolol, Ophthalmic
   Ocupress Ophthalmic)   Latanoprost (Xalatan)   (Timoptic)

Ophthalmic Antibiotics

Bacitracin, Ophthalmic   Bacitracin, Neomycin,   Neomycin and Dexa-
   (AK-Tracin   Polymyxin B, and   methasone (AK-Neo-
   Ophthalmic)   Hydrocortisone, Oph-   Dex Ophthalmic,
Bacitracin and   thalmic (AK Spore HC   NeoDecadron Oph-
   Polymyxin B,   Ophthalmic, Cor-   thalmic)
   Ophthalmic (AK Poly   tisporin Ophthalmic) Neomycin, Polymyxin
   Bac Ophthalmic,   Ciprofloxacin,   B, and Dexametha-
   Polysporin   Ophthalmic (Ciloxan)   sone (Maxitrol)
   Ophthalmic)   Erythromycin,   Neomycin, Polymyxin
Bacitracin, Neomycin,   Ophthalmic (Ilotycin   B, and Prednisolone
   and Polymyxin B (AK   Ophthalmic)   (Poly-Pred
   Spore Ophthalmic,   Gentamicin, Ophthalmic   Ophthalmic)
   Neosporin   (Garamycin, Genoptic, Ofloxacin (Floxin,
   Ophthalmic)   Gentacidin, Gentak)   Ocuflox Ophthalmic)

Silver Nitrate (Dey-Drop)
Sulfacetamide (Bleph-10, Cetamide, Sodium Sulamyd)

Sulfacetamide and Prednisolone (Blephamide)
Tobramycin, Ophthalmic (AKTob, Tobrex)

Tobramycin and Dexamethasone (TobraDex)
Trifluridine (Viroptic)

Other Ophthalmic Agents

Artificial Tears (Tears Naturale)
Cromolyn Sodium (Opticrom)
Cyclopentolate (Cyclogyl)
Dexamethasone, Ophthalmic (AK-Dex Ophthalmic, Decadron Ophthalmic)

Emedastine (Emadine)
Ketorolac, Ophthalmic (Acular)
Ketotifen (Zaditor)
Lodoxamide (Alomide)
Naphazoline and Antazoline (Albalon-A Ophthalmic)

Naphazoline and Pheniramine Acetate (Naphcon A)
Olopatadine (Patanol)
Pemirolast (Alamast)
Rimexolone (Vexol Ophthalmic)

GASTROINTESTINAL AGENTS

Antacids

Alginic Acid (Gaviscon)
Aluminum Hydroxide (Amphojel, AlternaGEL)
Aluminum Hydroxide with Magnesium Carbonate (Gaviscon)
Aluminum Hydroxide with Magnesium Hydroxide (Maalox)

Aluminum Hydroxide with Magnesium Hydroxide and Simethicone (Mylanta, Mylanta II, Maalox Plus)
Aluminum Hydroxide with Magnesium Trisilicate (Gaviscon, Gaviscon-2)

Calcium Carbonate (Tums, Alka-Mints)
Magaldrate (Riopan, Lowsium)
Simethicone (Mylicon)

Antidiarrheals

Bismuth Subsalicylate (Pepto-Bismol)
Diphenoxylate with Atropine (Lomotil)

Kaolin-Pectin (Kaodene, Kao-Spen, Kapectolin, Parepectolin)
Lactobacillus (Lactinex Granules)

Loperamide (Imodium)
Octreotide (Sandostatin, Sandostatin LAR)
Paregoric [Camphorated Tincture of Opium]

Antiemetics

Aprepitant (Emend)
Chlorpromazine (Thorazine)

Dimenhydrinate (Dramamine)
Dolasetron (Anzemet)

Dronabinol (Marinol)
Droperidol (Inapsine)
Granisetron (Kytril)

Meclizine (Antivert)
Metoclopramide (Reglan, Clopra, Octamide)
Ondansetron (Zofran)

Palonosetron (Aloxi)
Prochlorperazine (Compazine)
Promethazine (Phenergan)

Scopolamine (Scopace)
Thiethylperazine (Torecan)
Trimethobenzamide (Tigan)

Antiulcer Agents

Cimetidine (Tagamet)
Esomeprazole (Nexium)
Famotidine (Pepcid)
Lansoprazole (Prevacid)

Nizatidine (Axid)
Omeprazole (Prilosec)
Pantoprazole (Protonix)
Rabeprazole (Aciphex)

Ranitidine Hydrochloride (Zantac)
Sucralfate (Carafate)

Cathartics/Laxatives

Bisacodyl (Dulcolax)
Docusate Calcium (Surfak)
Docusate Potassium (Dialose)
Docusate Sodium (DOS, Colace)
Glycerin Suppository
Lactulose (Chronulac, Cephulac, Enulose)

Magnesium Citrate
Magnesium Hydroxide (Milk of Magnesia)
Mineral Oil
Polyethylene Glycol-Electrolyte Solution (GoLYTELY, CoLyte)

Psyllium (Metamucil, Serutan, Effer-Syllium)
Sodium Phosphate (Visicol)
Sorbitol

Enzymes

Pancreatin (Pancrease, Cotazym, Creon, Ultrase)

Miscellaneous GI Agents

Alosetron (Lotronex)
Balsalazide (Colazal)
Dexpanthenol (Ilopan-Choline Oral, Ilopan)
Dibucaine (Nupercainal)
Dicyclomine (Bentyl)
Hydrocortisone, Rectal (Anusol-HC Suppository, Cortifoam Rectal, Proctocort)

Hyoscyamine (Anaspaz, Cystospaz, Levsin)
Hyoscyamine, Atropine, Scopolamine, and Phenobarbital (Donnatal)
Infliximab (Remicade)
Mesalamine (Rowasa, Asacol, Pentasa)

Metoclopramide (Reglan, Clopra, Octamide)
Misoprostol (Cytotec)
Olsalazine (Dipentum)
Pramoxine (Anusol Ointment, Proctofoam-NS)
Pramoxine with Hydrocortisone (Enzone, Proctofoam-HC)

Propantheline (Pro-
  Banthine)
Sulfasalazine (Azulfidine)

Tegaserod Maleate
  (Zelnorm)

Vasopressin (Pitressin)

HEMATOLOGIC AGENTS

Anticoagulants

Ardeparin (Normiflo)
Argatroban (Acova)
Bivalirudin (Angiomax)
Dalteparin (Fragmin)

Enoxaparin (Lovenox)
Fondaparinux (Arixtra)
Heparin
Lepirudin (Refludan)

Protamine
Tinzaparin (Innohep)
Warfarin (Coumadin)

Antiplatelet Agents

Abciximab (ReoPro)
Aspirin (Bayer, Ecotrin,
  St. Joseph's)
Clopidogrel (Plavix)

Dipyridamole
  (Persantine)
Dipyridamole and
  Aspirin (Aggrenox)

Eptifibatide (Integrilin)
Reteplase (Retavase)
Ticlopidine (Ticlid)
Tirofiban (Aggrastat)

Antithrombotic Agents

Alteplase, Recombinant
  [tPA] (Activase)
Aminocaproic Acid
  (Amicar)
Anistreplase (Eminase)

Aprotinin (Trasylol)
Danaparoid (Orgaron)
Dextran 40
  (Rheomacrodex)
Reteplase (Retavase)

Streptokinase (Streptase,
  Kabikinase)
Tenecteplase (TNKase)
Urokinase (Abbokinase)

Hematopoietic Stimulants

Darbepoetin Alfa
  (Aranesp)
Epoetin Alfa [Erythro-
  poietin, EPO]
  (Epogen, Procrit)

Filgrastim [G-CSF]
  (Neupogen)
Oprelvekin (Neumega)
Pegfilgrastim (Neulasta)

Sargramostim
  [GM-CSF]
  (Prokine, Leukine)

Volume Expanders

Albumin (Albuminar,
  Buminate,
  Albutein)

Dextran 40
  (Rheomacrodex)
Hetastarch (Hespan)

Plasma Protein Fraction
  (Plasmanate)

Miscellaneous Hematologic Agents

Antihemophilic Factor
  VIII (Monoclate)

Desmopressin (DDAVP,
  Stimate)

Pentoxifylline (Trental)

IMMUNE SYSTEM AGENTS

Immunomodulators

Adalimumab (Humira)
Anakinra (Kineret)
Etanercept (Enbrel)
Interferon Alfa (Roferon-A, Intron A)

Interferon Alfacon-1 (Infergen)
Interferon Beta-1b (Betaseron)

Interferon Gamma-1b (Actimmune)
Peg Interferon Alfa-2b (PEG-Intron)

Immunosuppressive Agents

Azathioprine (Imuran)
Basiliximab (Simulect)
Cyclosporine (Sandimmune, NePO)
Daclizumab (Zenapax)

Lymphocyte Immune Globulin [Antithymocyte Globulin, ATG] (Atgam)
Muromonab-CD3 (Orthoclone OKT3)

Mycophenolate Mofetil (CellCept)
Sirolimus (Rapamune)
Steroids, Systemic (Table 4, page 271)
Tacrolimus (Prograf, Protopic)

Vaccines/Serums/Toxoids

Cytomegalovirus Immune Globulin [CMV-IG IV] (CytoGam)
Diphtheria, Tetanus Toxoids, and Acellular Pertussis Adsorbed, Hepatitis B (recombinant), and Inactivated Poliovirus Vaccine (IPV) Combined (Pediarix)
Haemophilus B Conjugate Vaccine (ActHIB, HibTITER, Pedvax-HIB, Prohibit)
Hepatitis A Vaccine (Havrix, Vaqta)

Hepatitis A (Inactivated) and Hepatitis B Recombinant Vaccine (Twinrix)
Hepatitis B Immune Globulin (HyperHep, H-BIG)
Hepatitis B Vaccine (Engerix-B, Recombivax HB)
Immune Globulin, IV (Gamimune N, Sandoglobulin, Gammar IV)
Influenza Vaccine (Fluzone, FluShield, Fluvirin)

Influenza Virus Vaccine Live, Intranasal (FluMist)
Meningococcal Polysaccharide Vaccine (Menomune)
Pneumococcal 7-Valent Conjugate Vaccine (Prevnar)
Pneumococcal Vaccine, Polyvalent (Pneumovax-23)
Tetanus Immune Globulin
Tetanus Toxoid
Varicella Virus Vaccine (Varivax)

MUSCULOSKELETAL AGENTS

Antigout Agents

Allopurinol (Zyloprim, Lopurin, Alloprim)

Colchicine
Probenecid (Benemid)

Sulfinpyrazone (Anturane)

Muscle Relaxants

Baclofen (Lioresal)
Carisoprodol (Soma)
Chlorzoxazone
  (Paraflex, Parafon
  Forte DSC)

Cyclobenzaprine
  (Flexeril)
Dantrolene (Dantrium)
Diazepam (Valium)
Metaxalone (Skelaxin)

Methocarbamol
  (Robaxin)
Orphenadrine (Norflex)

Neuromuscular Blockers

Atracurium (Tracrium)
Pancuronium (Pavulon)
Rocuronium (Zemuron)

Succinylcholine
  (Anectine, Quelicin,
  Sucostrin)

Vecuronium (Norcuron)

Miscellaneous Musculoskeletal Agents

Edrophonium (Tensilon)
Leflunomide (Arava)

Methotrexate (Folex,
  Rheumatrex)

OB/GYN AGENTS

Contraceptives

Estradiol Cypionate and
  Medroxyprogesterone
  Acetate (Lunelle)
Etonogestrel/Ethinyl
  Estradiol (NuvaRing)
Levonorgestrel Implant
  (Norplant)

Medroxyprogesterone
  (Provera, Depo-
  Provera)
Norgestrel (Ovrette)
Oral Contraceptives,
  Monophasic (Table 7,
  page 276)

Oral Contraceptives,
  Multiphasic (Table 7,
  page 276)
Oral Contraceptives,
  Progestin Only (Table
  7, page 276)

Emergency Contraceptives

Ethinyl Estradiol, and
  Levonorgestrel
  (Preven)

Levonorgestrel (Plan B)

Estrogen Supplementation Agents

Esterified Estrogens
  (Estratab,
  Menest)
Esterified Estrogens with
  Methyltestosterone
  (Estratest)

Estradiol (Estrace)
Estradiol, Transdermal
  (Estraderm, Climara,
  Vivelle)
Estrogen, Conjugated
  (Premarin)

Estrogen, Conjugated-
  Synthetic (Cenestin)
Estrogen, Conjugated
  with Medroxyproges-
  terone (Prempro,
  Premphase)

Estrogen, Conjugated with Methylprogesterone (Premarin with Methylprogesterone)

Estrogen, Conjugated with Methyltestosterone (Premarin with Methyltestosterone)

Ethinyl Estradiol (Estinyl, Feminone) Norethindrone Acetate/Ethinyl Estradiol (FemHRT)

Vaginal Preparations

Amino-Cerv pH 5.5 Cream
Miconazole (Monistat)

Nystatin (Mycostatin)
Terconazole (Terazol 7)

Tioconazole (Vagistat)

Miscellaneous Ob/Gyn Agents

Dinoprostone (Cervidil Vaginal Insert, Prepidil Vaginal Gel)
Gonadorelin (Lutrepulse)
Leuprolide (Lupron, Viadur, Eligard)

Magnesium Sulfate
Medroxyprogesterone (Provera, Depo-Provera)
Methylergonovine (Methergine)

Mifepristone [RU 486] (Mifeprex)
Oxytocin (Pitocin)
Terbutaline (Brethine, Bricanyl)

PAIN MEDICATIONS

Local Anesthetics

Benzocaine and Antipyrine (Auralgan)
Bupivacaine (Marcaine)
Capsaicin (Capsin, Zostrix)

Cocaine
Dibucaine (Nupercainal)
Lidocaine (Anestacon Topical, Xylocaine)

Lidocaine and Prilocaine (EMLA, LMX)
Pramoxine (Anusol Ointment, Proctofoam-NS)

Migraine Headache Medications

Acetaminophen with Butalbital w/wo Caffeine (Fioricet, Medigesic, Repan, Sedapap-10 Two-Dyne, Triapin, Axocet, Phrenilin Forte)

Almotriptan (Axert)
Aspirin and Butalbital Compound (Fiorinal)
Aspirin with Butalbital, Caffeine, and Codeine (Fiorinal with Codeine)

Frovatriptan (Frova)
Naratriptan (Amerge)
Serotonin Receptor Agonists (See Table 11, page 283)
Sumatriptan (Imitrex)
Zolmitriptan (Zomig)

Narcotics

Acetaminophen with Codeine (Tylenol No. 1, 2, 3, 4)

Alfentanil (Alfenta)
Aspirin with Codeine (Empirin No. 2, 3, 4)

Buprenorphine (Buprenex)
Butorphanol (Stadol)

Codeine
Dezocine (Dalgan)
Fentanyl (Sublimaze)
Fentanyl, Transdermal (Duragesic)
Fentanyl, Transmucosal (Actiq System)
Hydrocodone and Acetaminophen (Lorcet, Vicodin)
Hydrocodone and Aspirin (Lortab ASA)
Hydrocodone and Ibuprofen (Vicoprofen)
Hydromorphone (Dilaudid)

Levorphanol (Levo-Dromoran)
Meperidine (Demerol)
Methadone (Dolophine)
Morphine (Avinza XR, Duramorph, MS Contin, Kadian SR, Oramorph SR, Roxanol)
Nalbuphine (Nubain)
Oxycodone (OxyContin, OxyIR, Roxicodone)
Oxycodone and Acetaminophen (Percocet, Tylox)

Oxycodone and Aspirin (Percodan, Percodan-Demi)
Oxymorphone (Numorphan)
Pentazocine (Talwin)
Propoxyphene (Darvon)
Propoxyphene and Acetaminophen (Darvocet)
Propoxyphene and Aspirin (Darvon Compound-65, Darvon-N with Aspirin)

Nonnarcotic Agents

Acetaminophen [APAP] (Tylenol)
Aspirin (Bayer, Ecotrin, St. Joseph's)

Tramadol (Ultram)
Tramadol/Acetaminophen (Ultracet)

Nonsteroidal Antiinflammatory Agents

Celecoxib (Celebrex)
Diclofenac (Cataflam, Voltaren)
Diflunisal (Dolobid)
Etodolac (Lodine)
Fenoprofen (Nalfon)
Flurbiprofen (Ansaid)

Ibuprofen (Motrin, Rufen, Advil)
Indomethacin (Indocin)
Ketoprofen (Orudis, Oruvail)
Ketorolac (Toradol)
Meloxicam (Mobic)
Nabumetone (Relafen)

Naproxen (Aleve, Naprosyn, Anaprox)
Oxaprozin (Daypro)
Piroxicam (Feldene)
Rofecoxib (Vioxx)
Sulindac (Clinoril)
Tolmetin (Tolectin)
Valdecoxib (Bextra)

Miscellaneous Pain Medications

Amitriptyline (Elavil)

Imipramine (Tofranil)

Tramadol (Ultram)

RESPIRATORY AGENTS

Antitussives, Decongestants, and Expectorants

Acetylcysteine (Mucomyst)

Benzonatate (Tessalon Perles)

Codeine

Dextromethorphan (Mediquell, Benylin DM, PediaCare 1)

Guaifenesin (Robitussin)

Guaifenesin and Codeine (Robitussin AC, Brontex)

Guaifenesin and Dextromethorphan

Hydrocodone and Guaifenesin (Hycotuss Expectorant)

Hydrocodone and Homatropine (Hycodan, Hydromet)

Hydrocodone and Pseudoephedrine (Detussin, Histussin-D)

Hydrocodone, Chlorpheniramine, Phenylephrine, Acetaminophen, and Caffeine (Hycomine)

Potassium Iodide (SSKI, Thyro-Block)

Pseudoephedrine (Sudafed, Novafed, Afrinol)

Bronchodilators

Albuterol (Proventil, Ventolin, Volmax)

Albuterol and Ipratropium (Combivent)

Aminophylline

Bitolterol (Tornalate)

Ephedrine

Epinephrine (Adrenalin, Sus-Phrine, EpiPen)

Formoterol (Foradil Aerolizer)

Isoproterenol (Isuprel)

Levalbuterol (Xopenex)

Metaproterenol (Alupent, Metaprel)

Pirbuterol (Maxair)

Salmeterol (Serevent)

Terbutaline (Brethine, Bricanyl)

Theophylline (Theolair, Somophyllin)

Respiratory Inhalants

Acetylcysteine (Mucomyst)

Beclomethasone (Beconase, Vancenase Nasal Inhaler)

Beclomethasone (QVAR)

Beractant (Survanta)

Budesonide (Rhinocort, Pulmicort)

Calfactant (Infasurf)

Colfosceril Palmitate (Exosurf Neonatal)

Cromolyn Sodium (Intal, NasalCrom, Opticrom)

Dexamethasone, Nasal (Dexacort Phosphate Turbinaire)

Flunisolide (AeroBid, Nasalide)

Fluticasone, Oral, Nasal (Flonase, Flovent)

Fluticasone Propionate and Salmeterol Xinafoate (Advair Diskus)

Ipratropium (Atrovent)

Nedocromil (Tilade)

Tiotropium (Spiriva)

Triamcinolone (Azmacort)

Miscellaneous Respiratory Agents

Alpha$_1$-Protease Inhibitor (Prolastin)

Dornase Alfa (Pulmozyme)

Montelukast (Singulair)

Omalizumab (Xolair)

Zafirlukast (Accolate)

Zileuton (Zyflo)

URINARY/GENITOURINARY AGENTS

Alprostadil, Intracavernosal (Caverject, Edex)
Alprostadil, Urethral Suppository (Muse)
Ammonium Aluminum Sulfate [Alum]
Belladonna and Opium Suppositories (B & O Supprettes)
Bethanechol (Urecholine, Duvoid)
Dimethyl Sulfoxide [DMSO] (Rimso 50)
Flavoxate (Urispas)
Hyoscyamine (Anaspaz, Cystospaz, Levsin)

Methenamine (Hiprex, Urex)
Neomycin-Polymyxin Bladder Irrigant [Neosporin GU Irrigant]
Nitrofurantoin (Macrodantin, Furadantin, Macrobid)
Oxybutynin (Ditropan, Ditropan XL)
Oxybutynin Transdermal System (Oxytrol)
Pentosan Polysulfate (Elmiron)
Phenazopyridine (Pyridium)

Potassium Citrate (Urocit-K)
Potassium Citrate and Citric Acid (Polycitra-K)
Sildenafil (Viagra)
Sodium Citrate (Bicitra)
Tadalafil (Cialis)
Tolterodine (Detrol, Detrol LA)
Trimethoprim (Trimpex, Proloprim)
Trospium Chloride (Sanctura)
Vardenafil (Levitra)

Benign Prostatic Hyperplasia Medications

Alfuzosin (Uroxatral)
Doxazosin (Cardura)
Dutasteride (Avodart)

Finasteride (Proscar, Propecia)

Tamsulosin (Flomax)
Terazosin (Hytrin)

WOUND CARE

Becaplermin (Regranex Gel)

Silver Nitrate (Dey-Drop)

MISCELLANEOUS THERAPEUTIC AGENTS

Cilostazol (Pletal)
Drotrecogin Alfa (Xigris)
Megestrol Acetate (Megace)
Naltrexone (ReVia)
Nicotine Gum (Nicorette)

Nicotine Nasal Spray (Nicotrol NS)
Nicotine Transdermal (Habitrol, Nicoderm, Nicotrol)
Orlistat (Xenical)

Potassium Iodide [Lugol's Solution] (SSKI, Thyro-Block)
Sevelamer (Renagel)
Sodium Polystyrene Sulfonate (Kayexalate)
Talc (Sterile Talc Powder)

Commonly Used Medicinal Herbs

Arnica (*Arnica montana*)
Astragalus (*Astragalus membranaceus*)

Butcher's Broom (*Ruscus aculeatus*)

Black Cohosh (*Cimicifuga racemosa*)

Chamomile (*Matricaria recutita*)
Chondroitin Sulfate
Dong Quai (*Angelica polymorpha, sinensis*)
Echinacea (*Echinacea purpurea*)
Ephedra/Ma Huang
Feverfew (*Tanacetum parthenium*)
Garlic (*Allium sativum*)
Ginger (*Zingiber officinale*)
Ginkgo biloba

Ginseng (*Panax quinquefolius*)
Glucosamine Sulfate (chitosamine)
Hawthorn (*Crataegus laevigata*)
Kava Kava (*Piper methysticum*)
Licorice (*Glycyrrhiza glabra*)
Melatonin, (MEL)
Milk thistle (*Silybum marianum*)

Saw Palmetto (*Serenoa repens*)
Spirulina (*Spirulina* spp)
St. John's Wort (*Hypericum perforatum*)
Tea Tree (*Melaleuca alternifolia*)
Valerian (*Valeriana officinalis*)
Yohimbine (*Pausinystalia yohimbe*)

GENERIC DRUG DATA

Abacavir (Ziagen) **WARNING:** Hypersensitivity (fever, rash, fatigue, GI, resp) reported; lactic acidosis & hepatomegaly/steatosis reported **Uses:** *HIV infection* **Action:** Nucleoside RT inhibitor **Dose:** *Adults.* 300 mg PO bid **Peds.** 8 mg/kg bid **Caution:** [C, –] CDC recommends HIV-infected mothers not breast-feed due to risk of infant HIV transmission **Supplied:** Tabs 300 mg; soln 20 mg/mL **SE:** See Warning, ↑d LFTs, fat redistribution **Notes:** Numerous drug interactions **Interactions:** EtOH ↓ drug elimination and ↑ drug exposure **Labs:** Monitor LFTs, FBS, CBC & differential, BUN & creatinine, triglycerides **NIPE:** ⊘ EtOH; monitor & teach Pt about hypersensitivity Rxns; DC drug immediately if hypersensitivity Rxn occurs and ⊘ rechallenge; take w/ or w/o food

Abarelix (Plenaxis) **WARNING:** Immediate-onset systemic allergic Rxns (eg, hypotension & syncope), w/ initial & ↑d risk w/ subsequent doses possible. Following dose, observe for at least 30 min; allergic Rxns should be managed appropriately. Only physicians enrolled in the Plenaxis PLUS Program (Plenaxis User Safety Program) may prescribe (www.plenaxis.com). Effectiveness beyond 12 mo not established. Follow serum testosterone to document effectiveness. **Uses:** *Palliation of advanced symptomatic CAP where LHRH agonists are not appropriate* **Action:** GnRH antagonist; does not cause flare seen w/ agonists **Dose:** 100 mg IM (buttock) day 1, 15, 29 & q4wk. Check testosterone before day 29 dose & q8wk to confirm suppression **Caution:** [X, N/A] Body weight >225 lb, prolonged QT interval or liver dysfunction, w/ class IA or III antiarrhythmics **Contra:** Women or children **Supplied:** 100 mg inj vial **SE:** Immediate allergic Rxns (urticaria, pruritus, hypotension, syncope), gynecomastia, hot flashes, sleep disturbances, nipple tenderness **Interactions:** None known with drugs, herbs, or food **Labs:** ↑ AST, ALT, triglycerides; ↓ hgb **NIPE:** Use within 1 h of reconstitution, baseline EKG to measure QT interval

Abciximab (ReoPro) **Uses:** *Prevent acute ischemic complications in PTCA.* *MI* **Action:** Inhibits plt aggregation (glycoprotein IIb/IIIa inhibitor) **Dose:** 0.25 mg/kg bolus 10–60 min pre PTCA, then 0.125 μg/kg/min (max = 10 μg/min) cont inf × 12 h **Caution:** [C, ?/–] **Contra:** Active or recent (w/in 6 wk) internal hemorrhage, CVA w/in 2 y or CVA w/ significant neurologic deficit, bleeding diathesis or PO anticoagulants use w/in 7 d (unless PT ≥ 2× control), thrombocytopenia (<100,000 cells/μL), recent trauma or major surgery (w/in 6 wk), CNS tumor, AVM, aneurysm, severe uncontrolled HTN, vasculitis, use of dextran prior to or during PTCA, hypersensitivity to murine proteins **Supplied:** Inj 2 mg/mL **SE:** Al-

23

lergic Rxns, bleeding, thrombocytopenia possible **Notes:** Use w/ heparin **Interactions:** May ↑ bleeding w/ anticoagulants, antiplts, NSAIDs, thrombolytics **Labs:** Monitor CBC, PT, PTT, INR, guaiac stools, urine for blood **NIPE:** Monitor for ↑ bleeding & bruising; ⊘ shake vial or mix w/ another drug, contact sports ⊘

Acarbose (Precose) **Uses:** *Type 2 DM* **Action:** α-Glucosidase inhibitor; delays digestion of carbohydrates, to ↓ glucose **Dose:** 25–100 mg PO tid (w/ 1st bite each meal) **Caution:** [B, ?] ⊘ if CrCl <25 mL/min **Contra:** IBD, cirrhosis **Supplied:** Tabs 25, 50, 100 mg **SE:** Abdominal pain, diarrhea, flatulence, ↑ LFTs **Notes:** OK w/ sulfonylureas; can affect digoxin levels; check LFTs q3mo for 1st y **Interactions:** ↑ Hypoglycemic effect w/ sulfonylureas, juniper berries, ginseng, garlic, coriander, celery; ↓ effects w/ intestinal absorbents, digestive enzyme preps, diuretics, corticosteroids, phenothiazines, estrogens, phenytoin, INH, sympathomimetics, CCBs, thyroid hormones; ↓ conc of digoxin **Labs:** LFTs, FBS, HbA1c, LFTs, Hgb & Hct **NIPE:** Take drug tid w/ first bite of food, ↓ GI side effects by ↓ dietary starch, treat hypoglycemia w/ dextrose instead of sucrose, continue diet & exercise program

Acebutolol (Sectral) **Uses:** *HTN, arrhythmias* **Action:** Competitively blocks β-adrenergic receptors, β$_1$, & ISA **Dose:** 200–800 mg/d, ↓ if CrCl <50 mL/min **Caution:** [B, D in 2nd & 3rd tri, +] Can exacerbate ischemic heart Dz, ⊘ DC abruptly **Contra:** 2nd-, 3rd-degree heart block **Supplied:** Caps 200, 400 mg **SE:** Fatigue, HA, dizziness, bradycardia **Interactions:** ↓ Antihypertensive effect w/ NSAIDs, salicylates, thyroid preps, anesthetics, antacids, α-adrenergic stimulants, ma-huang, ephedra, licorice; ↓ hypoglycemic effect of glyburide; ↑ hypotensive response w/ other antihypertensives, nitrates, EtOH, diuretics, black cohash, hawthorn, goldenseal, parsley; ↑ bradycardia w/ digoxin, amiodarone; ↑ hypoglycemic effect of insulin **Labs:** Monitor lipids, uric acid, K⁺, FBS, LFTs, thyroxin, ECG **NIPE:** Teach Pt to monitor BP, pulse, S/Sxs CHF

Acetaminophen [APAP, N-acetyl-p-aminophenol] (Tylenol, other generic) [OTC] **Uses:** *Mild to moderate pain, HA, & fever* **Action:** Nonnarcotic analgesic; inhibits CNS synthesis of prostaglandins & hypothalamic heat-regulating center **Dose:** *Adults.* 650 mg PO or PR q4–6h or 1000 mg PO q6h; max 4 g/24 h. *Peds <12 y.* 10–15 mg/kg/dose PO or PR q4–6h; max 2.6 g/24 h. See quick dosing Table 1, page 263. Administer q6h if CrCl 10–50 mL/min & q8h if CrCl <10 mL/min **Caution:** [B, +] Hepatotoxic in elderly & w/ EtOH use w/ >4 g/day; alcoholic liver Dz **Contra:** G6PD deficiency **Supplied:** Tabs 160, 325, 500, 650 mg; chew tabs 80, 160 mg; liq 100 mg/mL, 120 mg/2.5 mL, 120 mg/5 mL, 160 mg/5 mL, 167 mg/5 mL, 325 mg/5 mL, 500 mg/15 mL; gtt 48 mg/mL, 60 mg/0.6 mL; supp 80, 120, 125, 300, 325, 650 mg **SE:** OD causes hepatotoxicity, Rx w/ N-acetylcysteine **Notes:** No antiinflammatory or plt-inhibiting action; ⊘ ETOH **Interactions:** ↑ Hepatotoxicity w/ ETOH, barbiturates, carbamazepine, INH, rifampin, phenytoin; ↑ risk of bleeding w/ NSAIDs, salicylates, warfarin, feverfew, ginkgo biloba, red clover; ↓ absorption w/ antacids, cholestyramine, colestipol **Labs:** Monitor LFTs, CBC, BUN, creatinine, PT, INR; false ↑ urine 5-HIAA, urine glucose, serum uric acid; false ↓ serum glucose, amylase **NIPE:** Delayed absorption if given w/ food, ⊘ EtOH, teach S/Sxs hepatotoxicity, consult health provider if temp ↑103° F/>3 d

Acetaminophen + Butalbital ± Caffeine (Fioricet, Medigesic, Repan, Sedapap-10, Two-Dyne, Triapin, Axocet, Phrenilin Forte) [C-III]

Uses: *Tension HA,* mild pain **Action:** Nonnarcotic analgesic w/ barbiturate **Dose:** 1–2 tabs or caps PO q4/6h PRN; ↓ dose in renal/hepatic impairment; 4 g/24 h APAP max **Caution:** [D, +] Alcoholic liver Dz **Contra:** G6PD deficiency **Supplied:** Caps *Medigesic, Repan, Two-Dyne:* butalbital 50 mg, caffeine 40 mg, + APAP 325 mg. Caps *Axocet, Phrenilin Forte:* butalbital 50 mg + APAP 650 mg; *Triapin:* butalbital 50 mg + APAP 325 mg. Tabs *Medigesic, Fioricet, Repan:* butalbital 50 mg, caffeine 40 mg, + APAP 325 mg; *Phrenilin:* butalbital 50 mg + APAP 325 mg; *Sedapap-10:* butalbital 50 mg + APAP 650 mg **SE:** Drowsiness, dizziness, "hangover" effect **Notes:** Butalbital is habit-forming; ⊘ ETOH intake **Interactions:** ↑ Effects of benzodiazepines, opioid analgesics, sedatives/hypnotics, ETOH, methylphenidate hydrochloride; ↓ effects of MAOIs, TCAs, corticosteroids, theophylline, oral contraceptives, BBs, doxycycline **NIPE:** ⊘ EtOH & CNS depressants, may impair coordination, monitor for depression, use barrier protection contraception

Acetaminophen + Codeine (Tylenol No. 1, No. 2, No. 3, No. 4) [C-III, C-V]

Uses: *Mild–moderate pain (No. 1, 2, 3); moderate–severe pain (No. 4)* **Action:** Combined APAP & a narcotic analgesic **Dose:** **Adults.** 1–2 tabs q3–4h PRN (max dose APAP = 4 g/d). **Peds.**APAP 10–15 mg/kg/dose; codeine 0.5–1 mg/kg dose q4–6h (dosing guide: 3–6 y, 5 mL/dose; 7–12 y, 10 mL/dose); ↓ in renal/hepatic impairment **Caution:** [C, +] Alcoholic liver Dz **Contra:** G6PD deficiency **Supplied:** Tabs 300 mg of APAP; caps 325 mg of APAP + codeine; helix, susp (C-V) APAP 120 mg + codeine 12 mg/5 mL **SE:** Drowsiness, dizziness, N/V **Notes:** Codeine in No. 1 = 7.5 mg, No. 2 = 15 mg, No. 3 = 30 mg, No. 4 = 60 mg **Interactions:** ↑ Effects of benzodiazepines, opioid analgesics, sedatives/hypnotics, ETOH, methylphenidate hydrochloride; ↓ effects of MAOIs, TCAs, corticosteroids, theophylline, oral contraceptives, BBs, doxycycline **NIPE:** ⊘ EtOH & CNS depressants, may impair coordination, monitor for depression, use barrier protection contraception

Acetazolamide (Diamox)

Uses: *Diuresis, glaucoma, prevent high altitude sickness, & refractory epilepsy* **Action:** Carbonic anhydrase inhibitor; ↓ renal excretion of hydrogen & ↑ renal excretion of Na^+, K^+, HCO_3^-, & H_2O **Dose:** **Adults.** *Diuretic:* 250–375 mg IV or PO q24h. *Glaucoma:* 250–1000 mg PO q24h in ÷ doses. *Epilepsy:* 8–30 mg/kg/d PO in ÷ doses. *Altitude sickness:* 250 mg PO q8–12h or SR 500 mg PO q12–24h start 24–48 h before ascent & 48 h after highest ascent. **Peds.** *Epilepsy:* 8–30 mg/kg/24 h PO in ÷ doses; max 1 g/d. *Diuretic:* 5 mg/kg/24 h PO or IV. *Alkalinization of urine:* 5 mg/kg/dose PO bid–tid. *Glau-*

coma: 5–15 mg/kg/24 h PO in ÷ doses; max 1 g/d; adjust in renal impairment; ⊘ if CrCl <10 mL/min **Caution:** [C, +] **Contra:** Renal/hepatic failure, sulfa hypersensitivity **Supplied:** Tabs 125, 250 mg; SR caps 500 mg; inj 500 mg/vial **SE:** Malaise, metallic taste, drowsiness, photosensitivity, hyperglycemia **Notes:** Follow Na⁺ & K⁺; SR forms ⊘ in epilepsy **Interactions:** Causes ↑ effects of amphetamines, quinidine, procainamide, TCAs, ephedrine; ↓ effects of Li, phenobarbital, salicylates, barbiturates; ↑ K⁺ loss w/ corticosteroids and amphotericin B **Labs:** Monitor serum electrolytes, FBS, CBC, creatinine, intraocular pressure; false + for urinary protein, urinary urobilinogen; ↓ I uptake; ↑ serum and urine glucose, uric acid, Ca²⁺, serum ammonia **NIPE:** ↓ GI distress w/ food, monitor for S/Sxs metabolic acidosis, ↑ fluid to ↓ risk of kidney stones

Acetic Acid & Aluminum Acetate (Otic Domeboro)

Uses: *Otitis externa* **Action:** Antiinfective **Dose:** 4–6 gtt in ear(s) q2–3h **Caution:** [C, ?] **Contra:** Perforated tympanic membranes **Supplied:** 2% otic soln **NIPE:** Burning w/ instillation or irrigation

Acetylcysteine (Mucomyst)

Uses: *Mucolytic* agent as adjuvant Rx for chronic bronchopulmonary Dzs & CF; *antidote to APAP hepatotoxicity* **Action:** Splits disulfide linkages between mucoprotein molecular complexes; protects liver by restoring glutathione in APAP OD **Dose:** *Adults & Peds. Nebulizer:* 3–5 mL of 20% soln diluted w/ equal vol of water or NS tid–qid. *Antidote:* PO or NG: 140 mg/kg load, then 70 mg/kg q4h for 17 doses. (Dilute 1:3 in carbonated beverage or orange juice; best if used w/in 24 h) **Caution:** [C, ?] **Supplied:** Soln 10%, 20% **SE:** Bronchospasm (inhalation), N/V, drowsiness **Notes:** Activated charcoal adsorbs acetylcysteine when given PO for acute APAP ingestion **Interactions:** Discolors rubber, Fe, Cu, Ag; incompatible w/ multiple antibiotics—administer drugs separately **Labs:** Monitor ABGs & pulse oximetry w/ bronchospasm **NIPE:** Inform Pt of ↑ productive cough, clear airway before aerosol administration, ↑ fluids to liquefy secretions, unpleasant odor will disappear & may cause N/V

Acitretin (Soriatane)

WARNING: Must not be used by females who are PRG or intend to become PRG during therapy or for up to 3 y following discontinuation of therapy; ⊘ EtOH during therapy or for 2 mo following cessation of therapy; ⊘ donate blood during or up to 3 y following cessation of therapy **Uses:** *Severe psoriasis*; other keratinization disorders (lichen planus, etc) **Action:** Retinoid-like activity **Dose:** 25–50 mg/d PO, w/ main meal; ↑ if no response by 4 wk to 75 mg/d **Caution:** [X, –] Renal/hepatic impairment; in women of reproductive potential **Contra:** See Warning **Supplied:** Caps 10, 25 mg **SE:** Cheilitis, skin peeling, alopecia, pruritus, rash, arthralgia, GI upset, photosensitivity, thrombocytosis, hypertriglyceridemia **Notes:** Follow LFTs; response often takes 2–3 mo; must sign a Pt agreement/informed consent prior to use **Interactions:** ↑ ½ life w/ EtOH use, ↑ hepatotoxicity w/ MRX, ↓ effects of progestin-only contraceptives **Labs:** Monitor LFTs, lipids, FBS, HbA1c **NIPE:** Use effective contraception, ⊘ donate blood for 3 y after Rx, teach Pt S/Sxs pancreatitis

Acyclovir (Zovirax) Uses: *Herpes simplex & zoster infections* Action: Interferes w/ viral DNA synthesis Dose: *Adults. PO: Initial genital herpes:* 200 mg PO q4h while awake, 5 caps/d × 10 d or 400 mg PO tid × 7–10 d. *Chronic suppression:* 400 mg PO bid. *Intermittent Rx:* As for initial Rx, except treat for 5 d, or 800 mg PO bid, at earliest prodrome. *Herpes zoster:* 800 mg PO 5×/d for 7–10 d. *IV:* 5–10 mg/kg/dose IV q8h. *Topical: Initial herpes genitalis:* Apply q3h (6×/d) for 7 d. *Peds.* 5–10 mg/kg/dose IV or PO q8h or 750 mg/m²/24 h ÷ q8h. *Chickenpox:* 20 mg/kg/dose PO qid; ↓ for CrCl <50 mL/min Caution: [C, +] Supplied: Caps 200 mg; tabs 400, 800 mg; susp 200 mg/5 mL; inj 500 mg/vial; oint 5% SE: Dizziness, lethargy, confusion, rash, inflammation at IV site Notes: PO better than topical for herpes genitalis Interactions: ↑ CNS SE w/ MRX & zidovudine, ↑ blood levels w/ probenecid Labs: Monitor BUN, SCr, LFTs, CBC NIPE: Start immediately w/ Sxs, ↑ hydration w/ IV dose, ↑ risk cervical cancer w/ genital herpes, ↑ length of Rx in immunocompromised Pts

Adalimumab (Humira) WARNING: Cases of TB have been observed; check tuberculin skin test prior to use Uses: *Moderate–severe RA w/ an inadequate response to one or more DMARDs* Action: TNF-α inhibitor Dose: 40 mg SQ every other week; may ↑ 40 mg qwk if not on MTX Caution: [B, ?/–] Serious infections & sepsis reported Supplied: Prefilled 1 mL (40 mg) syringe SE: Inj site Rxns, serious infections, neurologic events, malignancies Notes: Refrigerate prefilled syringe, rotate inj sites. OK w/ other DMARDs Interactions: ↑ Effects w/ MRX Labs: May ↑ lipids, alkaline phosphatase NIPE: ⊘ exposure to infection; ⊘ admin live-virus vaccines

Adefovir (Hepsera) WARNING: Acute exacerbations of hepatitis may occur on discontinuation of therapy (monitor LFTs); chronic administration may lead to nephrotoxicity especially in Pts w/ underlying renal dysfunction (monitor renal Fxn); HIV resistance may emerge; lactic acidosis & severe hepatomegaly w/ steatosis have been reported when used alone or in combination w/ other antiretrovirals Uses: *Chronic active hepatitis B virus* Action: Nucleotide analog Dose: CrCl > 50 mL/min: 10 mg PO qd; CrCl 20–49 mL/min: 10 mg PO q48h; CrCl 10–19 mL/min: 10 mg PO q72h; hemodialysis: 10 mg PO q7d post dialysis; adjust w/ CrCl < 50 mL/min Caution: [C, –] Supplied: Tabs 10 mg SE: Asthenia, HA, abdominal pain; see Warning Interactions: See Warning Labs: LFTs, BUN, creatinine, creatine kinase, amylase NIPE: Effects on fetus & baby not known—⊘ breast-feed; use barrier contraception

Adenosine (Adenocard) Uses: *PSVT;* including associated w/ WPW Action: Class IV antiarrhythmic; slows AV node conduction Dose: *Adults.* 6 mg IV bolus; may repeat in 1–2 min; max 12 mg IV. *Peds.* 0.05 mg/kg IV bolus; may repeat q1é2 min to 0.25 mg/kg max Caution: [C, ?] Contra: 2nd- or 3rd-degree AV block or SSS (w/o pacemaker); recent MI or cerebral hemorrhage Supplied: Inj 6 mg/2 mL SE: Facial flushing, HA, dyspnea, chest pressure, hypotension Notes: Doses >12 mg ⊘; can cause momentary asystole when administered. Inter-

actions: ↓ Effects w/ theophylline, caffeine, guarana; ↑ effects w/ dipyridamole; ↑ risk of hypotension & chest pain w/ nicotine; ↑ risk of bradycardia w/ BBs; ↑ risk of heart block w/ carbamazepine; ↑ risk of ventricular fibrillation w/ digitalis glycosides. **Labs:** Monitor ECG during administration; **NIPE:** Monitor BP & pulse during therapy, monitor resp status—↑ risk of bronchospasm in asthmatics, discard unused or unclear soln

Albumin (Albuminar, Buminate, Albutein)
Uses: *Plasma volume expansion for shock* (eg, burns, hemorrhage) **Action:** Maint of plasma colloid oncotic pressure **Dose:** *Adults.* Initially, 25 g IV; subsequent dose based on response; 250 g/48h max. *Peds.* 0.5–1 g/kg/dose; inf at 0.05–0.1 g/min **Caution:** [C, ?] Severe anemia; cardiac; renal, or hepatic insufficiency due to added protein load & possible hypervolemia **Contra:** Cardiac failure **Supplied:** Soln 5%, 25% **SE:** Chills, fever, CHF, tachycardia, hypotension, hypervolemia **Notes:** Contains 130–160 mEq Na/L; may precipitate pulmonary edema **Interactions:** Atypical Rxns w/ ACEI—withhold 24 h prior to plasma administration **Labs:** ↑ Alkaline phosphatase; monitor Hmg, Hct, electrolytes, serum protein **NIPE:** Monitor BP & DC if hypotensive, monitor intake & output, admin to all blood types

Albuterol (Proventil, Ventolin, Volmax)
Uses: *Asthma; prevent exercise-induced bronchospasm* **Action:** β-Adrenergic sympathomimetic bronchodilator; relaxes bronchial smooth muscle **Dose:** *Adults.* Inhaler: 2 inhal q4–6h PRN; 1 Rotacap inhaled q4–6h. *PO:* 2–4 mg PO tidóqid. *Neb:* 1.25–5 mg (0.25–1 mL of 0.5% soln in 2–3 mL of NS) tid-qid. *Peds. Inhaler:* 2 inhal q4–6h. *PO:* 0.1–0.2 mg/kg/dose PO; max 2–4 mg PO tid; *Neb:* 0.05 mg/kg (max 2.5 mg) in 2–3 mL of NS tid-qid **Caution:** [C, +] **Supplied:** Tabs 2, 4 mg; XR tabs 4, 8 mg; syrup 2 mg/5 mL; 90 (m)g/dose met-dose inhaler; Rotacaps 200 μg; soln for neb 0.083, 0.5% **SE:** Palpitations, tachycardia, nervousness, GI upset **Interactions:** ↑ Effects w/ other sympathomimetics; ↑ CV effects w/ MAOI, TCA, inhaled anesthetics; ↓ effects w/ BBs; ↑ effectiveness of insulin, oral hypoglycemics, digoxin **Labs:** Transient ↑ in serum glucose after inhalation; transient ↓ K⁺ after inhalation **NIPE:** Monitor HR, BP, ABGs, s&s bronchospasm & CNS stimulation; instruct on use of inhaler, must use as 1st inhaler, & rinse mouth after use

Albuterol & Ipratropium (Combivent)
Uses: *COPD* **Action:** Combination of β-adrenergic bronchodilator & quaternary anticholinergic compound **Dose:** 2 inhal qid **Caution:** [C, +] **Contra:** Allergy to peanut/soybean **Supplied:** Met-dose inhaler, 18 μg ipratropium/103 μg albuterol/puff **SE:** Palpitations, tachycardia, nervousness, GI upset, dizziness, blurred vision **Interactions:** ↑ Effects w/ anticholinergics, including ophthalmic meds; ↓ effects w/ herb jaborandi tree, pill-bearing spurge **NIPE:** See Albuterol; may cause transient blurred vision/irritation or urinary changes

Aldesleukin [IL-2] (Proleukin)
WARNING: Use restricted to Pts w/ normal pulmonary & cardiac Fxn **Uses:** *Metastatic RCC, melanoma* **Action:**

Acts via IL-2 receptor; numerous immunomodulatory effects **Dose:** 600,000 IU/kg q8h × 14 doses (FDA-approved dose/schedule for RCC). Multiple cont inf & alternate schedules (including "high dose" using $24 × 10^6$ IU/m^2 IV q8h on days 1–5 & 12–16) **Caution:** [C, ?/–] **Contra:** Organ allografts **Supplied:** Inj 1.1 mg/mL ($22 × 10^6$ IU) **SE:** Flu-like syndrome (malaise, fever, chills), N/V/D, ↑ bilirubin; capillary leak syndrome w/ ↓ BP, pulmonary edema, fluid retention, & weight gain; renal toxicity & mild hematologic toxicity (anemia, thrombocytopenia, leukopenia) & secondary eosinophilia; cardiac toxicity (myocardial ischemia, atrial arrhythmias); neurologic toxicity (CNS depression, somnolence, rarely coma, delirium). Pruritic rashes, urticaria, & erythroderma common. **Notes:** Cont inf Rx less likely to cause severe hypotension & fluid retention **Interactions:** May ↑ toxicity of cardiotoxic, hepatotoxic, myelotoxic, & nephrotoxic drugs; ↑ hypotension w/ antihypertensive drugs; ↓ effects w/ corticosteroids; acute Rxn w/ iodinated contrast media up to several months after inf; CNS effects w/ psychotropics **Labs:** May cause ↑ alkaline phosphatase, bilirubin, BUN, SCr, LFTs. **NIPE:** Thoroughly explain serious SE of drug & that some SE are expected; ⊘ EtOH, NSAIDs, ASA

Alefacept (Amevive) **WARNING:** Must monitor CD4 before each dose; w/hold if <250; DC if <250 × 1 month **Uses:** *Moderate/severe chronic plaque psoriasis* **Action:** Fusion protein inhibitor **Dose:** 7.5 mg IV or 15 mg IM once weekly × 12 wk **Caution:** [B, ?/–] PRG registry; associated w/ serious infections **Contra:** Lymphopenia **Supplied:** 7.5-, 15-mg vials **SE:** Pharyngitis, myalgia, inj site Rxn, malignancy **Notes:** IV or IM different formulations; may repeat course 12 wk later if CD4 acceptable **Interactions:** No studies performed **Labs:** Monitor WBCs, CD4+ T lymphocyte counts **NIPE:** ↑ Risk of infection; ⊘ exposure to infections; inj site inflammation; rotate sites

Alendronate (Fosamax) **Uses:** *Rx & prevention of osteoporosis, Rx of steroid-induced osteoporosis & Paget's Dz* **Action:** ↓ Normal & abnormal bone resorption **Dose:** *Osteoporosis Rx:* 10 mg/d PO or 70 mg qwk. *Steroid-induced osteoporosis Rx:* 5 mg/d PO. *Prevention:* 5 mg/d PO or 35 mg qwk. *Paget's Dz:* 40 mg/d PO qwk **Caution:** [C, ?] ⊘ if CrCl <35 mL/min; w/ NSAID use **Contra:** Abnormalities of the esophagus, inability to sit or stand upright for 30 min, hypocalcemia **Supplied:** Tabs 5, 10, 35, 40, 70 mg **SE:** GI disturbances, HA, pain **Notes:** Take 1st thing in AM w/ water (8 oz) > 30 min before 1st food/beverage of the day. ⊘ Lie down for 30 min after. Adequate Ca^{2+} & vitamin D suppl necessary **Interactions:** ↓ Absorption w/ antacids, Ca suppls, Fe, food; ↑ risk of upper GI bleed w/ ASA & NSAIDs **Labs:** May cause transient ↑ serum Ca & phosphate **NIPE:** Adequate Ca & vitamin D suppl needed, ↑ weight-bearing activity, ↓ smoking, EtOH use

Alfentanil (Alfenta) [C-II] **Uses:** *Adjunct in the maint of anesthesia; analgesia* **Action:** Short-acting narcotic analgesic **Dose:** *Adults & Peds >12 y.* 3–75 µg/kg IV inf; total depends on duration of procedure **Caution:** [C, +/–] ↑ ICP, resp depression **Supplied:** Inj 500 µg/mL **SE:** Bradycardia, hypotension, cardiac arrhythmias, peripheral vasodilation, ↑ ICP, drowsiness, resp depression **Interactions:** ↓ Effect w/ phenothiazines; ↑ effects w/ BBs, CNS depressants, erythromycin **NIPE:** Monitor HR, BP, resp rate

Alfuzosin (Uroxatral) **WARNING:** May prolong QTc interval **Uses:** *Benign prostatic hypertrophy* **Action:** α-Blocker **Dose:** 10 mg PO daily immediately after the same meal **Caution:** [B, –] **Contra:** Concomitant CYP3A4 inhibitors; moderate/severe hepatic impairment **Supplied:** Tabs 10 mg **SE:** Postural hypotension, dizziness, HA, fatigue **Notes:** XR tablet—◎ cut or crush; fewest reports of ejaculatory disorders compared w/ other drugs in class **Interactions:** ↑ Effects w/ atenolol, azole antifungals, cimetidine, ritonavir; ↑ effects of antihypertensives **NIPE:** Not indicated for use in women or children; take w/ food; ↑ risk of postural hypotension; ◎ take other meds that prolong QT interval

Alginic Acid + Aluminum Hydroxide & Magnesium Trisilicate (Gaviscon) [OTC] **Uses:** *Heartburn*; pain from hiatal hernia **Action:** Forms protective layer to block gastric acid **Dose:** 2–4 tabs or 15–30 mL PO qid followed by water; **Caution:** [B, –] ◎ in renal impairment or w/ Na-restricted diet **Supplied:** Tabs, susp **SE:** Diarrhea, constipation **Interactions:** ↓ Absorption of tetracyclines

Allopurinol (Zyloprim, Lopurin, Alloprim) **Uses:** *Gout, hyperuricemia of malignancy, & uric acid urolithiasis* **Action:** Xanthine oxidase inhibitor; ↓ uric acid production **Dose:** *Adults. PO:* Initial 100 mg/d; usual 300 mg/d; max 800 mg/d. *IV:* 200–400 mg/m²/d (max 600 mg/24 h) (take after meal w/ plenty of fluid). *Peds.* Use only for treating hyperuricemia of malignancy in <10 y: 10 mg/kg/24 h PO or 200 mg/m²/d IV ÷ q6–8h (max 600 mg/24 h); ↓ in renal impairment **Caution:** [C, M] **Supplied:** Tabs 100, 300 mg; inj 500 mg/30 mL (Aloprim) **SE:** Skin rash, N/V, renal impairment, angioedema **Notes:** Aggravates acute gout; begin after acute attack resolves; IV dose of 6 mg/mL final conc as single daily inf or ÷ 6-, 8-, or 12-h intervals **Interactions:** ↑ Effect of theophylline, oral anticoagulants; ↑ hypersensitivity Rxns w/ ACEIs, thiazide diuretics; ↑ risk of rash w/ ampicillin/amoxicillin; ↑ bone marrow depression w/ cyclophosphamide, azathioprine, mercaptopurine; ↓ effects w/ EtOH **Labs:** ↑ Alkaline phosphatase, bilirubin, LFTs **NIPE:** ↑ fluids to 2–3 L/day, take pc, may ↑ drowsiness

Almotriptan (Axert) See Table 11, page 283

Alosetron (Lotronex) **WARNING:** Serious GI side effects, some fatal, including ischemic colitis, have been reported. May be prescribed only through participation in the prescribing program for Lotronex **Uses:** *Severe diarrhea-predominant IBS in women who have failed conventional therapy* **Action:** Selective 5-HT₃ receptor antagonist **Dose:** *Adults.* 1 mg PO qd × 4 wk; titrate to max of 1 mg bid; DC after 4 wk at max dose if IBS Sxs not controlled **Caution:** [B, ?/–] **Contra:** Hx chronic or severe constipation, GI obstruction, strictures, toxic megacolon, GI perforation, adhesions, ischemic colitis, Crohn's Dz, ulcerative colitis, diverticulitis, thrombophlebitis, or hypercoagulable state. **Supplied:** Tabs 1 mg

SE: Constipation, abdominal pain, nausea **Notes:** DC immediately if constipation or Sxs of ischemic colitis develop; must sign a Pt agreement/informed consent prior to use. **Interactions:** ↑ Risk constipation w/ other drugs that ↓ GI motility, inhibits *N*-acetyltransferase & may influence metabolism of INH, procainamide, hydralazine **NIPE:** Administer w/o regard to food, eval effectiveness >4 w

Alpha₁-Protease Inhibitor (Prolastin)   **Uses:** *α₁-Antitrypsin deficiency*; panacinar emphysema **Action:** Replace human α₁-protease inhibitor **Dose:** 60 μg/kg IV once/wk **Caution:** [C, ?] **Contra:** Selective IgA deficiencies w/ known IgA antibodies **Supplied:** Inj 500 mg/20 mL, 1000 mg/40 mL **SE:** Fever, dizziness, flu-like Sxs, allergic Rxns **NIPE:** Infuse over 30 min, ∅ mix w/ other drugs, use w/in 3 h of reconstitution

Alprazolam (Xanax) [C-IV]   **Uses:** *Anxiety & panic disorders,* anxiety w/ depression **Action:** Benzodiazepine; antianxiety agent **Dose:** *Anxiety:* Initially, 0.25–0.5 mg tid; ↑ to a max of 4 mg/d in ÷ doses. *Panic:* Initially, 0.5 mg tid; may gradually ↑ to desired response; ↓ dose in elderly, debilitated, & hepatic impairment **Caution:** [D, –] **Contra:** Narrow-angle glaucoma, concomitant itra-/ketoconazole **Supplied:** Tabs 0.25, 0.5, 1, 2 mg; soln 1 mg/mL **SE:** Drowsiness, fatigue, irritability, memory impairment, sexual dysfunction **Notes:** ∅ abrupt discontinuation after prolonged use **Interactions:** ↑ CNS depression w/ EtOH, other CNS depressants, narcotics, MAOIs, anesthetics, antihistamines, theophylline, & herbs: kava kava, valerian; ↑ effect w/ oral contraceptives, cimetidine, INH, disulfiram, omeprazole, valproic acid, ciprofloxacin, erythromycin, clarithromycin, phenytoin, verapamil, grapefruit juice; ↑ risk of ketoconazole, itraconazole, & digitalis toxicity; ↓ effectiveness of levodopa; ↓ effect w/ carbamazepine, rifampin, rifabutin, barbiturates, cigarette smoking **Labs:** ↑ Alkaline phosphatase, may cause ↓ Hct & neutropenia **NIPE:** Monitor for resp depression

Alprostadil [Prostaglandin E₁] (Prostin VR)   **Uses:** *Any state in which blood flow must be maintained through the ductus arteriosus* to sustain either pulmonary or systemic circulation until surgery can be performed (eg, pulmonary atresia, pulmonary stenosis, tricuspid atresia, transposition, severe tetralogy of Fallot) **Action:** Vasodilator, plt aggregation inhibitor; smooth muscle of the ductus arteriosus is especially sensitive **Dose:** 0.05 μg/kg/min IV; ↓ dose to lowest that maintains response **Caution:** [X, –] **Contra:** Neonatal resp distress syndrome **Supplied:** Injectable forms **SE:** Cutaneous vasodilation, Sz-like activity, jitteriness, ↑ temp, hypocalcemia, apnea, thrombocytopenia, ↓ BP; may cause apnea **Notes:** Keep intubation kit at bedside if Pt is not intubated **Interactions:** ↑ Effects of anticoagulants & antihypertensives, ↓ effects of cyclosporine **Labs:** ↓ fibrinogen **NIPE:** Dilute drug before administration, refrigerate & discard >24 h, apnea & bradycardia indicates drug overdose, central line preferred, flushing indicates catheter malposition

Alprostadil, Intracavernosal (Caverject, Edex)   **Uses:** *Erectile dysfunction* **Action:** Relaxes smooth muscles, dilates cavernosal arteries, ↑s lacu-

nar spaces & entrapment of blood by compressing venules against tunica albuginea **Dose:** 2.5–60 µg intracavernosal; adjusted to individual **Caution:** [X, –] **Contra:** Conditions predisposing to priapism; anatomic deformities of the penis; penile implants; men in whom sexual activity is inadvisable **Supplied:** *Caverject:* 6–10 or 6–20 µg vials w/wo diluent syringes. *Caverject Impulse:* Self-contained syringe (29 gauge) 10 & 20 µg. *Edex:* 5, 10, 20, 40 µg vials w/ syringes **SE:** Local pain w/ inj **Notes:** Counsel Pts about possible priapism, penile fibrosis, & hematoma; titrate dose at health care provider's office **Interactions:** ↑ Effects of anticoagulants & antihypertensives, ↓ effects of cyclosporine **Labs:** ↓ Fibrinogen **NIPE:** Vaginal itching and burning in female partners, ⊘ inj >3×/wk or closer than 24 h/dose

Alprostadil, Urethral Suppository (Muse) Uses: *Erectile dysfunction* **Action:** Alprostadil (PGE₁) absorbed through urethral mucosa; vasodilator & smooth muscle relaxant of corpus cavernosa **Dose:** 125–1000 µg system 5–10 min prior to sexual activity **Caution:** [X, –] **Contra:** Conditions predisposing to priapism; anatomic deformities of the penis; penile implants; men in whom sexual activity is inadvisable **Supplied:** 125, 250, 500, 1000 µg w/ a transurethral delivery system **SE:** ↓ BP, dizziness, syncope, penile pain, testicular pain, urethral burning/bleeding, priapism **Notes:** Dose titration under health care provider's supervision **Interactions:** ↑ effects of anticoagulants & antihypertensives, ↓ effects of cyclosporine **Labs:** ↓ Fibrinogen **NIPE:** No more than 2 supp/24 h, urinate prior to use

Alteplase, Recombinant [tPA] (Activase) Uses: *AMI, PE, acute ischemic stroke, & CV cath occlusion* **Action:** Thrombolytic; initiates local fibrinolysis by binding to fibrin in the thrombus **Dose:** *AMI & PE:* 100 mg IV over 3 h (10 mg over 2 min, then 50 mg over 1 h, then 40 mg over 2 h). *Stroke:* 0.9 mg/kg (max 90 mg) inf over 60 min. *Cath occlusion:* 10–29 kg 1 mg/mL, ≥30 kg 2 mg/mL **Caution:** [C, ?] **Contra:** Active internal bleeding; uncontrolled HTN (systolic BP = 185 mm Hg/diastolic = 110 mm Hg); recent (w/in 3 mo) CVA, GI bleed, trauma, surgery, prolonged external cardiac massage; intracranial neoplasm, suspected aortic dissection, AVM/aneurysm, bleeding diathesis, hemostatic defects, Sz at the time of stroke, suspicion of subarachnoid hemorrhage **Supplied:** Powder for inj 50, 100 mg **SE:** Bleeding, bruising (especially from venipuncture sites), hypotension **Notes:** Give heparin to prevent reocclusion; in AMI doses of >150 mg associated w/ intracranial bleeding **Interactions:** ↑ Risk of bleeding w/ heparin, ASA, NSAIDs, abciximab, dipyridamole, eptifibatide, tirofiban; ↓ effects w/ nitroglycerine **Labs:** ↓ Fibrinogen **NIPE:** Compress venipuncture site at least 30 min, monitor PT/PTT, bed rest during inf

Altretamine (Hexalen) Uses: *Epithelial ovarian CA* **Action:** Unknown; cytotoxic agent, possibly alkylating agent; inhibits nucleotide incorporation into DNA/RNA **Dose:** 260 mg/m²/d in 4 ÷ doses for 14–21 d of a 28-d Rx cycle; dose ↑ to 150 mg/m²/d for 14 d in multiagent regimens (see specific protocols) **Caution:** [D, ?/–]. **Contra:** Preexisting BM depression or neurologic toxicity **Supplied:** Caps 50, 100 mg **SE:** Vomiting, diarrhea, & cramps; neurologic (peripheral neuropathy, CNS depression); minimally myelosuppressive **Interactions:** ↓ Effect w/ phenobarbital, ↓ antibody response w/ live virus vaccines, ↑ risk of toxicity w/ cimetidine & hypotension w/ MAOIs, ↑ bone marrow depression w/ radiation **Labs:** ↑ Alkaline phosphatase, BUN, & SCr **NIPE:** Use barrier contraception, take w/ food, monitor CBC

Aluminum Hydroxide (Amphojel, AlternaGEL) [OTC]

Uses: *Relief of heartburn, upset or sour stomach, or acid indigestion*; suppl to Rx of hyperphosphatemia **Action:** Neutralizes gastric acid; binds phosphate **Dose:** *Adults.* 10–30 mL or 2 tabs PO q4–6h. *Peds.* 5–15 mL PO q4–6h or 50–150 mg/kg/24 h PO q4–6h (hyperphosphatemia) **Caution:** [C, ?] **Supplied:** Tabs 300, 600 mg; chew tabs 500 mg; susp 320, 600 mg/5 mL **SE:** constipation **Notes:** OK in renal failure **Interactions:** ↓ Absorption & effects of allopurinol, benzodiazepines, corticosteroids, chloroquine, cimetidine, digoxin, INH, phenytoin, quinolones, ranitidine, tetracycline **Labs:** ↑ Serum gastrin, ↓ serum phosphate **NIPE:** Separate other drug administration by 2 h, ↑ effectiveness of liquid form

Aluminum Hydroxide + Magnesium Carbonate (Gaviscon) [OTC]

Uses: *Relief of heartburn, acid indigestion* **Action:** Neutralizes gastric acid **Dose:** *Adults.* 15–30 mL PO pc & hs. *Peds.* 5–15 mL PO qid or PRN; ⊘ in renal impairment **Caution:** [C, ?] **Supplied:** Liq w/ Al hydroxide 95 mg + Mg carbonate 358 mg/15 mL **SE:** May cause ↑ Mg^{2+} (w/ renal insufficiency), constipation, diarrhea **Notes:** Doses qid are best given pc & hs; may affect absorption of some drugs **Interactions:** In addition to Al hydroxide ↓ effects of histamine blockers, hydantoins, nitrofurantoin, phenothiazines, ticlopidine, ↑ effects of quinidine, sulfonylureas **NIPE:** ⊘ Concurrent drug use & separate by 2 h, ↑ fiber

Aluminum Hydroxide + Magnesium Hydroxide (Maalox) [OTC]

Uses: *Hyperacidity* (peptic ulcer, hiatal hernia, etc) **Action:** Neutralizes gastric acid **Dose:** *Adults.* 10–60 mL or 2–4 tabs PO qid or PRN. *Peds.* 5–15 mL PO qid or PRN **Caution:** [C, ?] **Supplied:** Tabs, susp **SE:** May cause ↑ Mg^{2+} in renal insufficiency, constipation, diarrhea **Notes:** Doses qid best given pc & hs **Interactions:** In addition to Al hydroxide, ↓ effects of digoxin, quinolones, phenytoin, Fe suppl, and ketoconazole **NIPE:** ⊘ Concurrent drug use; separate by 2 h

Aluminum Hydroxide + Magnesium Hydroxide & Simethicone (Mylanta, Mylanta II, Maalox Plus) [OTC]

Uses: *Hyperacidity w/ bloating* **Action:** Neutralizes gastric acid & defoaming **Dose:** *Adults.* 10–60 mL or 2–4 tabs PO qid or PRN. *Peds.* 5–15 mL PO qid or PRN; ⊘ in renal impairment **Caution:** [C, ?] **Supplied:** Tabs, susp **SE:** Hypermagnesemia in renal insufficiency, diarrhea, constipation **Notes:** Mylanta II contains twice the Al & Mg hydroxide of Mylanta; may affect absorption of some drugs **Interactions:** In addition to Al hydroxide, ↓ effects of digoxin, quinolones, phenytoin, Fe suppl, and ketoconazole **NIPE:** ⊘ Concurrent drug use; separate by 2 h

Aluminum Hydroxide + Magnesium Trisilicate (Gaviscon, Gaviscon-2) [OTC]

Uses: *Relief of heartburn, upset or sour stomach, or acid indigestion* **Action:** Neutralizes gastric acid **Dose:** Chew 2–4 tabs qid; ⊘ in renal impairment **Caution:** [C, ?] **Contra:** Mg sensitivity **Supplied:** *Gaviscon:* Al hydroxide 80 mg & Mg trisilicate 20 mg; *Gaviscon-2:* Al hydroxide 160 mg & Mg trisilicate 40 mg **SE:** Hypermagnesemia in renal insufficiency, constipation, diarrhea **Notes:** Concomitant administration may affect absorption of some drugs **Interactions:** In addition to Al hydroxide, ↓ effects of digoxin, quinolines, phenytoin, Fe suppl, and ketoconazole **NIPE:** ⊘ Concurrent drug use; separate by 2 h

Amantadine (Symmetrel)

Uses: *Rx or prophylaxis for influenza A viral infections, parkinsonism, & drug-induced EPS* **Action:** Prevents release of infectious viral nucleic acid into the host cell; releases dopamine from intact dopaminergic terminals **Dose:** *Adults. Influenza A:* 200 mg/d PO or 100 mg PO bid. *Parkinsonism:* 100 mg PO daily or bid. *Peds.* 1–9 y: 4.4–8.8 mg/kg/24 h to 150 mg/24 h max ÷ doses qd–bid. *10–12 y:* 100–200 mg/d in 1–2 ÷ doses; reduce dose in renal impairment **Caution:** [C, M] **Supplied:** Caps 100 mg; tabs 100 mg; soln 50 mg/5 mL **SE:** Orthostatic hypotension, edema, insomnia, depression, irritability, hallucinations, dream abnormalities **Interactions:** ↑ Effects w/ HCTZ, triamterene, amiloride, pheasant's eye herb, scopolia root, benztropine **Labs:** ↑ BUN, SCr, CPK, alkaline phosphatase, bilirubin, LDH, AST, ALT **NIPE:** ⊘ Discontinue abruptly, take at least 4 h before sleep if insomnia occurs, eval for mental status changes, take w/ meals, ⊘ EtOH

Amifostine (Ethyol)

Uses: *Xerostomia prophylaxis during RT (head & neck, ovarian, or non-small-cell lung CA). Reduces renal toxicity associated w/ repeated administration of cisplatin* **Action:** Prodrug, dephosphorylated by alkaline phosphatase to the pharmacologically active thiol metabolite **Dose:** 910 mg/m²/d as a 15-min IV inf 30 min prior to chemotherapy **Caution:** [C, +/–] **Supplied:** 500-mg vials of lyophilized drug w/ 500 mg of mannitol, reconstituted in sterile NS **SE:** Transient hypotension in >60%, N/V, flushing w/ hot or cold chills, dizziness, hypocalcemia, somnolence, & sneezing. **Notes:** Does not reduce the effectiveness of cyclophosphamide plus cisplatin chemotherapy **Interactions:** ↑ Effects w/ antihypertensives **Labs:** ↓ Calcium levels **NIPE:** Monitor BP, ensure adequate hydration, infuse over 15 min w/Pt supine

Amikacin (Amikin)

Uses: *Serious infections caused by gram(–) bacteria* & mycobacteria **Action:** Aminoglycoside antibiotic; inhibits protein synthesis *Spectrum:* Good gram(–) bacterial coverage including *Pseudomonas* sp; *Mycobacterium* sp **Dose:** *Adults & Peds.* 5–7.5 mg/kg/dose ÷ q8–24h based on renal Fxn. *Neonates <1200 g, 0–4 wk:* 7.5 mg/kg/dose q12h–18h. *Postnatal age <7 d, 1200–2000 g:* 7.5 mg/kg/dose q12h; *>2000 g:* 10 mg/kg/dose q12h. *Postnatal age >7 d, 1200–2000 g:* 7 mg/kg/dose q8h; *>2000 g:* 7.5–10 mg/kg/dose q8h **Caution:** [C, +/–] **Supplied:** Inj 100, 500 mg/2 mL **SE:** Nephrotoxicity, ototoxicity, neurotoxicity; $\varnothing$ use w/ potent diuretics **Notes:** May be effective against gram(−) bacteria resistant to gentamicin & tobramycin; monitor renal Fxn carefully for dosage adjustments; monitor serum levels (see Table 2, page 265) **Interactions:** ↑ Risk of ototoxicity and nephrotoxicity w/ acyclovir, amphotericin B, cephalosporins, cisplatin, loop diuretics, methoxyflurane, polymyxin B, vancomycin; ↑ neuromuscular blocking effect w/ muscle relaxants & anesthetics **Labs:** ↑ BUN, SCr, AST, ALT, serum alkaline phosphatase, bilirubin, LDH **NIPE:** ↑ Fluid consumption

Amiloride (Midamor)
Uses: *HTN, CHF, & thiazide-induced hypokalemia* **Action:** K-sparing diuretic; interferes w/ K^+/Na^+ exchange in distal tubules **Dose:** *Adults.* 5–10 mg PO qd. *Peds.* 0.625 mg/kg/d; ↓ dose in renal impairment **Caution:** [B, ?] **Contra:** Hyperkalemia, SCr > 1.5 BUN > 30 **Supplied:** Tabs 5 mg **SE:** Hyperkalemia possible; monitor serum K⁺ levels; HA, dizziness, dehydration, impotence **Interactions:** ↑ Risk of hyperkalemia w/ ACE-I, K-sparing diuretics, NSAIDs, & K salt substitutes; ↑ effects of Li, digoxin, antihypertensives, amantadine; ↑ risk of hyperkalemia w/ licorice **NIPE:** Take w/ food, I&O, daily weights, $\varnothing$ salt substitutes, bananas, & oranges

Aminocaproic Acid (Amicar)
Uses: *Excessive bleeding from systemic hyperfibrinolysis & urinary fibrinolysis* **Action:** Inhibits fibrinolysis via inhibition of tPA substances **Dose:** *Adults.* 5 g IV or PO (1st h) then by 1–1.25 g/h IV or PO. *Peds.* 100 mg/kg IV (1st h) (max dose/d: 30 g), then 1 g/m²/h; max 18 g/m²/d; ↓ in renal failure **Caution:** [C, ?] Hematuria of upper urinary tract **Contra:** Disseminated intravascular coagulation **Supplied:** Tabs 500 mg; syrup 250 mg/mL; inj 250 mg/mL **SE:** ↓ BP, bradycardia, dizziness, HA, fatigue, rash, GI disturbance, ↓ plt Fxn **Notes:** Administer for 8 h or until bleeding is controlled; not for upper urinary tract bleeding **Interactions:** ↑ Coagulation w/ estrogens & oral contraceptives **Labs:** ↑ K⁺ levels, false ↑ urine amino acids **NIPE:** Creatine kinase monitoring w/ long-term use, eval for thrombophlebitis & difficulty urinating

Amino-Cerv pH 5.5 Cream
Uses: *Mild cervicitis,* postpartum cervicitis/cervical tears, postcauterization, postcryosurgery, & postconization **Action:** Hydrating agent; removes excess keratin in hyperkeratotic conditions **Dose:** 1 Applicatorful intravaginally hs for 2–4 wk **Caution:** [C, ?] Use in viral skin infection **Supplied:** Vaginal cream **SE:** Transient stinging, local irritation **Notes:** AKA carbamide or urea; contains 8.34% urea, 0.5% sodium propionate, 0.83% methionine, 0.35% cystine, 0.83% inositol, & benzalkonium chloride

Aminoglutethimide (Cytadren)
Uses: Adrenocortical carcinoma, *Cushing's syndrome,* breast CA & CAP **Action:** Inhibits adrenal steroidogenesis & conversion of androgens to estrogens **Dose:** 750–1500 mg/d in ÷ doses plus hydrocortisone 20–40 mg/d; ↓ dose in renal insufficiency **Caution:** [D, ?] **Supplied:** Tabs 250 mg **SE:** Adrenal insufficiency ("medical adrenalectomy"), hypothyroidism, masculinization, hypotension, vomiting, rare hepatotoxicity, rash, myalgia, fever **Interactions:** ↓ Effects w/ dexamethasone & hydrocortisone, ↓ effects

of warfarin, theophylline, medroxyprogesterone **NIPE:** Masculinization reversible after DC drug. ⊘ PRG

Aminophylline **Uses:** *Asthma, COPD* & bronchospasm **Action:** Relaxes smooth muscle of the bronchi, pulmonary blood vessels; stimulates diaphragm **Dose:** *Adults.* *Acute asthma:* Load 6 mg/kg IV, then 0.4–0.9 mg/kg/h IV cont inf. *Chronic asthma:* 24 mg/kg/24 h PO or PR ÷ q6h. *Peds.* Load 6 mg/kg IV, then 1 mg/kg/h IV cont inf; ↓ in hepatic insufficiency & w/ certain drugs (macrolide & quinolone antibiotics, cimetidine, & propranolol) **Caution:** [C, +] Uncontrolled arrhythmias, hyperthyroidism, peptic ulcers, uncontrolled Sz disorder **Supplied:** Tabs 100, 200 mg; soln 105 mg/5 mL; supp 250, 500 mg; inj 25 mg/mL **SE:** N/V, irritability, tachycardia, ventricular arrhythmias, & Szs **Notes:** Individualize dosage; follow serum levels (as theophylline, Table 2, page 265; aminophylline is about 85% theophylline; erratic absorption w/ rectal doses **Interactions:** ↓ Effects of Li, phenytoin, adenosine; ↓ effects w/ phenobarbital, aminoglutethamide, barbiturates, rifampin, ritonavir, thyroid meds; ↑ effects w/ cimetidine, ciprofloxacin, erythromycin, INH, oral contraceptives, verapamil, tobacco, charcoal-broiled foods, St. John's wort **Labs:** ↑ Uric acid levels, falsely ↑ levels w/ furosemide, probenecid, acetaminophen, coffee, tea, cola, chocolate **NIPE:** ⊘ Chew or crush time-released capsules & take on empty stomach, immediate release can be taken w/ food, ↑ fluids 2 L/d, tobacco ↑ drug elimination

Amiodarone (Cordarone, Pacerone) **Uses:** *Recurrent VF or hemodynamically unstable VT,* supraventricular arrhythmias, AF **Action:** Class III antiarrhythmic **Dose:** *Adults.* *Ventricular arrhythmias:* *IV:* 15 mg/min for 10 min, then 1 mg/min for 6 h, then maint 0.5 mg/min cont. inf or *PO:* Load: 800–1600 mg/d PO for 1–3 wk. Maint: 600–800 mg/d PO for 1 mo, then 200–400 mg/d. *Supraventricular arrhythmias:* *IV:* 300 mg IV over 1 h, then 20 mg/kg for 24 h, then 600 mg PO qd for 1 wk, then maint 100–400 mg qd or *PO:* Load: 600–800 mg/d PO for 1–4 wk. Maint: Gradually ↓ to 100–400 mg q day. *Peds.* 10–15 mg/kg/24 h ÷ q12h PO for 7–10 d, then 5 mg/kg/24 h ÷ q12h or qd (infants/neonates require a higher loading dose); ↓ in severe liver insufficiency **Caution:** [D, –] **Contra:** Sinus node dysfunction, 2nd- or 3rd-degree AV block, sinus bradycardia (w/o pacemaker) **Supplied:** Tabs 200 mg; inj 50 mg/mL **SE:** Pulmonary fibrosis, exacerbation of arrhythmias, prolongs QT interval; CHF, arrhythmias, hypo-/hyperthyroidism, ↑ LFTs, liver failure, corneal microdeposits, optic neuropathy/neuritis, peripheral neuropathy, photosensitivity **Notes:** Half-life is 53 d; IV conc of >0.2 mg/mL administered via a central catheter; alters digoxin levels, may require reduced digoxin dose **Interactions:** ↑ Serum levels of digoxin, quinidine, procainamide, flecainide, phenytoin, warfarin, theophylline, cyclosporine; ↑ levels w/ cimetidine, indinavir, ritonavir; ↓ levels w/ cholestyramine, rifampin, St. John's wort; ↑ cardiac effects w/ BBs, CCB **Labs:** ↑ T_4 & RT_3, ANA titer, ↓ T_3 **NIPE:** Monitor cardiac rhythm, BP, LFTs, thyroid Fxn, ophthalmologic exam; ↑ photosensitivity—use sunscreen; take w/ food

Amitriptyline (Elavil) **Uses:** *Depression,* peripheral neuropathy, chronic pain, & tension HAs **Action:** TCA; inhibits reuptake of serotonin & norepinephrine by the presynaptic neurons **Dose:** *Adults.* Initially, 30–50 mg PO hs; may ↑ to 300 mg hs. *Peds.* ⊘ if <12 y unless for chronic pain; initially 0.1 mg/kg PO hs, advance over 2–3 wk to 0.5–2 mg/kg PO hs; caution in hepatic impairment; taper when discontinuing **Caution:** [D, +/–] Narrow-angle glaucoma **Contra:** W/ MAOIs, during acute recovery following MI **Supplied:** Tabs 10, 25, 50, 75, 100, 150 mg; inj 10 mg/mL **SE:** Strong anticholinergic SEs; OD may be fatal; urine retention & sedation, ECG changes, photosensitivity **Interactions:** ↓ Dffects w/ carbamazepine, phenobarbital, rifampin, cholestyramine, colestipol, tobacco; ↑ effects w/ cimetidine, quinidine, indinavir, ritonavir, CNS depressants, SSRIs, haloperidol, oral contraceptives, BBs, phenothiazines, EtOH, evening primrose oil; ↑ effects of amphetamines, anticholinergics, epinephrine, hypoglycemics, phenylephrine **Labs:** ↑ Glucose, false ↑ carbamazepine levels **NIPE:** ↑ photosensitivity—use sunscreen, appetite, & craving for sweets, ⊘ DC abruptly, may turn urine blue-green

Amlodipine (Norvasc) **Uses:** *HTN & stable or unstable angina* **Action:** CCB; relaxes coronary vascular smooth muscle **Dose:** 2.5–10 mg/d PO **Caution:** [C, ?] **Supplied:** Tabs 2.5, 5, 10 mg **SE:** Peripheral edema, HA, palpitations, flushing **Notes:** May be taken w/out regard to meals

Amlodipine/Atorvastatin (Caduet) **Uses:** * HTN, chronic stable angina, vasospastic angina, control ↑d cholesterol & triglycerides* **Action:** CCB & HMG-CoA reductase inhibitor **Dose:** Amlodipine 5–10 mg PO daily/ Atorvastatin 10–80 mg PO daily **Caution:** [X, –] **Contra:** Active liver Dz, unexplained elevation of serum transaminases **Supplied:** Tabs amlodipine/atorvastatin: 5/10, 5/20, 5/40, 5/80, 10/10, 10/20, 10/40, 10/80 mg **SE:** Peripheral edema, HA, palpitations, flushing, myopathy, arthralgia, myalgia, GI upset **Interactions:** ↑ Hypotension w/ fentanyl, nitrates, EtOH, quinidine, other antihypertensives, grapefruit juice; ↑ effects w/ diltiazem, erythromycin, H₂ blockers, proton pump inhibitors, quinidine; ↓ effects w/ NSAIDs, barbiturates, rifampin **Labs:** Monitor LFTs **NIPE:** ⊘ DC abruptly, ↑ photosensitivity—use sunscreen

Ammonium Aluminum Sulfate [Alum] [OTC] **Uses:** *Hemorrhagic cystitis when bladder irrigation fails* **Action:** Astringent **Dose:** 1–2% soln used w/ constant bladder irrigation w/ NS **Caution:** [+/–] **Supplied:** Powder for reconstitution **SE:** Encephalopathy possible; obtain Al levels, especially in renal insufficiency; can precipitate & occlude catheters **Notes:** Safe to use w/out anesthesia & w/ vesicoureteral reflux

Amoxicillin (Amoxil, Polymox) **Uses:** *Ear, nose, & throat, lower resp, skin, urinary tract infections resulting from susceptible gram(+) bacteria (streptococci) & gram(–) bacteria (H. influenzae, E. coli, P. mirabilis), H. pylori,* endocarditis prophylaxis **Action:** β-Lactam antibiotic; inhibits cell wall synthesis from *Spectrum:* Gram(+) including *Streptococcus* sp, *Enterococcus* sp; some gram(−) including *H. influenzae, E. coli, N. gonorrhoeae,* & *P. mirabilis* **Dose:** *Adults.* 250–500 mg PO tid or 500–875 mg bid. *Peds.* 25–100 mg/kg/24 h PO ÷ q8h. 200–400 mg PO bid (equivalent to 125–250 mg tid); ↓ dose in renal impairment **Caution:** [B, +] **Supplied:** Caps 250, 500 mg; chew tabs 125, 200, 250, 400 mg; susp 50 mg/mL, 125, 250 mg/5 mL; tabs 500, 875 mg **SE:** Diarrhea; skin rash common **Notes:** Cross-hypersensitivity w/ penicillin; many hospital strains of *E. coli*-resistant **Interactions:** ↑ Effects of warfarin, ↑ effects w/ probenecid, disulfiram, ↑ risk of rash w/ allopurinol, ↓ effects of oral contraceptives, ↓ effects w/ tetracyclines, chloramphenicol **Labs:** ↑ Serum alkaline phosphatase, LDH, LFTs, false + direct Coombs test **NIPE:** Space meds over 24/h, eval for superinfection, use barrier contraception

Amoxicillin & Clavulanic Acid (Augmentin, Augmentin 600 ES, Augmentin XR)

Uses: *Ear, lower resp, sinus, urinary tract, skin infections caused by β-lactamase-producing *H. influenzae, S. aureus,* & *E. coli** **Action:** Combination of a β-lactam antibiotic & a β-lactamase inhibitor. *Spectrum:* Gram(+) coverage same as amoxicillin alone, MSSA; gram(−) coverage as w/ amoxicillin alone, β-lactamase-producing *H. influenzae, Klebsiella* sp, *M. catarrhalis* **Dose:** *Adults.* 250–500 mg PO q8h or 875 mg q12h; XR 2000 mg PO q12h. *Peds.* 20–40 mg/kg/d as amoxicillin PO ÷ q8h or 45 mg/kg/d ÷ q12h; ↓ in renal impairment (take w/ food) **Caution:** [B, ?] **Supplied** (expressed as amoxicillin/clavulanic acid): Tabs 250/125, 500/125, 875/125 mg; chew tabs 125/31.25, 200/28.5, 250/62.5, 400/57 mg; susp 125/31.25, 250/62.5, 200/28.5, 400/57 mg/5 mL; 600-ES 600/42.9 mg tab; XR tab 1000/62.5 mg **SE:** Abdominal discomfort, N/V/D, allergic Rxn, vaginitis **Notes:** ○ Substitute two 250-mg tabs for one 500-mg tab or an OD of clavulanic acid will occur **Interactions:** ↑ Effects of warfarin, ↑ effects w/ probenecid, disulfiram, ↑ risk of rash w/ allopurinol, ↓ effects of oral contraceptives, ↓ effects w/ tetracyclines, chloramphenicol **Labs:** ↑ Serum alkaline phosphatase, LDH, LFTs, false + direct Coombs' test **NIPE:** Space meds over 24/h, eval for superinfection, use barrier contraception

Amphotericin B (Fungizone)

Uses: *Severe, systemic fungal infections; oral & cutaneous candidiasis* **Action:** Binds ergosterol in the fungal membrane, altering membrane permeability **Dose:** *Adults & Peds.* 1 mg adults or 0.1 mg/kg to 1 mg in children, then 0.25–1.5 mg/kg/24 h IV over 2–6 h (range 25–50 mg/d or qod). Total dose varies w/ indication. *PO:* 1 mL qid. *Topical:* Apply bid–qid for 1–4 wk depending on infection; ↓ dose in renal impairment **Caution:** [B, ?] **Supplied:** Powder for inj 50 mg/vial; PO susp 100 mg/mL; cream, lotion, oint 3% **SE:** Reduced K⁺/Mg²⁺ from renal wasting; anaphylaxis reported **Notes:** Monitor renal Fxn/LFTs; pretreatment w/ APAP & antihistamines (Benadryl) minimizes adverse effects w/ IV inf (eg, fever, chills, HA, nephrotoxicity, hypotension, anemia) **Interactions:** ↑ Nephrotoxic effects w/ antineoplastics, cyclosporine, furosemide, vancomycin, aminoglycosides, ↑ hypokalemia w/ corticosteroids, skeletal muscle relaxants **Labs:** ↑ Serum bilirubin, serum cholesterol **NIPE:** Monitor CNS effects & ⊘ take hs; topical cream discolors skin

Amphotericin B Cholesteryl (Amphotec)   Uses: *Aspergillosis in Pts intolerant or refractory to conventional amphotericin B,* systemic candidiasis **Action:** Binds sterols in the cell membrane, alters membrane permeability **Dose: Adults & Peds.** Test dose 1.6–8.3 mg, over 15–20 min, then 3–4 mg/kg/d; 1 mg/kg/d inf: ↓ in renal insufficiency **Caution:** [B, ?] **Supplied:** Powder for inj 50 mg, 100 mg/vial (final conc 0.6 mg/mL) **SE:** Anaphylaxis reported; fever, chills, HA, ↓ K⁺, ↓ Mg²⁺, nephrotoxicity, ↓ BP, anemia **Notes:** ⊘ Use in-line filter; monitor LFT & electrolytes **Interactions:** See Amphotericin B

Amphotericin B Lipid Complex (Abelcet)   Uses: *Refractory invasive fungal infection in Pts intolerant to conventional amphotericin B* **Action:** Binds sterols in cell membrane, alters membrane permeability **Dose: Adults & Peds.** 5 mg/kg/d IV as a single daily dose; 2.5 mg/kg/h inf **Caution:** [B, ?] **Supplied:** Inj 5 mg/mL **SE:** Anaphylaxis reported; fever, chills, HA, ↓ K⁺, ↓ Mg²⁺, nephrotoxicity, hypotension, anemia **Notes:** Filter soln w/ a 5-mm filter needle; ⊘ mix in electrolyte-containing solns; if inf >2 h, manually mix bag **Interactions:** See Amphotericin B

Amphotericin B Liposomal (AmBisome)   Uses: *Refractory invasive fungal infection in Pts intolerant to conventional amphotericin B, cryptococcal meningitis in HIV, empiric Rx for febrile neutropenia, visceral leishmaniasis* **Action:** Binds to sterols in the cell membrane, resulting in changes in membrane permeability **Dose: Adults & Peds.** 3–5 mg/kg/d, inf 60–120 min; ↓ in renal insufficiency **Caution:** [B, ?] **Supplied:** Powder for inj 50 mg **SE:** Anaphylaxis reported; fever, chills, HA, ↓ K⁺, ↓ Mg²⁺ nephrotoxicity, hypotension, anemia **Notes:** Filter w/ no less than 1-μm filter **Interactions:** See Amphotericin B

Ampicillin (Amcill, Omnipen)   Uses: *Resp tract, GU tract, GI tract infections & meningitis due to susceptible gram(–) & gram(+) bacteria; endocarditis prophylaxis* **Action:** β-Lactam antibiotic; inhibits cell wall synthesis. *Spectrum:* Gram(+) coverage, including *Streptococcus* sp, *Staphylococcus* sp, *Listeria*; gram(–) coverage, including *Klebsiella* sp, *E. coli, H. influenzae, P. mirabilis, Shigella* sp, *Salmonella* sp **Dose: Adults.** 500 mg–2 g IM or IV q6h or 250–500 mg PO q6h. **Peds.** *Neonates <7 d:* 50–100 mg/kg/24 h IV ÷ q8h. *Term infants:* 75–150 mg/kg/24 h ÷ q6–8h IV or PO. *Children >1 mo:* 100–200 mg/kg/24 h ÷ q4–6h IM or IV; 50–100 mg/kg/24 h ÷ q6h PO up to 250 mg/dose. *Meningitis:* 200–400 mg/kg/24 h ÷ q4–6h IV; ↓ in renal impairment (take on an empty stomach) **Caution:** [B, M] Cross-hypersensitivity w/ penicillin **Supplied:** Caps 250, 500 mg; susp 100 mg/mL (reconstituted as drops), 125 mg/5 mL, 250 mg/5 mL, 500 mg/5 mL; powder for inj 125 mg, 250 mg, 500 mg, 1 g, 2 g, 10 g/vial **SE:** Diarrhea, skin rash, allergic Rxn **Notes:** Many hospital strains of *E. coli* now resistant **Interactions:** ↓ Effects of oral contraceptives & atenolol, ↓ effects w/ chloramphenicol,

erythromycin, tetracycline, & food; ↑ effects of anticoagulants & MRX; ↑ risk of rash w/ allopurinal; ↑ effects w/ probenecid & disulfiram **Labs:** ↑ LFTs, serum protein, serum theophylline, serum uric acid; ↓ serum estrogen, serum cholesterol, serum folate; false + direct Coombs' test, urine glucose, & urine amino acids **NIPE:** Take on empty stomach & around the clock; may cause candidal vaginitis; use barrier contraception

Ampicillin–Sulbactam (Unasyn)

Uses: *Gynecologic, intraabdominal, skin infections caused by β-lactamase-producing strains of *S. aureus, Enterococcus, H. influenzae, P. mirabilis,* & *Bacteroides* sp* **Action:** Combination of a β-lactam antibiotic & a β-lactamase inhibitor. *Spectrum:* Gram(+) coverage as ampicillin alone, gram(−) coverage as ampicillin alone; also *Enterobacter, Acinetobacter, Bacteroides* **Dose:** *Adults.* 1.5–3 g IM or IV q6h. *Peds.* 100–200 mg ampicillin/kg/d (150–300 mg Unasyn) q6h; ↓ in renal failure **Caution:** [B, M] **Supplied:** Powder for inj 1.5, 3.0 g/vial **SE:** Hypersensitivity Rxns, rash, diarrhea, pain at inj site **Notes:** A 2:1 ratio of ampicillin:sulbactam **Interactions:** See Ampicillin

Amprenavir (Agenerase)

WARNING: PO soln contra in children <4 y due to potential toxicity from large volume of excipient polypropylene glycol in the formulation **Uses:** *HIV infection* **Action:** Protease inhibitor; prevents the maturation of the virion to mature viral particle **Dose:** *Adults.* 1200 mg bid. *Peds.* 20 mg/kg bid or 15 mg/kg tid up to 2400 mg/d **Caution:** [C, ?] CDC recommends HIV-infected mothers not breast-feed due to risk of transmission of HIV to infant; previous allergic Rxn to sulfonamides **Contra:** CYP3A4 substrates (ergot derivatives, midazolam, triazolam, etc); soln < 4 y, PRG, hepatic or renal failure, disulfram, or metronidazole **Supplied:** Caps 50, 150 mg; soln 15 mg/mL **SE:** Life-threatening rash, hyperglycemia, hypertriglyceridemia, fat redistribution, N/V/D, depression **Notes:** Caps & soln contain vitamin E exceeding RDA intake amounts; ⊘ high-fat meals w/ administration; many drug interactions **Interactions:** ↑ Effects w/ abacavir, cimetidine, delavirdine, indinavir, itraconazole, ketoconazole, macrolides, ritonavir, zidovudine, grapefruit juice; ↑ effects of cisapride, clozapine, ergotamine, loratadine, nelfinavir, dapsone, pimozide, rifabutin, saquinavir, sildenafil, terfenadine, triazolam, warfarin, zidovudine, HMG-CoA reductase inhibitors; ↓ effects w/ antacids, barbiturates, carbamazepine, nevirapine, phenytoin, rifampin, St. John's wort, high-fat food; ↓ effects of oral contraceptives **Labs:** ↑ Serum glucose, cholesterol, & triglyceride levels **NIPE:** Use barrier contraception, may take w/ food other than high-fat food, ⊘ take vitamin E

Anakinra (Kineret)

WARNING: Associated w/ ↑ incidence of serious infections; DC w/ serious infection **Uses:** *Reduce signs & Sxs of moderately to severely active RA, failed 1 or more Dz-modifying antirheumatic drugs* **Action:** Human IL-1 receptor antagonist **Dose:** 100 mg SQ qd **Caution:** [B, ?] **Contra:** Hypersensitivity to *E. coli*-derived proteins, active infection, <18 y **Supplied:** 100-mg prefilled syringes **SE:** Neutropenia especially when used w/ TNF-blocking agents, inj site Rxns, infections **Interactions:** ↓ Effects of immunizations; ↑ risk of infections if combined w/ TNF-blocking drugs **Labs:** ↓ WBCs, plts, absolute neutrophil count **NIPE:** Store drug in refrigerator, ⊘ light exposure, & discard any unused portion; ⊘ use soln if discolored or has particulate matter

Anastrozole (Arimidex)
Uses: *Breast CA: postmenopausal women w/ metastatic breast CA, adjuvant Rx of postmenopausal women w/ early hormone-receptor-+ breast CA* **Action:** Selective nonsteroidal aromatase inhibitor, ↓ circulating estradiol **Dose:** 1 mg/d **Caution:** [C, ?] **Contra:** PRG **Supplied:** Tabs 1 mg **SE:** May ↑ cholesterol; diarrhea, hypertension, flushing, ↑d bone & tumor pain, HA, somnolence **Notes:** No effect on adrenal corticosteroids or aldosterone **Interactions:** None noted **Labs:** ↑ GTT, LFTs, alkaline phosphatase, total & LDL cholesterol **NIPE:** May ↓ fertility & cause fetal damage, eval for pain & administer adequate analgesia, may cause vaginal bleeding first few weeks

Anistreplase (Eminase)
Uses: *AMI* **Action:** Thrombolytic; activates conversion of plasminogen to plasmin, promoting thrombolysis **Dose:** 30 units IV over 2–5 min **Caution:** [C, ?] **Contra:** Active internal bleeding, Hx CVA, recent (<2 mo) intracranial or intraspinal surgery or trauma, intracranial neoplasm, AVM, aneurysm, bleeding diathesis, severe uncontrolled HTN **Supplied:** Vials w/30 units **SE:** Bleeding, hypotension, hematoma **Notes:** May not be effective if readministered >5 d after the previous dose of anistreplase or streptokinase, or streptococcal infection, because of the production of antistreptokinase antibody **Interactions:** ↑ Risk of hemorrhage w/ warfarin, oral anticoagulants, ASA, NSAIDs, dipyridamole; ↓ effectiveness w/ aminocaproic acid **Labs:** ↑ Plasminogen & fibrinogen, ↑ transaminase level, thrombin time, APTT & PT **NIPE:** Store powder in refrigerator & use w/in 30 min of reconstitution, initiate therapy ASAP after MI, monitor S/Sxs internal bleeding

Anthralin (Anthra-Derm)
Uses: *Psoriasis* **Action:** Keratolytic **Dose:** Apply qd **Caution:** [C, ?] **Contra:** Acutely inflamed psoriatic eruptions, erythroderma **Supplied:** Cream, oint 0.1, 0.2, 0.25, 0.4, 0.5, 1% **SE:** Irritation; discoloration of hair, fingernails, skin **Interactions:** ↑ Toxicity if used immediately after long-term topical corticosteroid therapy **NIPE:** May stain fabric; external use only; ⊘ sunlight-medicated areas

Antihemophilic Factor [AHF, Factor VIII] (Monoclate)
Uses: *Classic hemophilia A, von Willebrand's Dz* **Action:** Provides factor VIII needed to convert prothrombin to thrombin **Dose:** *Adults & Peds.* 1 AHF unit/kg ↑ factor VIII level ≈2%. Units required = (kg) (desired factor VIII ↑ as % normal) × (0.5). Prophylaxis of spontaneous hemorrhage = 5% normal. Hemostasis after trauma/surgery = 30% normal. Head injuries, major surgery, or bleeding = 80–100% normal. Determine Pt's % of normal factor VIII before dosing **Caution:** [C, ?] **Supplied:** Check each vial for units contained **SE:** Rash, fever, HA, chills, N/V **Interactions:** None **Labs:** Monitor CBC & direct Coombs' test **NIPE:** ⊘ ASA, immunize against Hep B, DC if tachycardic

Antithymocyte Globulin [ATG] (ATGAM) **Uses:** *RX allograft rejection in transplant Pts* **Action:** Reduces the number of circulating, thymus-dependent lymphocytes **Dose:** 10–15 mg/kg/d **Caution:** [C, ?/–] **Contra:** ⊘ Use w/ a Hx of severe systemic Rxn to other equine gamma globulin prep **Supplied:** Inj 50 mg/mL **SE:** Thrombocytopenia, leukopenia **Notes:** DC if severe thrombocytopenia/leucopenia **Interactions:** ↑ Risk of infection with antineoplastics, corticosteroids, cyclosporines **Labs:** Baseline hematopoietic function & periodically during drug therapy **NIPE:** Refrigerate & keep out of light, reconstitute at room temperature, soln stable for 4 h after reconstitution, 1st dose infused over 6 h

Apomorphine (Apokyn) **WARNING:** ⊘ Administer IV **Uses:** *Acute, intermittent hypomobility ("off") episodes of Parkinson's Dz* **Action:** Dopamine agonist **Dose:** *Adults.* 0.2-mL SQ test dose under medical supervision; if BP OK, initial 0.2 mL SQ during "off" periods; only 1 dose per "off" period; requires careful titration; 0.6 mL max single doses; requires concomitant antiemetic; ↓ in renal impairment **Caution:** [C, +/–] ⊘ EtOH; antihypertensives, vasodilators, cardio or cerebrovascular Dz, hepatic impairment **Contra:** 5HT₃ antagonists, sulfite hypersensitivity **Supplied:** Inj 10 mg/mL, 3-mL prefilled pen cartridges; 2-mL amp **SE:** Emesis, syncope, QT interval prolongation, orthostatic hypotension, somnolence, ischemia, inj site Rxn, abuse potential, dyskinesia, fibrotic conditions, priapism **Notes:** Potential for daytime somnolence may limit Pts activities; trimethobenzamide 300 mg tid PO or other non-5HT₃ antagonist antiemetic given 3 d prior to & up to 2 mo following initiation **Interactions:** ↑ Risk of hypotension with alosetron, dolasetron, granisetron, ondansetron, palonosetron **Labs:** ECG–monitor for prolongation of QT interval **NIPE:** Start antiemetic 3 d before therapy and for 2 mo after therapy ends

Apraclonidine (Iopidine) **Uses:** *Glaucoma, postop intraocular HTN* **Action:** α₂-Adrenergic agonist **Dose:** 1–2 gtt of 0.5% tid **Caution:** [C, ?] **Contra:** MAOI use **Supplied:** 0.5, 1% soln **SE:** Ocular irritation, lethargy, xerostomia **Interactions:** ↓ Intraocular pressure w/ pilocarpine or topical BBs **NIPE:** Monitor CV status of Pts w/ CAD, potential for dizziness

Aprepitant (Emend) **Uses:** *Prevents N/V assoc w/ highly emetogenic CA chemotherapy (eg, cisplatin) (used in combination w/ other antiemetic agents)* **Action:** Substance P/neurokinin 1(NK₁) receptor antagonist **Dose:** 125 mg PO day 1, 1 h before chemo, then 80 mg q ᴀᴍ on days 2 & 3 **Caution:** [B, ?/–]; substrate & moderate inhibitor of CYP3A4; inducer of CYP2C9 **Contra:** Use w/ pimozide **Supplied:** Caps 80, 125 mg **SE:** Fatigue, asthenia, hiccups **Notes:** ↓ Effectiveness of PO contraceptives; ↓ anticoagulant effect of warfarin **Interactions:** ↑ Effects w/ clarithromycin, diltiazem, itraconazole, ketoconazole, nefazodone, nelfinavir, ritonavir, troleandomycin; ↑ effects of alprazolam, astemizole, cisapride, dexamethasone, methylprednisolone, midazolam, pimozide, terfenadine, triazolam and chemotherapeutic agents eg docetaxel, etoposide, ifosfamide, imatinib, irinotecan, paclitaxel, vinblastine, vincristine, vinorelbine; ↓ effects w/

paroxetine, rifampin; ↓ effects of oral contraceptives, paroxetine, phenytoin, tolbutamide, warfarin **Labs:** ↑ ALT, AST, BUN, alkaline phosphatase, leukocytes **NIPE:** Use barrier contraception, take w/o regard to food

Aprotinin (Trasylol) Uses: *↓/Prevents blood loss in Pts undergoing CABG* **Action:** Protease inhibitor, antifibrinolytic **Dose:** 1-mL IV test dose. *High dose:* 2 million KIU load, 2 million KIU to prime pump, then 500,000 KIU/h until surgery ends. *Low dose:* 1 million KIU load, 1 million KIU to prime pump, then 250,000 KIU/h until surgery ends; 7 million KIU max total **Caution:** [B, ?] Thromboembolic Dz requiring anticoagulants or blood factor administration **Supplied:** Inj 1.4 mg/mL (10,000 KIU/mL) **SE:** AF, MI, HF, dyspnea, postop renal dysfunction **Notes:** 1000/KIU = 0.14 mg of aprotinin **Interactions:** ↑ Clotting time w/ heparin, ↓ effects of fibrinolytics, captopril **Labs:** Monitor aPTT, ACT, CBC, BUN, creatinine **NIPE:** Monitor cardiac and pulmonary status during inf

Ardeparin (Normiflo) Uses: *Prevents DVT/PE following knee replacement* **Action:** LMW heparin **Dose:** 35–50 units/kg SQ q12h. Begin day of surgery, continue up to 14 d; caution in ↓ renal Fxn **Caution:** [C, ?] **Contra:** Active hemorrhage; hypersensitivity to pork products **Supplied:** Inj 5000, 10,000 IU/0.5 mL **SE:** Bleeding, bruising, thrombocytopenia, pain at inj site, ↑ serum transaminases **Notes:** Lab monitoring usually not necessary

Argatroban (Acova) Uses: *Prophylaxis or Rx of thrombosis in HIT, PCI in Pts w/ risk of HIT* **Action:** Anticoagulant, direct thrombin inhibitor **Dose:** 2 µg/kg/min IV; adjust until aPTT 1.5–3× baseline not to exceed 100 s; 10 µg/kg/min max; ↓ dose in hepatic impairment. **Caution:** [B, ?] ⊘ PO anticoagulants, ↑ bleeding risk; ⊘ concomitant use of thrombolytics **Contra:** Overt major bleed **Supplied:** Inj 100 mg/mL **SE:** AF, cardiac arrest, cerebrovascular disorder, hypotension, VT, N/V/D, sepsis, cough, renal toxicity, ↓ Hgb **Interactions:** ↑ Risk of bleeding w/ anticoagulants, feverfew, garlic, ginger, ginkgo, ↑ risk of intracranial bleed w/ thrombolytics **Labs:** ↑ aPTT, PT, INR, ACT, thrombin time **NIPE:** Report ↑ bruising & bleeding, ⊘ breast-feed

Aripiprazole (Abilify) Uses: *Schizophrenia* **Action:** Dopamine & serotonin antagonist **Dose:** *Adults.* 10–15 mg PO qd; ↓ when used w/ potent CYP3A4 or CYP2D6 inhibitors; ↑ when used in combination w/ inducer of CYP3A4 **Caution:** [C, –] **Supplied:** Tabs 10, 15, 20, 30 mg **SE:** Neuroleptic malignant syndrome, tardive dyskinesia, orthostatic hypotension, cognitive & motor impairment **Interactions:** ↑ Effects w/ ketoconazole, quinidine, fluoxetine, paroxetine, ↓ effects w/ carbamazepine **NIPE:** ⊘ Breast-feed, consume EtOH, or use during PRG; use barrier contraception; ↑ fluid intake

Artificial Tears (Tears Naturale) [OTC] Uses: *Dry eyes* **Action:** Ocular lubricant **Dose:** 1–2 gtt tid–qid **Caution:** N/A **Supplied:** OTC soln **SE:** N/A

L-Asparaginase (Elspar, Oncaspar) Uses: *ALL* (in combination w/ other agents) **Action:** Protein synthesis inhibitor **Dose:** 500–20,000 IU/m^2/d for

1–14 d (see specific protocols) **Caution:** [C, ?] **Contra:** Active/Hx pancreatitis **Supplied:** Inj 10,000 IU **SE:** Hypersensitivity Rxn in 20–35% (spectrum of urticaria to anaphylaxis); test dose recommended; rare GI toxicity (mild nausea/anorexia, pancreatitis) **Interactions:** ↑ Effects w/ prednisone, vincristine; ↓ effects of MRX, sulfonylureas, insulin **Labs:** ↑ T_4 & T_4-binding globulin, serum albumin, total cholesterol, plasma fibrinogen; ↑ BUN, glucose, uric acid, LFTs, alkaline phosphatase **NIPE:** ↑ Fluid intake, monitor for bleeding, monitor I&O and weight, ⊘ EtOH or ASA

Aspirin (Bayer, Ecotrin, St. Joseph's) [OTC]

Uses: *Angina, CABG, PTCA, carotid endarterectomy, ischemic stroke, TIA, MI, arthritis, pain,* HA, *fever,* * inflammation, Kawasaki Dz **Action:** Prostaglandin inhibitor **Dose:** **Adults.** Pain, fever: 325–650 mg q4–6h PO or PR. *RA:* 3–6 g/d PO in ÷ doses. *Plt inhibitor:* 81–325 mg PO qd. *Prevent MI:* 81–325 mg PO qd. **Peds.** Antipyretic: 10–15 mg/kg/dose PO or PR q4h up to 80 mg/kg/24 h. *RA:* 60–100 mg/kg/24 h PO ÷ q4–6h (keep levels between 15 & 30 mg/dL); ⊘ w/ CrCl <10 mL/min, in severe liver Dz **Caution:** [C, M] Use linked to Reye's syndrome; ⊘ w/ viral illness in children **Contra:** Allergy to ASA, chickenpox or flu Sxs, syndrome of nasal polyps, asthma, rhinitis **Supplied:** Tabs 325, 500 mg; chew tabs 81 mg; EC tabs 165, 325, 500, 650, 975 mg; SR tabs 650, 800 mg; effervescent tabs 325, 500 mg; supp 120, 200, 300, 600 mg **SE:** GI upset & erosion **Notes:** DC 1 wk prior to surgery to ⊘ postoperative bleeding; ⊘ or limit EtOH intake **Interactions:** ↑ Effects w/ anticoagulants, ammonium chloride, antibiotics, ascorbic acid, furosemide, methionine, nizatidine, NSAIDs, verapamil, EtOH, feverfew, garlic, ginkgo biloba, horse chestnut, kelpware (black-tang), prickly ash, red clover; ↓ effects w/ antacids, activated charcoal, corticosteroids, griseofulvin, $NaHCO_3$, ginseng, food; ↑ effects of ACEI, hypoglycemics, insulin, Li, MRX, phenytoin, sulfonamides, valproic acid; ↓ effects of BBs, probenecid, spironolactone, sulfinpyrazone **Labs:** False – results of urinary glucose & urinary ketone tests, serum albumin, total serum phenytoin, T_3 & T_4 **NIPE:** Chronic ASA use may result in ↓ folic acid, Fe-deficiency anemia, & hypernatremia; ⊘ foods ↑ salicylate, eg curry powder, paprika, licorice, prunes, raisins, tea; take ASA w/ food or milk; report S/Sxs bleeding/GI pain/ringing in ears

Aspirin & Butalbital Compound (Fiorinal) [C-III]

Uses: *Tension HA,* pain **Action:** Combination barbiturate & analgesic **Dose:** 1–2 PO q4h PRN, max 6 tabs/d; ⊘ use w/ CrCl <10 mL/min & in severe liver Dz **Caution:** [C (D if used for prolonged periods or high doses at term), ?] **Contra:** Allergy to ASA, GI ulceration, bleeding disorder, porphyria, syndrome of nasal polyps, angioedema, & bronchospasm to NSAIDs **Supplied:** Caps Fiorgen PF, Fiorinal. Tabs Fiorinal, Lanorinal: ASA 325 mg/butalbital 50 mg/caffeine 40 mg **SE:** Drowsiness, dizziness, GI upset, ulceration, bleeding **Notes:** Butalbital habit-forming; ⊘ or limit EtOH intake See Aspirin. **Additional Interactions:** ↑ Effect of benzodiazepines,

CNS depressants, chloramphenicol, methylphenidate, propoxyphene, valproic acid; ↓ effects of BBs, corticosteroids, chloramphenicol, cyclosporines, doxycycline, griseofulvin, haloperidol, oral contraceptives, phenothiazines, quinidine, TCAs, theophylline, warfarin **NIPE:** Use barrier contraception, ⊘ EtOH

Aspirin + Butalbital, Caffeine, & Codeine (Fiorinal + Codeine) [C-III]

Uses: Mild *pain*, HA, especially when associated w/ stress **Action:** Sedative analgesic, narcotic analgesic **Dose:** 1–2 tabs (caps) PO q4–6h PRN **Caution:** [D, ?] **Contra:** Allergy to ASA **Supplied:** Cap/tab contains 325 mg ASA, 40 mg caffeine, 50 mg of butalbital, 30 mg of codeine **SE:** Drowsiness, dizziness, GI upset, ulceration, bleeding See Aspirin + Butalbital **Additional Interactions:** ↑ Effects w/ narcotic analgesics, MAOIs, neuromuscular blockers, ↓ effects w/ tobacco smoking; ↑ effects of digitoxin, phenytoin, rifampin; ↑ resp & CNS depression w/ cimetidine **Labs:** ↑ Plasma amylase & lipase **NIPE:** May cause constipation, ↑ fluids & fiber, take w/ milk to ↓ GI distress

Aspirin + Codeine (Empirin No. 2, No. 3, No. 4) [C-III]

Uses: Mild to *moderate pain* **Action:** Combined effects of ASA & codeine **Dose:** *Adults.* 1–2 tabs PO q4–6h PRN. *Peds.* ASA 10 mg/kg/dose; codeine 0.5–1.0 mg/kg/dose q4h **Caution:** [D, M] **Contra:** Allergy to ASA/codeine, PUD, bleeding, anticoagulant Rx, children w/ chickenpox or flu Sxs **Supplied:** Tabs 325 mg of ASA & codeine (Codeine in No. 2 = 15 mg, No. 3 = 30 mg, No. 4 = 60 mg) **SE:** Drowsiness, dizziness, GI upset, ulceration, bleeding See Aspirin. **Additional Interactions** ↑ Effects w/ narcotic analgesics, MAOIs, neuromuscular blockers, Ø effects w/ tobacco smoking; ↑ effects of digitoxin, phenytoin, rifampin; ↑ resp & CNS depression w/ cimetidine **Labs:** ↑ Plasma amylase & lipase **NIPE:** May cause constipation, ↑ fluids & fiber, take w/ milk to ↓ GI distress

Atazanavir (Reyataz)

WARNING: Hyperbilirubinemia may require drug discontinuation **Uses:** *HIV-1 infection* **Action:** Protease inhibitor **Dose:** 400 mg PO daily w/ food; when given w/ efavirenz 600 mg, administer atazanavir 300 mg + ritonavir 100 mg once/d; separate doses from buffered didanosine administration; ↓ in hepatic impairment **Caution:** [B, –]; ↑ levels of statins, sildenafil, antiarrhythmics, warfarin, cyclosporine, tricyclics; atazanavir conc ↓ by St. John's wort **Contra:** Concomitant use of midazolam, triazolam, ergots, cisapride, pimozide **Supplied:** 100-mg, 150-mg, 200-mg caps **SE:** Headache, N/V/D, rash, abdominal pain, DM, photosensitivity; ↑ PR interval **Notes:** May have ↓ effects on cholesterol profile **Interactions:** ↑ Effects w/ amprenavir, clarithromycin, indinavir, lamivudine, lopinavir, ritonavir, saquinavir, stavudine, tenofovir, zalcitabine, zidovudine; ↑ effects of amiodarone, atorvastatin, CCBs, clarithromycin, cyclosporine, diltiazem, irinotecan, lidocaine, lovastatin, oral contraceptives, rifabutin, quinidine, saquinavir, sildenafil, simvastatin, sirolimus, tacrolimus, TCAs, warfarin; ↓ effects w/ antacids, antimycobacterials, efavirenz, esomeprazole, H2 receptor antagonists, lansoprazole, omeprazole, rifampin, St. John's wort **Labs:** ↑

ALT, AST, total bilirubin, amylase, lipase, serum glucose, ↓ Hgb, neutrophils **NIPE:** Take w/ food; will not cure HIV or ↓ risk of transmission; use barrier contraception; ↑ risk of skin and/or scleral yellowing

Atenolol (Tenormin)
Uses: *HTN, angina, MI* **Action:** Competitively blocks β-adrenergic receptors, β₁ **Dose:** *HTN & angina:* 50–100 mg/d PO. *AMI:* 5 mg IV ×2 over 10 min, then 50mg PO bid if tolerated; ↓ in renal impairment **Caution:** [D, M] DM, bronchospasm; abrupt DC can exacerbate angina & MI risk **Contra:** Bradycardia, cardiogenic shock, cardiac failure, 2nd- or 3rd- degree AV block **Supplied:** Tabs 25, 50, 100 mg; inj 5 mg/10 mL **SE:** Bradycardia, ↓ BP, 2nd- or 3rd-degree AV block, dizziness, fatigue **Interactions:** ↑ Effects w/ other antihypertensives especially diltiazem & verapamil, nitrates, EtOH; ↑ bradycardia w/ adenosine, digitalis glycosides, dipyridamole, physostigmine, tacrine; ↓ effects w/ ampicillin, antacids, NSAIDs, salicylates; ↑ effects of lidocaine; ↓ effects of dopamine, glucagons, insulin, sulfonylureas **Labs:** ↑ ANA titers, BUN, glucose, serum lipoprotein, K⁺, triglyceride, uric acid levels; ↓ HDL **NIPE:** May mask S/Sxs hypoglycemia, may ↑ sensitivity to cold, may ↑ depression, wheezing, orthostatic hypotension

Atenolol & Chlorthalidone (Tenoretic)
Uses: *HTN* **Action:** β-Adrenergic blockade w/ diuretic **Dose:** 50–100 mg/d PO; ↓ in renal impairment **Caution:** [D, M] DM, bronchospasm **Contra:** See atenolol; anuria **Supplied:** *Tenoretic 50:* Atenolol 50 mg/chlorthalidone 25 mg; *Tenoretic 100:* Atenolol 100 mg/chlorthalidone 25 mg **SE:** Bradycardia, ↓ BP, 2nd- or 3rd-degree AV block, dizziness, fatigue, ↓ K⁺, photosensitivity See Atenolol. **Additional Interactions:** ↑ Effects w/ other antihypertensives; ↓ effects w/ cholestyramine, NSAIDs; ↑ effects of Li, digoxin, ↓ effects of sulfonylureas **Labs:** False ↓ urine esriol; ↑ CPK, serum ammonia, amylase, Ca²⁺, Cl⁻, cholesterol, glucose; ↓ serum Cl⁻, Mg²⁺, K⁺, Na⁺ **NIPE:** Take in AM to prevent nocturia, use sunblock >SPF 15, monitor S/Sxs gout

Atomoxetine (Strattera)
Uses: *ADHD* **Action:** Selective norepinephrine reuptake inhibitor **Dose:** *Adults & children >70kg.* 40 mg × 3 days, titrate ↑ to 80–100 mg ÷ qd–bid. *Peds < 70 kg:* 0.5 mg/kg × 3 d, then titrate to max of 1.2 mg/kg given qd or bid **Caution:** [C, ? /–] **Contra:** Narrow-angle glaucoma, use w/ or w/in 2 wk of DC an MAOI **Supplied:** Caps 10, 18, 25, 40, 60 mg **SE:** ↑ BP, tachycardia, weight loss, sexual dysfunction **Notes:** ↓ Dose w/ hepatic insufficiency, ↓ dose in combination w/ inhibitors of CYP2D6

Atorvastatin (Lipitor)
Uses: *↑ Cholesterol & triglycerides* **Action:** HMG-CoA reductase inhibitor **Dose:** Initial dose 10 mg/d, may be ↑ to 80 mg/d **Caution:** [X, –] **Contra:** Active liver Dz, unexplained ↑ of serum transaminases **Supplied:** Tabs 10, 20, 40, 80 mg **SE:** May cause myopathy, HA, arthralgia, myalgia, GI upset **Notes:** monitor LFTs regularly **Interactions:** ↑ Effects w/ azole antifungals, erythromycin, nefazodone, protease inhibitors, grapefruit juice; ↓ effects w/ antacids, bile acid sequestrants; ↑ effects of digoxin, levothyroxine, oral contra-

ceptives **Labs:** ↑ LFTs, CPK, ↓ lipid levels **NIPE:** ⊘ EtOH, breast-feeding, or while PRG

Atovaquone (Mepron) **Uses:** *Rx & prevention PCP* **Action:** ↓ Nucleic acid & ATP synthesis **Dose:** *Rx:* 750 mg PO bid for 21 d. *Prevention:* 1500 mg PO once/d (w/ meals) **Caution:** [C, ?] **Supplied:** Suspension 750 mg/5 mL **SE:** Fever, HA, anxiety, insomnia, rash, N/V **Interactions:** ↓ Effects w/ metoclopramide, rifabutin, rifampin, tetracycline **NIPE:** ↑ Absorption w/ meal esp ↑ fat, monitor LFTs w/ long-term use

Atovaquone/Proguanil (Malarone) **Uses:** *Prevention or Rx Pseudomonas falciparum malaria* **Action:** Antimalarial **Dose:** *Adults:* Prevention: 1 tab PO 2 d before, during, & 7 d after leaving endemic region; *Rx:* 4 tabs PO single dose qd ×3 d. *Peds.* See insert **Caution:** [C, ?] **Contra:** CrCl < 30 mL/min **Supplied:** Tab atovaquone 250 mg/proguanil 100 mg; pediatric 62.5/25 mg **SE:** HA, fever, myalgia. See Atovaquone

Atracurium (Tracrium) **Uses:** *Adjunct to anesthesia to facilitate ET intubation* **Action:** Nondepolarizing neuromuscular blocker **Dose:** *Adults & Peds.* 0.4–0.5 mg/kg IV bolus, then 0.08–0.1 mg/kg q20–45 min PRN **Caution:** [C, ?] **Supplied:** Inj 10 mg/mL **SE:** Flushing **Notes:** Pt must be intubated & on controlled ventilation; use adequate amounts of sedation & analgesia **Interactions:** ↑ Effects w/ general anesthetics, aminoglycosides, bacitracin, BBs, β agonists, clindamycin, CCBs, diuretics, lidocaine, Li, Mg sulfate, narcotic analgesics, procainamide, quinidine, succinylcholine, trimethaphan, verapamil; ↓ effects w/ Ca, carbamazepine, phenytoin, theophylline, caffeine **Labs:** Monitor BUN, creatinine, LFTs **NIPE:** Drug does not effect consciousness or pain, inability to speak until drug wears off

Atropine **Uses:** *Preanesthetic; symptomatic bradycardia & asystole* **Action:** Antimuscarinic agent; blocks acetylcholine at parasympathetic sites **Dose:** *Adults.* ECC: 0.5–1 mg IV q3–5min. *Preanesthetic:* 0.3–0.6 mg IM. *Peds.* ECC: 0.01–0.03 mg/kg IV q2–5min, max 1 mg, min dose 0.1 mg. *Preanesthetic:* 0.01 mg/kg/dose SC/IV (max 0.4 mg) **Caution:** [C, +] **Contra:** Glaucoma **Supplied:** Tabs 0.3, 0.4, 0.6 mg; inj 0.05, 0.1, 0.3, 0.4, 0.5, 0.8, 1 mg/mL; ophthalmic 0.5, 1, 2% **SE:** Blurred vision, urinary retention, constipation, dried mucous membranes **Interactions:** ↑ Effects w/ amantadine, antihistamines, disopyramide, procainamide, quinidine, TCA, thiazides, betel palm, squaw vine; ↓ effects w/ antacids, levodopa; ↓ effects of phenothiazines **Labs:** ↓ Gastric motility & emptying may effect results of upper GI series **NIPE:** Monitor I&O, ↑ fluids & oral hygiene, wear dark glasses to ↓ photophobia

Azathioprine (Imuran) **Uses:** *Adjunct to prevent rejection following kidney transplantation, RA,* SLE **Action:** Immunosuppressive; antagonizes purine metabolism **Dose:** *Adults & Peds.* 1–3 mg/kg/d IV or PO (↓ in renal failure) **Caution:** [D, ?] **Contra:** PRG **Supplied:** Tabs 50 mg; inj 100 mg/20 mL **SE:** GI intol-

erance, fever, chills, leukopenia, thrombocytopenia; chronic use may ↑ neoplasia **Notes:** Handle inj w/ cytotoxic precautions; interaction w/ allopurinol; ⊘ administer live vaccines to a Pt taking azathioprine **Interactions:** ↑ Effects w/ allopurinol; ↑ effects of antineoplastic drugs, cyclosporine, myelosuppressive drugs, MRX; ↑ risk of severe leucopenia w/ ACEI; ↓ effects of nondepolarizing neuromuscular blocking drugs, warfarin **Labs:** Monitor BUN, creatinine, CBC, LFTs during therapy **NIPE:** ⊘ PRG, breast-feeding, immunizations, take w/ or pc

Azelastine (Astelin, Optivar) Uses: *Allergic rhinitis (rhinorrhea, sneezing, nasal pruritus); allergic conjunctivitis* **Action:** Histamine H_1-receptor antagonist **Dose:** *Nasal:* 2 sprays/nostril bid. *Ophthalmic:* 1 gt into each affected eye bid **Caution:** [C, ?/–] **Contra:** Component sensitivity **Supplied:** Nasal spray 137 μg/spray; ophthalmic soln 0.05% **SE:** Somnolence, bitter taste **Interactions:** ↑ Effects with cimetidine; ↑ effects of EtOH, CNS depressants **Labs:** ↑ AST, ↓ skin reactions to antigen skin tests **NIPE:** Systemically absorbed; clear nares before admin; prime pump before use

Azithromycin (Zithromax) Uses: *Community-acquired pneumonia, pharyngitis, otitis media, skin infections, nongonococcal urethritis, & PID; Rx & prevention of MAC in HIV* **Action:** Macrolide antibiotic; inhibits protein synthesis. *Spectrum: Chlamydia, Haemophilus ducreyi, H. influenzae, Legionella, Moraxella catarrhalis, Mycoplasma pneumoniae, M. hominis, Neisseria gonorrhoeae, Staphylococcus aureus, Streptococcus agalactiae, S. pneumoniae, S. pyogenes* **Dose:** *Adults. PO: Resp tract infections:* 500 mg day 1, then 250 mg/d PO ×4 d or 500 mg/d PO × 3 days. *Nongonococcal urethritis:* 1 g single dose. *Prevention of MAC:* 1200 mg PO once/wk. *IV:* 500 mg ×2 d, then 500 mg PO ×7–10 d. *Peds. Otitis media:* 10 mg/kg PO day 1, then 5 mg/kg/d days 2–5. *Pharyngitis:* 12 mg/kg/d PO ×5 d (take susp on an empty stomach; tabs may be taken w/wo food) **Caution:** [B, +] **Supplied:** Tabs 250, 600 mg; Z-Pack (5-day regimen); Tri-Pak (500-mg tabs × 3); susp 1-g single-dose packet; susp 100, 200 mg/5 mL; inj 500 mg **SE:** GI upset **Interactions:** ↓ Effects w/ Al- & Mg-containing antacids, atovaquone, food (suspension); ↑ effects of alfentanil, barbiturates, bromocriptine, carbamazepine, cyclosporine, digoxin, disopyramide, ergot alkaloids, phenytoin, pimozide, terfenadine, theophylline, triazolam, warfarin; ↓ effects of penicillins **Labs:** May ↑ serum bilirubin, alkaline phosphatase, BUN, creatinine, CPK, glucose, K+, LFTs, LDH, PT; may ↓ WBC, plt count, serum folate **NIPE:** Monitor S/Sxs superinfection, use sunscreen & protective clothing

Aztreonam (Azactam) Uses: *Aerobic gram(–) UTIs, lower resp, intraabdominal, skin, gynecologic infections & septicemia* **Action:** Monobactam antibiotic; inhibits cell wall synthesis. *Spectrum:* Gram(–) coverage including *Pseudomonas, E. coli, Klebsiella, H. influenzae, Serratia, Proteus, Enterobacter, Citrobacter* **Dose:** *Adults.* 1–2 g IV/IM q6–12h. *Peds. Premature:* 30 mg/kg/dose IV q12h. *Term, children:* 30 mg/kg/dose q6–8h; ↓ in renal impairment **Caution:** [B, +] **Supplied:** Inj 500 mg, 1 g, 2 g **SE:** N/V/D, rash, pain at inj site **Notes:** No gram(+) or anaerobic activity; OK in penicillin-allergic Pts **Interactions:** ↑ Effects w/ probenecid, aminoglycosides, β-lactam antibiotics; ↓ effects w/ cefoxitin, chloramphenicol, imipenem **Labs:** ↑ LFTs, alkaline phosphatase, SCr, PT, PTT, & + Coombs' test **NIPE:** Monitor S/Sxs superinfection, taste changes w/ IV administration

Bacitracin, Ophthalmic (AK-Tracin Ophthalmic); Bacitracin & Polymyxin B, Ophthalmic (AK Poly Bac Ophthalmic, Polysporin Ophthalmic); Bacitracin, Neomycin, & Polymixin B, Ophthalmic (AK Spore Ophthalmic, Neosporin Ophthalmic); Bacitracin, Neomycin, Polymyxin B, & Hydrocortisone, Ophthalmic (AK Spore HC Ophthalmic, Cortisporin Ophthalmic) Uses: *Steroid-responsive inflammatory ocular conditions* **Action:** Topical antibiotic plus antiinflammatory components **Dose:** Apply q3–4h into conjunctival sac **Caution:** [C, ?] **Contra:** Viral, mycobacterial, or fungal eye infection **Supplied:** See Bacitracin, Topical equivalents, below **Interactions:** ↑ Effects w/ neuromuscular blocking agents, anesthetics, nephrotoxic drugs **NIPE:** May cause blurred vision

Bacitracin, Topical (Baciguent); Bacitracin & Polymyxin B, Topical (Polysporin); Bacitracin, Neomycin, & Polymyxin B, Topical (Neosporin Ointment); Bacitracin, Neomycin, Polymyxin B, & Hydrocortisone, Topical (Cortisporin); Bacitracin, Neomycin, Polymyxin B, & Lidocaine, Topical (Clomycin) Uses: *Prevent/Rx of *minor skin infections* **Action:** Topical antibiotic w/ added effects based on components (antiinflammatory & analgesic) **Dose:** Apply sparingly bid–qid **Caution:** [C, ?] **Supplied:** Bacitracin 500 U/g oint; Bacitracin 500 U/polymyxin B sulfate 10,000 U/g oint & powder; Bacitracin 400 U/neomycin 3.5 mg/polymyxin B 5000 U/g oint (for Neosporin Cream, see page 178); Bacitracin 400 U/neomycin 3.5 mg/polymyxin B/10,000 U/hydrocortisone 10 mg/g oint; Bacitracin 500 U/neomycin 3.5 g/ polymyxin B 5000 U/lidocaine 40 mg/g oint **SE:** N/A **Notes:** Systemic & irrigation forms of bacitracin available but not generally used due to potential toxicity

Baclofen (Lioresal) Uses: *Spasticity secondary to severe chronic disorders such as MS, ALS, or spinal cord lesions,* trigeminal neuralgia, hiccups **Action:** Centrally acting skeletal muscle relaxant; inhibits transmission of both monosynaptic & polysynaptic spinal cord reflexes **Dose:** *Adults.* Initial, 5 mg PO tid; ↑ q3d to effect; max 80 mg/d. *Intrathecal:* Through implantable pump *Peds* 2–7 y: 10–15 mg/d ÷ q8h; titrate, max of 40 mg/d. >8 y: Max of 60 mg/d. *IT:* Through implantable pump; ↓ in renal impairment; ⊘ abrupt withdrawal; take w/ food or milk **Caution:** [C, +] Epilepsy & neuropsychiatric disturbances; withdrawal may occur w/ abrupt discontinuation **Supplied:** Tabs 10, 20 mg; IT inj 10 mg/20 mL, 10 mg/5 mL **SE:** Dizziness, drowsiness, insomnia, ataxia, weakness, hypotension **Interactions:** ↑ CNS depression w/ CNS depressants, MAOIs, EtOH, antihistamines, opioid analgesics, sedatives, hypnotics; ↑ effects of antihypertensives, clindamycin, guanabenz; ↑ risk of resp paralysis & renal failure w/ aminoglycosides **Labs:** ↑ Serum glucose, AST, ammonia, alkaline phosphatase; ↓ bilirubin **NIPE:** Take oral meds w/ food

Balsalazide (Colazal) **Uses:** *Ulcerative colitis* **Action:** 5-Aminosalicylic acid derivative, antiinflammatory, ↓ leukotriene synthesis **Dose:** 2.25 g (3 caps) tid ×8–12 wk **Caution:** [B, ?] Severe renal/hepatic failure **Contra:** Hypersensitivity to mesalamine or salicylates **Supplied:** Caps 750 mg **SE:** Dizziness, HA, nausea, agranulocytosis, pancytopenia, renal impairment, allergic Rxns **Notes:** Each daily dose of 6.75 g is equivalent to 2.4 g of mesalamine **Interactions:** Oral antibiotics may interfere w/ mesalamine release in the colon **Labs:** ↑ Bilirubin, CPK, LFTs, LDH, plasma fibrinogen; ↓ Ca²⁺, K⁺, protein **NIPE:** ⊘ if ASA allergy, take w/ food & swallow capsule whole

Basiliximab (Simulect) **Uses:** *Prevention of acute organ transplant rejections* **Action:** IL-2 receptor antagonists **Dose:** *Adults.* 20 mg IV 2 h before transplant, then 20 mg IV 4 d posttransplant. *Peds.* 12 mg/m² ↑ to max of 20 mg 2 h prior to transplant; the same dose IV 4 d posttransplant **Caution:** [B, ?/–] **Contra:** Known hypersensitivity to murine proteins **Supplied:** Inj 20 mg **SE:** Edema, HTN, HA, dizziness, fever, pain, infection, GI effects, electrolyte disturbances **Notes:** Murine/human monoclonal antibody **Interactions:** May ↑ immunosuppression w/ other immunosuppressive drugs **Labs:** ↑ Serum cholesterol, BUN, creatinine, uric acid; ↓ serum Mg phosphate, plts; ↑ or ↓ in Hgb, Hct, serum glucose, K⁺, Ca²⁺ **NIPE:** Monitor for infection, hypersensitivity Rxns, IV dose over 20–30 min

BCG [Bacillus Calmette-Guérin] (TheraCys, Tice BCG) **Uses:** *Bladder carcinoma (superficial).* TB prophylaxis **Action:** Immunomodulator **Dose:** Bladder CA, 1 vial prepared & instilled in bladder for 2 h. Repeat once/wk for 6 wk; then maint 3/wk at 3, 6, 12, 18, & 24 mo after initial therapy **Caution:** [C, ?] Asthma, ⊘ administer w/ traumatic catheterization or UTI **Contra:** Immunosuppression, UTI steroid use, acute illness, fever of unknown origin **Supplied:** Inj 81 mg (10.5 ± 8.7 × 10⁸ CFU vial) (TheraCys), 1–8 × 10⁸ CFU/vial (Tice BCG) **SE:** *Intravesical:* Hematuria, urinary frequency, dysuria, bacterial UTI, rare BCG sepsis **Notes:** Routine US adult BCG immunization ⊘; occasionally used in high-risk children who are PPD– & cannot take INH **Interactions:** ↓ Effects w/ antimicrobials, immunosuppressives, radiation **Labs:** Prior BCG may cause false + PPD **NIPE:** Monitor for S/Sxs systemic infection, report persistent pain on urination or blood in urine

Becaplermin (Regranex Gel) **Uses:** Adjunct to local wound care in *diabetic foot ulcers* **Action:** Recombinant PDGF, enhances formation of granulation tissue **Dose:** Based on lesion; 1⅓-in. ribbon from 2-g tube, ⅔-in. ribbon from 7.5- or 15-g tube/in.² of ulcer; apply & cover w/moist gauze; rinse after 12h; ⊘ reapply; repeat in 12 h **Caution:** [C, ?] **Contra:** Neoplasm or active infection at site **Supplied:** 0.01% gel in 2-, 7.5-, 15-g tubes **SE:** Erythema, local pain **Notes:** Use along w/ good wound care; wound must be vascularized **Interactions:** None known **NIPE:** Dosage recalculated q1–2wk

Beclomethasone (Beconase, Vancenase Nasal Inhaler)
Uses: Allergic *rhinitis* refractory to antihistamines & decongestants; *nasal polyps* **Action:** Inhaled steroid **Dose:** *Adults.* 1 spray intranasally bid–qid. *Aqueous inhal:* 1–2 sprays/nostril daily–bid. *Peds 6–12 y:* 1 spray intranasally tid **Caution:** [C, ?] **Supplied:** Nasal met-dose inhaler **SE:** Local irritation, burning, epistaxis **Notes:** Nasal spray delivers 42 µg/dose & 84 µg/dose **Interactions:** None noted **NIPE:** Prior use of decongestant nasal gtt if edema or secretions, may take several days for full steroid effect

Beclomethasone (QVAR)
Uses: Chronic *asthma* **Action:** Inhaled corticosteroid **Dose:** *Adults & Peds.* 1–4 inhal bid (Rinse mouth/throat after use) **Caution:** [C, ?] **Contra:** Acute asthma **Supplied:** PO met-dose inhaler; 40, 80 µg/inhal **SE:** HA, cough, hoarseness, oral candidiasis **Notes:** Not effective for acute asthmatic **Interactions:** None noted **NIPE:** Use inhaled bronchodilator prior to inhaled steroid, rinse mouth after inhaled steroid

Belladonna & Opium Suppositories (B & O Supprettes) [C-II]
Uses: *Bladder spasms; moderate/severe pain* **Action:** Antispasmodic, analgesic **Dose:** 1 supp PR q6h PRN; 15A = 30 mg powdered opium/16.2 mg belladonna extract; 16A = 60 mg powdered opium/16.2 mg belladonna extract **Caution:** [C, ?] **Supplied:** Supp 15A, 16A **SE:** Anticholinergic side effects (sedation, urinary retention, & constipation) **Interactions:** ↑ Effects w/ CNS depressants, TCAs; ↓ effects w/ phenothiazines **Labs:** ↑ LFTs **NIPE:** ⊘ Refrigerate, moisten finger & supp before insertion, may cause blurred vision

Benazepril (Lotensin)
Uses: *HTN,* *HTN,* DN, CHF **Action:** ACEI **Dose:** 10–40 mg/d PO **Caution:** [C (1st tri), D (2nd & 3rd tri), +] **Contra:** Angioedema, Hx edema **Supplied:** Tabs 5, 10, 20, 40 mg **SE:** Symptomatic ↓ BP w/ diuretics; dizziness, HA, ↓ K⁺, nonproductive cough **Interactions:** ↑ Effects w/ α-blockers, diuretics, capsaicin; ↓ effects w/ NSAIDs, ASA; ↑ effects of insulin, Li; ↑ risk of hyperkalemia w/ trimethoprim & K-sparing diuretics **Labs:** ↑ BUN, SCr, K⁺; ↓ hemoglobin; ECG changes **NIPE:** Persistent cough and/or taste changes may develop, ⊘ PRG, DC if angioedema

Benzocaine & Antipyrine (Auralgan)
Uses: *Analgesia in severe otitis media* **Action:** Anesthetic w/local decongestant **Dose:** Fill the ear & insert a moist cotton plug; repeat 1–2 h PRN **Caution:** [C, ?] **Contra:** ⊘ Use w/ perforated eardrum **Supplied:** Soln **SE:** Local irritation **Interactions:** May ↓ effects of sulfonamides

Benzonatate (Tessalon Perles)
Uses: Symptomatic relief of *cough* **Action:** Anesthetizes the stretch receptors in the resp passages **Dose:** *Adults & Peds >10 y.* 100 mg PO tid **Caution:** [C, ?] **Supplied:** Caps 100 mg **SE:** Sedation, dizziness, GI upset **Notes:** ⊘ Chew or puncture the caps **Interactions:** ↑ CNS de-

pression w/ antihistamines, EtOH, hypnotics, opioids, sedatives **NIPE:** ↑ Fluid intake to liquefy secretions

Benztropine (Cogentin)
Uses: *Parkinsonism & drug-induced extrapyramidal disorders* **Action:** Partially blocks striatal cholinergic receptors **Dose:** *Adults.* 0.5–6 mg PO, IM, or IV in ÷ doses/d. *Peds >3 y.* 0.02–0.05 mg/kg/dose 1–2/d **Caution:** [C, ?] **Contra:** < 3 y **Supplied:** Tabs 0.5, 1, 2 mg; inj 1 mg/mL **SE:** Anticholinergic side effects **Notes:** Physostigmine 1–2 mg SC/IV to reverse severe Sxs **Interactions:** ↑ Sedation and depressant effects w/ EtOH & CNS depressants; ↑ anticholinergic effects w/ antihistamines, phenothiazines, quinidine, disopyramide, TCAs, MAOIs; ↑ effect of digoxin; ↓ effect of levodopa; ↓ effects w/ antacids and antidiarrheal drugs **NIPE:** May ↑ susceptibility to heat stroke, take w/ meals to avoid GI upset

Bepridil (Vascor)
Uses: Chronic stable angina **Action:** CCB agent **Dose:** 200–400 mg/d PO **Caution:** [C, ?] **Contra:** QT interval prolongation, Hx ventricular arrhythmias, sick sinus syndrome, hypotension (DBP <90 mm Hg) **Supplied:** Tabs 200, 300, 400 mg **Notes/SE:** Dizziness, nausea, agranulocytosis, bradycardia, and serious ventricular arrhythmias, including torsades de pointes **Interactions:** ↑ Effects w/ amprenavir, ritonavir, moxifloxacin, gatifloxacin, sparfloxacin; ↑ effects of digitalis glycoside, cyclosporine, BBs; ↑ QT prolongation w/ procainamide, quinidine, TCAs **Labs:** ↑ LFTs, CPK, LDH **NIPE:** Take w/ food if GI upset, monitor K^+ & ECG

Beractant (Survanta)
Uses: *Prevention & Rx of RDS in premature infants* **Action:** Replaces pulmonary surfactant **Dose:** 100 mg/kg via ET tube; may repeat 3× q6h; max 4 doses/48 h **Caution:** [N/A, N/A] **Supplied:** Suspension 25 mg of phospholipid/mL **SE:** Transient bradycardia, oxygen desaturation, apnea **Notes:** Administer via 4-quadrant method **Interactions:** None noted **NIPE:** ↑ Risk of nosocomial sepsis after Rx w/ this drug

Betaxolol (Kerlone)
Uses: *HTN* **Action:** Competitively blocks β-adrenergic receptors, $β_1$ **Caution:** [C (1st tri), D (2nd or 3rd tri), +/–] **Contra:** Sinus bradycardia, AV conduction abnormalities, cardiac failure **Dose:** 10–20 mg/d **Supplied:** Tabs 10, 20 mg **SE:** Dizziness, HA, bradycardia, edema, CHF **Interactions:** ↑ Effects w/ anticholinergics, verapamil, general anesthetics; ↓ effects w/ thyroid drugs, amphetamine, cocaine, ephedrine, epinephrine, norepinephrine, phenylephrine, pseudoephedrine, NSAIDs; ↑ effects of insulin, digitalis glycosides; ↓ effects of theophylline, dopamine, glucagon **Labs:** ↑ BUN, serum lipoprotein, glucose, K^+, triglyceride, uric acid, ANA titers **NIPE:** May ↑ sensitivity to cold, ⊘ DC abruptly

Betaxolol, Ophthalmic (Betoptic)
Uses: Glaucoma **Action:** Competitively blocks β-adrenergic receptors, $β_1$ **Dose:** 1 gt bid **Caution:** [C (1st tri), D (2nd or 3rd tri), ?/–] **Supplied:** Soln 0.5%; susp 0.25% **SE:** Local irritation. See Betaxolol + **NIPE:** Use sunglasses to ⊘ exposure, may cause photophobia, review installation procedures

Bethanechol (Urecholine, Duvoid, others) Uses: *Neurogenic bladder atony w/ retention,* acute *postoperative* & postpartum functional *(nonobstructive) urinary retention* Action: Stimulates cholinergic smooth muscle receptors in bladder & GI tract Dose: *Adults.* 10–50 mg PO tid–qid or 2.5–5 mg SQ tid–qid & PRN. *Peds.* 0.6 mg/kg/24 h PO ÷ tid–qid or 0.15–2 mg/kg/d SQ ÷ 3–4× (take on empty stomach) Caution: [C, ?/–] Contra: Bladder outlet obstruction, PUD, epilepsy, hyperthyroidism, bradycardia, COPD, AV conduction defects, parkinsonism, hypotension, vasomotor instability Supplied: Tabs 5, 10, 25, 50 mg; inj 5 mg/mL SE: Abdominal cramps, diarrhea, salivation, hypotension Notes: ⊘ use IM/IV Interactions: ↑ Effects w/ BBs, tacrine, cholinesterase inhibitors; ↓ effects w/ atropine, anticholinergic drugs, procainamide, quinidine, epinephrine Labs: ↑ In serum AST, ALT, amylase, lipase, bilirubin NIPE: May cause blurred vision, monitor I&O, take on an empty stomach

Bevacizumab (Avastin) WARNING: Associated w/ GI perforation, wound dehiscence, & fatal hemoptysis Uses: *Colorectal metastatic carcinoma, w/ 5-FU* Action: Vascular endothelial growth factor inhibitor Dose: *Adults.* 5 mg/kg IV q14d. 1st dose over 90 min; 2nd over 60 min, 3rd over 30 min if tolerated Caution: [C, –] Contra: ⊘ Use w/in 28 d of surgery if time for separation of drug & anticipated surgical procedures is unknown; DC w/ serious adverse events Supplied: 100 mg/4 mL, 400 mg/16 mL vials SE: Wound dehiscence, GI perforation, hemoptysis, hemorrhage, hypertension, proteinuria, CHF, inf Rxns, diarrhea, leucopenia, thromboembolism Labs: Monitor for ↑ BP & proteinuria

Bicalutamide (Casodex) Uses: *Advanced CAP* (w/ GnRH agonists [eg, leuprolide, goserelin]) Action: Nonsteroidal antiandrogen Dose: 50 mg/d Caution: [X, ?] Contra: Women Supplied: Caps 50 mg SE: Hot flashes, loss of libido, impotence, diarrhea, N/V, gynecomastia, & LFT elevation Interactions: ↑ Effects of anticoagulants, TCAs, phenothiazides; ↓ effects of antipsychotic drugs Labs: ↑ LFTs, alkaline phosphatase, bilirubin, BUN, creatinine; ↓ Hgb, WBCs NIPE: Monitor PSA, may experience hair loss

Bicarbonate (See Sodium Bicarbonate, page 219)

Bisacodyl (Dulcolax) [OTC] Uses: *Constipation; preop bowel prep* Action: Stimulates peristalsis Dose: *Adults.* 5–15 mg PO or 10 mg PR PRN. *Peds* <2 y: 5 mg PR PRN. >2 y: 5 mg PO or 10 mg PR PRN (⊘ chew tabs; ⊘ give w/in 1 h of antacids or milk) Caution: [B, ?] Contra: Acute abdomen or bowel obstruction, appendicitis, gastroenteritis Supplied: EC tabs 5 mg; supp 10 mg SE: Abdominal cramps, proctitis, & inflammation w/ suppositories Interactions: Antacids & milk ↑ dissolution of enteric coating causing abdominal irritation Labs: False ↓ urine glucose NIPE: ↑ Fluid intake & high-fiber foods, ⊘ take w/ milk or antacids

Bismuth Subsalicylate (Pepto-Bismol) [OTC] Uses: Indigestion, nausea, & *diarrhea;* combination for Rx of *H. pylori infection* Action: Antisecretory & antiinflammatory effects Dose: *Adults.* 2 tabs or 30 mL PO PRN (max 8

doses/24 h). **Peds.** *3–6 y:* ⅛ tab or 5 mL PO PRN (max 8 doses/24 h). *6–9 y:* ⅜ tab or 10 mL PO PRN (max 8 doses/24 h). *9–12 y:* 1 tab or 15 mL PO PRN (max 8 doses/24 h) **Caution:** [C, D (3rd tri), –] ⊘ in renal failure **Contra:** Influenza or chickenpox (↑ risk of Reye's syndrome), ASA allergy **Supplied:** Chew tabs 262 mg; liq 262, 524 mg/15 mL **Interactions:** ↑ Effects of ASA, MRX, valproic acid; ↓ effects of tetracyclines, quinolones, probenecid; ↓ effects w/ corticosteroids **Labs:** False ↑ uric acid, AST; may interfere w/ GI tract x-rays; ↓ K⁺, T₃, & T₄ **NIPE:** May darken tongue & stool, chew tab, ⊘ swallow whole

Bisoprolol (Zebeta) **Uses:** *HTN* **Action:** Competitively blocks β₁-adrenergic receptors **Dose:** 5–10 mg/d (max dose 20 mg/d); ↓ in renal impairment **Caution:** [C (D 2nd & 3rd tri), +/–] **Contra:** Sinus bradycardia, AV conduction abnormalities, cardiac failure **Supplied:** Tabs 5, 10 mg **SE:** Fatigue, lethargy, HA, bradycardia, edema, CHF **Notes:** Not dialyzed **Interactions:** ↑ Bradycardia w/ adenosine, amiodarone, digoxin, dipyridamole, neostigmine, physostigmine, tacrine; ↑ effects w/ cimetidine, fluoxetine, prazosin; ↓ effects w/ NSAIDs, rifampin; ↓ effects of theophylline, glucagon **Labs:** ↑ T₄, cholesterol, glucose, triglycerides, uric acid; ↓ HDL **NIPE:** ⊘ DC abruptly, may mask S/Sxs hypoglycemia, take w/o regard to food

Bitolterol (Tornalate) **Uses:** Prophylaxis & Rx of *asthma* & reversible bronchospasm **Action:** Sympathomimetic bronchodilator; stimulates β₂-adrenergic receptors in the lungs **Dose:** *Adults & Peds >12 y.* 2 inhal q8h **Caution:** [C, ?] **Supplied:** Aerosol 0.8% **SE:** Dizziness, nervousness, trembling, HTN, palpitations **Interactions:** ↑ Cardiac effects of theophylline; ↑ hypokalemia w/ furosemide; ↑ effects w/ other β-adrenergic bronchodilators, MAOIs, TCAs, inhaled anesthetics; ↓ effects w/ β-adrenergic blockers; **Labs:** ↑ AST, ↓ plts, WBCs, proteinuria **NIPE:** Wait 15 min after use of this drug before using an adrenocorticoid inhaler. Shake inhaler well before use

Bivalirudin (Angiomax) **Uses:** *Anticoagulant w/ASA in unstable angina undergoing PTCA* **Action:** Anticoagulant, thrombin inhibitor **Dose:** 1 mg/kg IV bolus, then 2.5 mg/kg/h over 4 h; PRN, use 0.2 mg/kg/h for up to 20 h (give w/ ASA 300–325 mg/d; start pre-PTCA) **Caution:** [B, ?] **Contra:** Major bleeding **Supplied:** Powder for inj **SE:** Bleeding, back pain, nausea, HA **Interactions:** ↑ Cardiac effects of theophylline; ↑ hypokalemia w/ furosemide; ↑ effects w/ other β-adrenergic bronchodilators, MAOIs, TCAs, inhaled anesthetics; ↓ effects w/ β-adrenergic blockers; **Labs:** ↑ AST, ↓ plts, WBCs, proteinuria **NIPE:** Wait 15 min after use of this drug before using an adrenocorticoid inhaler. Shake inhaler well before use

Bleomycin Sulfate (Blenoxane) **Uses:** *Testis CA; Hodgkin's & NHLs; cutaneous lymphomas; & squamous cell CA (head & neck, larynx, cervix, skin, penis); sclerosing agent for malignant pleural effusion* **Action:** Induces breakage (scission) of single-/double-stranded DNA **Dose:** 10–20 mg (U)/m² 1–2/wk (refer to specific protocols); ↓ in renal impairment **Caution:** [D, ?] Severe pulmonary Dz **Supplied:** Inj 15 mg (15 U) **SE:** Hyperpigmentation (skin staining) & hypersensitivity (rash to anaphylaxis); fever in 50%; lung toxicity (idiosyncratic & dose-related); pneumonitis may progress to fibrosis; Raynaud's phenomenon, N/V **Notes:** Test dose 1 mg (U) recommended, especially in lymphoma Pts; lung toxicity w/total dose >400 mg (U) **Interactions:** ↑ Effects w/ cisplatin & other antineoplastic drugs; ↓ effects of digoxin & phenytoin **Labs:** Monitor CBC, LFTs, BUN, creatinine; pulmonary Fxn tests **NIPE:** ⊘ Immunizations, breast-feeding; use contraception method

Bortezomib (Velcade) **WARNING:** May worsen preexisting neuropathy **Uses:** *Progression of multiple myeloma despite two previous Rxs* **Action:** Proteasome inhibitor **Dose:** 1.3 mg/m² bolus IV 2×/wk × 2 wk, w/ 10-day rest period (= 1 cycle); ↓ dose for hematologic toxicity, neuropathy **Caution:** [D, ?/–] **Supplied:** 3.5-mg vial **SE:** Asthenia, GI upset, anorexia, dyspnea, headache, orthostatic hypotension, edema, insomnia, dizziness, rash, pyrexia, arthralgia, neuropathy **Notes:** May interact w/ drugs metabolized via CYP450 system **Interactions:** ↑ Risk of peripheral neuropathy and/or hypotension w/ amiodarone, antivirals, INH, nitrofurantoin, statins **Labs:** Monitor for ↑ uric acid, ↓ K⁺, Ca²⁺, neutrophils, plts **NIPE:** ⊘ PRG or breast-feeding; use contraception; caution w/ driving due to fatigue/dizziness; ↑ fluids if C/O N/V

Brimonidine (Alphagan) **Uses:** *Open-angle glaucoma, ocular HTN* **Action:** α₂-Adrenergic agonist **Dose:** 1 gt in eye(s) tid (wait 15 min to insert contacts) **Caution:** [B, ?] **Contra:** MAOI therapy **Supplied:** 0.2% soln **SE:** Local irritation, HA, fatigue **Interactions:** ↑ Effects of antihypertensives, BBs, cardiac glycosides, CNS depressants; ↓ effects w/ TCAs **NIPE:** ⊘ EtOH, insert soft contact lenses 15 + min after drug use

Brinzolamide (Azopt) **Uses:** *Open-angle glaucoma, ocular HTN* **Action:** Carbonic anhydrase inhibitor **Dose:** 1 gt in eye(s) tid **Caution:** [C, ?] **Supplied:** 1% susp **SE:** Blurred vision, dry eye, blepharitis, taste disturbance **Interactions:** ↑ Effects w/ oral carbonic anhydrase inhibitors **Labs:** Check LFTs, BUN, creatinine **NIPE:** ⊘ Use drug if ↓ renal & hepatic studies or allergies to sulfonamides; shake well before use; insert soft contact lenses 15 + min after drug use; wait 10 min before use of other topical ophthalmic drugs

Bromocriptine (Parlodel) **Uses:** *Parkinson's Dz, hyperprolactinemia, acromegaly, pituitary tumors* **Action:** Direct-acting on the striatal dopamine receptors; inhibits prolactin secretion **Dose:** Initial, 1.25 mg PO bid; titrate to effect **Caution:** [C, ?] **Contra:** Severe ischemic heart Dz or PVD **Supplied:** Tabs 2.5 mg; caps 5 mg **SE:** ↓ BP, Raynaud's phenomenon, dizziness, nausea, hallucinations **Interactions:** ↑ Effects w/ erythromycin, fluvoxamine, nefazodone, sympathomimetics; ↓ effects w/ phenothiazines, antipsychotics; **Labs:** ↑ BUN, AST, ALT, CPK, alkaline phosphatase, uric acid **NIPE:** ⊘ Breast-feeding, PRG, oral contraceptives; drug may cause intolerance to EtOH, return of menses & suppression of galactorrhea may take 6–8 wk

Budesonide (Rhinocort, Pulmicort) Uses: *Allergic & nonallergic rhinitis, asthma* **Action:** Steroid **Dose:** *Intranasal:* 2 sprays/nostril bid or 4 sprays/nostril/d. *Aqueous:* 1 spray/nostril/d. *PO inhaled:* 1–4 inhal bid. *Peds:* 1–2 inhal bid (Rinse mouth after PO use) **Caution:** [C, ?/–] **Supplied:** Met-dose Turbuhaler, nasal inhaler, & aqueous spray **SE:** HA, cough, hoarseness, *Candida* infection, epistaxis **Interactions:** ↑ Effects w/ ketoconazole, itraconazole, ritonavir, indinavir, saquinavir, erythromycin, & grapefruit juice **NIPE:** Shake inhaler well before use, rinse mouth & wash inhaler after use, swallow capsules whole, ⊘ exposure chickenpox or measles.

Bumetanide (Bumex) Uses: *Edema from CHF, hepatic cirrhosis, & renal Dz* **Action:** Loop diuretic; inhibits reabsorption of Na & Cl in the ascending loop of Henle & the distal renal tubule **Dose:** *Adults.* 0.5–2 mg/d PO; 0.5–1 mg IV q8–24h (max 10 mg/d). *Peds.* 0.015–0.1 mg/kg/d PO, IV, or IM ÷ q6–24h **Caution:** [D, ?] **Contra:** Anuria, hepatic coma, severe electrolyte depletion **Supplied:** Tabs 0.5, 1, 2 mg; inj 0.25 mg/mL **SE:** ↓ K⁺, ↓ Na⁺, ↑ creatinine, ↑ uric acid, dizziness, ototoxicity **Notes:** Monitor fluid & electrolytes **Interactions:** ↑ Effects w/ antihypertensives, thiazides, nitrates, EtOH, clofibrate; ↑ effects of Li, warfarin, thrombolytic drugs, anticoagulants; ↑ K⁺ loss w/ carbenoxolone, corticosteroids, terbutaline; ↑ ototoxicity w/ aminoglycosides, cisplatin; ↓ effects w/ cholestyramine, colestipol, NSAIDs, probenecid, barbiturates, phenytoin **Labs:** ↑ T₄, T₃, BUN, serum glucose, creatinine uric acid; ↓ serum K⁺, Ca²⁺, Mg²⁺ **NIPE:** Take drug w/ food, take early to prevent nocturia, daily weights

Bupivacaine (Marcaine) Uses: *Local, regional, & spinal anesthesia, local & regional analgesia* **Action:** Local anesthetic **Dose:** *Adults & Peds.* Dose-dependent on procedure (ie, tissue vascularity, depth of anesthesia, etc) **Caution:** [C, ?] **Contra:** Severe bleeding, severe hypotension, shock & arrhythmias, local infections at anesthesia site, septicemia **Supplied:** Inj 0.25, 0.5, 0.75% **SE:** ↓ BP, bradycardia, dizziness, anxiety **Interactions:** ↑ Effects w/ BBs, hyaluronidase, ergot-type oxytocics, MAOI, TCAs, phenothiazines, vasopressors, CNS depressants; ↓ effects w/ chloroprocaine **NIPE:** Anesthetized area has temporary loss of sensation & Fxn

Buprenorphine (Buprenex) [C-V] Uses: *Moderate/severe pain* **Action:** Opiate agonist–antagonist **Dose:** 0.3–0.6 mg IM or slow IV push q6h PRN **Caution:** [C, ?] **Supplied:** Inj 0.324 mg/mL (= 0.3 mg of buprenorphine) **SE:** Sedation, ↓ BP, resp depression **Notes:** May induce withdrawal syndrome in opioid-dependent Pts **Interactions:** ↑ Effects of resp & CNS depression w/ EtOH, opiates, benzodiazepines, TCAs, MAOIs, other CNS depressants **Labs:** ↑ Eerum amylase and lipase **NIPE:** ⊘ EtOH & other CNS depressants

Bupropion (Wellbutrin, Wellbutrin SR, Wellbutrin XL, Zyban) Uses: *Depression, adjunct to smoking cessation* **Action:** Weak inhibitor of neuronal uptake of serotonin & norepinephrine; inhibits the neuronal re-uptake of dopamine **Dose:** *Depression:* 100–450 mg/d ÷ bid–tid; SR 100–200 mg bid; XL 150–300 mg daily. *Smoking cessation:* 150 mg/d × 3 d, then 150 mg bid ×8–12 wk; ↓ in renal/hepatic impairment **Caution:** [B, ?/–] **Contra:** Sz disorder, prior diagnosis of anorexia nervosa or bulimia, MAOI, abrupt discontinuation of EtOH or sedatives **Supplied:** Tabs 75, 100 mg; SR tabs 100, 150, 200 mg; XL tabs 150, 300 mg **SE:** Associated w/ Szs; agitation, insomnia, HA, tachycardia **Notes:** ⊘ Use of EtOH & other CNS depressants **Interactions:** ↑ Effects w/ cimetidine, levodopa, MAOIs; ↑ risk of Szs w/ EtOH, phenothiazines, antidepressants, theophylline, TCAs, or abrupt withdrawal of corticosteroids, benzodiazepines **Labs:** ↓ Prolactin level **NIPE:** Drug may cause Szs, take 3–4 wk for full effect, ⊘ EtOH or abrupt DC

Buspirone (BuSpar) **WARNING:** Closely monitor for worsening depression or emergence of suicidality **Uses:** Short-term relief of *anxiety* *Action:* Antianxiety; selectively antagonizes CNS serotonin receptors **Dose:** 5–10 mg PO tid; ↑ to desired response; usual 20–30 mg/d; max 60 mg/d; ↓ in severe hepatic/renal insufficiency **Caution:** [B, ?/–] **Supplied:** Tabs 5, 10, 15, 30 mg ÷ dose **SE:** Drowsiness, dizziness; HA, nausea **Notes:** No abuse potential or physical or psychologic dependence **Interactions:** ↑ Effects w/ erythromycin, clarithromycin, itraconazole, ketoconazole, diltiazem, verapamil, grapefruit juice; ↓ effects w/ carbamazepine, rifampin, phenytoin, dexamethasone, phenobarbital, fluoxetine **Labs:** ↑ AST, ALT, growth hormone, prolactin **NIPE:** ↑ Sedation w/ EtOH, therapeutic effects may take up to 4 wk

Busulfan (Myleran, Busulfex) **Uses:** *CML,* preparative regimens for allogeneic & ABMT in high doses **Action:** Alkylating agent **Dose:** 4–12 mg/d for several wks; 16 mg/kg once or 4 mg/kg/d for 4 d w/ another agent in transplant regimens. Refer to specific protocol **Caution:** [D, ?] **Supplied:** Tabs 2 mg, inj 60 mg/10 mL **SE:** Myelosuppression, pulmonary fibrosis, nausea (high-dose therapy), gynecomastia, adrenal insufficiency, & skin hyperpigmentation **Interactions:** ↑ Effects w/ acetaminophen; ↑ bone-marrow suppression w/ antineoplastic drugs & radiation therapy; ↑ uric acid levels w/ probenecid & sulfinpyrazone; ↓ effects w/ itraconazole, phenytoin **Labs:** ↑ Uric acid; monitor CBC, LFTs **NIPE:** ⊘ Immunizations, PRG, breast-feeding; ↑ fluids; use barrier contraception; ↑ risk of hair loss, rash, darkened skin pigment; ↑ susceptibility to infection

Butorphanol (Stadol) [C-IV] **Uses:** *Anesthesia adjunct, pain* & migraine HA **Action:** Opiate agonist–antagonist w/ central analgesic actions **Dose:** 1–4 mg IM or IV q3–4h PRN. *HA:* 1 spray in 1 nostril; may repeat ×1 if pain not relieved in 60–90 min; ↓ dose in renal impairment **Caution:** [C (D if high doses or prolonged periods at term), +] **Supplied:** Inj 1, 2 mg/mL; nasal spray 10 mg/mL **SE:** Drowsiness, dizziness, nasal congestion **Notes:** May induce withdrawal in opioid dependency **Interactions:** ↑ Effects w/ EtOH, antihistamines, cimetidine, CNS depressants, phenothiazines, barbiturates, skeletal-muscle relaxants, MAOIs; ↓ effects of opioids **Labs:** ↑ Serum amylase & lipase **NIPE:** ⊘ EtOH or other CNS depressants

Calcipotriene (Dovonex) **Uses:** *Plaque psoriasis* **Action:** Keratolytic **Dose:** Apply bid **Caution:** [C, ?] **Contra:** ↑ Ca^{2+}; vitamin D toxicity; ⊘ apply to face **Supplied:** Cream; oint; soln 0.005% **SE:** Skin irritation, dermatitis **Interactions:** None noted **Labs:** Monitor serum Ca **NIPE:** Wash hands after application or wear gloves to apply, DC drug if ↑ Ca

Calcitonin (Cibacalcin, Miacalcin) **Uses:** *Paget's Dz of bone, hypercalcemia,* osteogenesis imperfecta, *postmenopausal osteoporosis* **Action:** Polypeptide hormone **Dose:** *Paget's salmon form:* 100 units/d IM/SC initially, 50 units/d or 50–100 units q1–3d maint. *Paget's human form:* 0.5 mg/d initially; maint 0.5 mg 2–3 ×/wk or 0.25 mg/d, max 0.5 mg bid. *Hypercalcemia salmon calcitonin:* 4 units/kg IM/SC q12h; ↑ to 8 units/kg q12h, max q6h. *Osteoporosis salmon calcitonin:* 100 units/d IM/SQ; intranasal 200 units = 1 nasal spray/d **Caution:** [C, ?] **Supplied:** Spray, nasal 200 units/activation; inj, human (Cibacalcin) 0.5 mg/vial, salmon 200 units/mL (2 mL) **SE:** Facial flushing, nausea, edema at inj site, nasal irritation, polyuria **Notes:** Human (Cibacalcin) & salmon forms; human only approved for Paget's bone Dz **Interactions:** None noted **Labs:** ↓ Serum Li **NIPE:** Allergy skin test prior to use

Calcitriol (Rocaltrol) **Uses:** *Reduction of ↑ PTH levels, ↓ Ca^{2+} on dialysis* **Action:** 1,25-Dihydroxycholecalciferol (vitamin D analogue) **Dose:** *Adults. Renal failure:* 0.25 µg/d PO, ↑ 0.25 µg/d q4–6wk PRN; 0.5 µg 3×/wk IV, ↑ PRN. *Hyperparathyroidism:* 0.5–2 µg/d. *Peds. Renal failure:* 15 ng/kg/d, ↑ PRN; maint 30–60 ng/kg/d. *Hyperparathyroidism:* <5 y. 0.25–0.75 µg/d. >6 y. 0.5–2 µg/d **Caution:** [C, ?] **Contra:** ↑ Ca^{2+}; vitamin D toxicity **Supplied:** Inj 1, 2 µg/mL (in 1-mL); caps 0.25, 0.5 µg **SE:** ↑ Ca^{2+} possible **Notes:** Monitor dose to keep Ca^{2+} WNL **Interactions:** ↑ Effect w/ thiazide diuretics; ↓ effect w/ cholestyramine, colestipol **Labs:** ↑ Ca^{2+}, cholesterol, Mg^{2+}, BUN, AST, ALT; ↓ alkaline phosphatase; **NIPE:** ⊘ Mg-containing antacids or suppls

Calcium Acetate (Calphron, Phos-Ex, PhosLo) **Uses:** *ESRD-associated hyperphosphatemia* **Action:** Ca suppl to treat hyperphosphatemia w/o Al **Dose:** 2–4 tabs PO w/ meals **Caution:** [C, ?] **Contra:** ↑ Ca^{2+} **Supplied:** Caps Phos-Ex 500 mg (125 mg Ca); tabs Calphron & PhosLo 667 mg (169 mg Ca) **SE:** Can cause ↑ Ca^{2+}, hypophosphatemia, constipation **Notes:** Monitor Ca^{2+} **Interactions:** ↑ Effects of quinidine, ↓ effects w/ large intake of dietary fiber, spinach, rhubarb; ↓ effects of atenolol, CCB, etidronate, tetracyclines, fluoroquinolones, phenytoin, Fe salts **Labs:** ↑ Ca^{2+}; ↓ Mg^{2+} **NIPE:** ⊘ EtOH, caffeine, tobacco; separate Ca suppls and other meds by 1–2 h

Calcium Carbonate (Tums, Alka-Mints) [OTC] **Uses:** *Hyperacidity associated w/ peptic ulcer Dz, hiatal hernia,* etc **Action:** Neutralizes gastric acid **Dose:** 500 mg–2 g PO PRN; ↓ in renal impairment **Caution:** [C, ?] **Supplied:** Chew tabs 350, 420, 500, 550, 750, 850 mg; susp **SE:** ↑ Ca^{2+}, hypophosphatemia, constipation **Interactions:** ↓ Effect of tetracyclines, fluoroquinolones, Fe salts, and ASA; ↓ Ca absorption w/ high intake of dietary fiber **Labs:** ↑ Ca^{2+}, ↓ Mg^{2+} **NIPE:**

↑ Fluids, may cause constipation, ⊘ EtOH, caffeine, tobacco; separate Ca suppls and other meds by 1–2 h, chew tablet well

Calcium Glubionate (Neo-Calglucon) [OTC]
Uses: *Rx & prevent Ca deficiency* Action: Ca suppl Dose: *Adults.* 6–18 g/d ÷ doses. *Peds.* 600–2000 mg/kg/d ÷ qid (9 g/d max); ↓ in renal impairment Caution: [C, ?] Contra: ↑ Ca²⁺ Supplied: OTC syrup 1.8 g/5 mL = Ca 115 mg/5 mL SE: Hypercalcemia, hypophosphatemia, constipation Interactions: ↑ Effects of quinidine; ↓ effect of tetracyclines; ↓ Ca absorption w/ high intake of dietary fiber; Labs: ↑ Ca²⁺, ↓ Mg²⁺ NIPE: ⊘ EtOH, caffeine, tobacco, separate Ca suppls and other meds by 1–2 h, chew tab well

Calcium Salts (Chloride, Gluconate, Gluceptate)
Uses: *Ca replacement,* VF, Ca blocker toxicity, Mg intoxication, tetany, *hyperphosphatemia in ESRD* Action: Ca suppl/replacement Dose: *Adults. Replacement:* 1–2 g/d PO. *Cardiac emergencies:* CaCl 0.5–1 g IV q 10 min or Ca gluconate 1–2 g IV q 10 min. *Tetany:* 1 g CaCl over 10–30 min; repeat in 6 h PRN. *Peds. Replacement:* 200–500 mg/kg/24 h PO or IV ÷ qid. *Cardiac emergency:* 100 mg/kg/dose IV of gluconate salt q 10 min. *Tetany:* 10 mg/kg CaCl over 5–10 min; repeat in 6 h or use inf (200 mg/kg/d max). *Adult & Peds. Hypocalcemia due to citrated blood inf:* 0.45 mEq Ca/100 mL citrated blood inf (↓ in renal impairment) Caution: [C, ?] Contra: Hypercalcemia Supplied: CaCl inj 10% = 100 mg/mL = Ca 27.2 mg/mL = 10-mL amp; Ca gluconate inj 10% = 100 mg/mL = Ca 9 mg/mL; tabs 500 mg = 45 mg Ca, 650 mg = 58.5 mg Ca, 975 mg = 87.75 mg Ca, 1 g = 90 mg Ca; Ca gluceptate inj 220 mg/mL = 18 mg/mL Ca SE: Bradycardia, cardiac arrhythmias, ↑ Ca²⁺ Notes: CaCl 270 mg (13.6 mEq) elemental Ca/g, & Ca gluconate 90 mg (4.5 mEq) Ca/g. *RDA for Ca:* Adults = 800 mg/d; Peds = <6 mo 360 mg/d, 6 mo–1 y 540 mg/d, 1–10 y 800 mg/d, 10–18 y 1200 mg/d Interactions: ↑ Effects of quinidine and digitalis; ↓ effects of tetracyclines, quinolones, verapamil, CCBs, Fe salts, ASA, atenolol; ↓ Ca absorption w/ high intake of dietary fiber Labs: ↑ Ca²⁺, ↓ Mg²⁺ NIPE: ⊘ EtOH, caffeine, tobacco; separate Ca suppls and other meds by 1–2 h, chew tablet well

Calfactant (Infasurf)
Uses: *Prevention & Rx of RSD in infants* Action: Exogenous pulmonary surfactant Dose: 3 mL/kg instilled into lungs. Can retreat for a total of 3 doses given 12 h apart Caution: [?, ?] Supplied: Intratracheal susp 35 mg/mL SE: Monitor for cyanosis, airway obstruction, bradycardia during administration Interactions: None noted NIPE: ⊘ Reconstitute, dilute, or shake vial; refrigerate & keep away from light; no need to warm soln prior to use

Candesartan (Atacand)
Uses: *HTN,* DN, CHF Action: Angiotensin II receptor antagonists Dose: 2–32 mg/d (usual 16 mg/d) Caution: [X, –] Contra: Primary hyperaldosteronism; bilateral renal artery stenosis Supplied: Tabs 4, 8, 16, 32 mg SE: Dizziness, HA, flushing, angioedema Interactions: ↑ Effects w/ cimetidine; ↑ risk of hyperkalemia w/ amiloride, spironolactone, triamterene, K suppls, trimethoprim; ↑ effects of Li; ↓ effects w/ phenobarbital, rifampin Labs: ↑

Creatine phosphatase; monitor for albuminuria, hyperglycemia, triglyceridemia, uricemia. **NIPE:** ⊘ Breast-feeding or PRG, use barrier contraception, may take 4–6 wk for full effect, adequate fluid intake, take w/o regard to food

Capsaicin (Capsin, Zostrix, others) [OTC] Uses: Pain due to *postherpetic neuralgia,* chronic neuralgia, *arthritis, diabetic neuropathy,* postoperative pain, psoriasis, intractable pruritus **Action:** Topical analgesic **Dose:** Apply tid–qid **Caution:** [?. ?] **Supplied:** OTC creams; gel; lotions; roll-ons **SE:** Local irritation, neurotoxicity, cough **Interactions:** May ↑ cough w/ ACEIs **NIPE:** External use only, ⊘ contact w/ eyes or broken/irritated skin, apply w/ gloves, transient stinging/burning

Captopril (Capoten, others) Uses: *HTN, CHF, MI.* *LVD, DN Action:** ACEI **Dose:** *Adults. HTN:* Initially, 25 mg PO bid–tid; ↑ to maint q1–2wk by 25-mg increments/dose (max 450 mg/d) to effect. *CHF:* Initially, 6.25–12.5 mg PO tid; titrate PRN *LVD:* 50 mg PO tid. *DN:* 25 mg PO tid. **Peds.** Infants <2 mo: 0.05–0.5 mg/kg/dose PO q8–24h. Children: Initially, 0.3–0.5 mg/kg/dose PO; ↑ to 6 mg/kg/d max (Take 1 h ac) **Caution:** [C (1st tri); D (2nd & 3rd tri); ? in renal impairment +] **Contra:** Hx angioedema **Supplied:** Tabs 12.5, 25, 50, 100 mg **SE:** Rash, proteinuria, cough, ↑ K+ **Interactions:** ↑ Effects w/ antihypertensives, diuretics, nitrates, probenecid, black catechu; ↓ effects w/ antacids, ASA, NSAIDs, food; ↑ effects of digoxin, insulin, oral hypoglycemics, Li **Labs:** False + urine acetone; may ↑ urine protein, serum BUN, creatinine, K+, prolactin, LFTs; may ↓ FBS **NIPE:** ⊘ PRG, breast-feeding, K-sparing diuretics; take w/o food, may take 2 wk for full therapeutic effect

Carbamazepine (Tegretol) WARNING: Aplastic anemia & agranulocytosis have been reported w/ carbamazepine **Uses:** *Epilepsy, trigeminal neuralgia.* EtOH withdrawal **Action:** Anticonvulsant **Dose:** *Adults.* Initially, 200 mg PO bid; ↑ by 200 mg/d; usual 800–1200 mg/d ÷ doses. *Peds.* <6 y: 5 mg/kg/d, ↑ to 10–20 mg/kg/d ÷ in 2–4 doses. 6–12 y: Initial, 100 mg PO bid or 10 mg/kg/24 h PO ÷ qd–bid; ↑ to maint 20–30 mg/kg/24 h ÷ tid–qid; ↓ dose in renal impairment (take w/ food) **Caution:** [D. +] **Contra:** MAOI use, Hx bone marrow depression **Supplied:** Tabs 200 mg: chew tabs 100 mg: XR tabs 100, 200, 400 mg; susp 100 mg/5 mL **SE:** Drowsiness, dizziness, blurred vision, N/V, rash, ↓ Na+, leukopenia, agranulocytosis **Notes:** Monitor CBC & serum levels (see Table 2, page 265); generic products not interchangeable **Interactions:** ↑ Effects w/ cimetidine, clarithromycin, danazol, diltiazem, felbamate, fluconazole, fluoxetine, fluvoxamine, INH, itraconazole, ketoconazole, macrolides, metronidazole, propoxyphene, protease inhibitors, valproic acid, verapamil, grapefruit juice; ↑ effects of Li, MAOIs; ↓ effects w/ phenobarbital, phenytoin, primidone, plantain; ↓ effects of benzodiazepines, corticosteroids, cyclosporine, doxycycline, felbamate, haloperidol, oral contraceptives, phenytoin, theophylline, thyroid hormones, TCAs, warfarin **Labs:** ↑ BUN, LFTs, bilirubin, alkaline phosphatase; ↓ Ca2+, T3, T4, Na; false – PRG test & uric acid **NIPE:** Take w/ food, may cause photosensitivity—use sunscreen, use barrier contraception, abrupt withdrawal may cause Szs, ⊘ breast-feeding or PRG

Carbidopa/Levodopa (Sinemet) Uses: *Parkinson's Dz* Action: ↑ CNS levels of dopamine Dose: 25/100 mg bid–qid; ↑ as needed (max 200/2000 mg/d) Caution: [C, ?] Contra: Narrow-angle glaucoma, suspicious skin lesion (may activate melanoma), melanoma, MAOI use Supplied: Tabs (mg carbidopa/mg levodopa) 10/100, 25/100, 25/250; tabs SR (mg carbidopa/mg levodopa) 25/100, 50/200 SE: Psychiatric disturbances, orthostatic hypotension, dyskinesias, & cardiac arrhythmias Interactions: ↑ Effects w/ antacids; ↓ effects w/ anticonvulsants, benzodiazepines, haloperidol, Fe, methionine, papaverine, phenothiazines, phenytoin, pyridoxine, spiramycin, tacrine, thioxanthenes, high protein food Labs: ↑ Urine amino acids, serum acid phosphatase, aspartate aminotransferase; ↓ serum bilirubin, BUN, creatinine, glucose, uric acid NIPE: Darkened urine & sweat may result, ⊘ crush or chew sustained release tabs, take w/o food

Carboplatin (Paraplatin) Uses: *Ovarian, lung, head & neck, testicular, urothelial,* & brain *CA, NHL* & allogeneic & ABMT in high doses Action: DNA cross-linker; forms DNA-platinum adducts Dose: 360 mg/m^2 (ovarian carcinoma); AUC dosing 4–7 mg/mL (using Culvert's formula: mg = AUC × [25 + calculated GFR]); adjusted based on pretreatment plt count, CrCl, & BSA (Egorin's formula); up to 1500 mg/m^2 used in ABMT setting (refer to specific protocols) Caution: [D, ?] Contra: Severe bone marrow suppression, excessive bleeding Supplied: Inj 50, 150, 450 mg SE: Myelosuppression, N/V/D, nephrotoxicity, hematuria, neurotoxicity, ↑ LFTs Notes: Physiologic dosing based on either Culvert's or Egorin's formula allows ↑ doses to reduce toxicity Interactions: ↑ Myelosuppression w/ myelosuppressive drugs; ↑ hemotologic effects w/ bone-marrow suppressants; ↑ bleeding w/ ASA; ↑ nephrotoxicity w/ nephrotoxic drugs; ↓ effects of phenytoin; ↓ effects w/ food and w/ Al Labs: ↓ Mg^{2+}, K$^+$, Na$^+$, Ca^{2+}; ↑ LFTs NIPE: ⊘ Use w/ Al needles or IV administration sets, PRG, breast-feeding; antiemetics prior to admin may prevent N/V, maintain adequate food & fluid intake

Carisoprodol (Soma) Uses: *Adjunct to sleep & physical therapy for the relief of painful musculoskeletal conditions* Action: Centrally acting muscle relaxant Dose: 350 mg PO tid–qid Caution: [C, M] Tolerance may result; caution in renal/hepatic impairment Contra: Hypersensitivity to meprobamate; acute intermittent porphyria Supplied: Tabs 350 mg SE: CNS depression, drowsiness, dizziness, tachycardia Notes: ⊘ EtOH & other CNS depressants; available in combination w/ ASA or codeine. Interactions: ↑ Effects w/ CNS depressants, phenothiazines, EtOH NIPE: ⊘ Breast-feeding, take w/ food if GI upset

Carmustine [BCNU] (BiCNU, Gliadel) Uses: *Primary brain tumors, melanoma, Hodgkin's lymphoma & NHLs, multiple myeloma, & induction for allogeneic & ABMT in high doses; adjunct to surgery in Pts w/ recurrent glioblastoma multiforme* Action: Alkylating agent; nitrosourea forms DNA cross-links; inhibits DNA Dose: 150–200 mg/m^2 q6–8wk single or ÷ dose daily inj over 2d; 20–65 mg/m^2 q4–6wk; 300–900 mg/m^2 in BMT (see specific protocols); ↓ dose in

hepatic impairment **Caution:** [D, ?] In ↓ WBC, RBC, plt counts, renal or hepatic impairment **Contra:** Myelosuppression, PRG **Supplied:** Inj 100 mg/vial; wafer: 7.7 mg **SE:** Hypotension, N/V, myelosuppression (WBC & plt), phlebitis, facial flushing, hepatic & renal dysfunction, pulmonary fibrosis, & optic neuroretinitis; hematologic toxicity may persist up to 4–6 wk after dose **Notes:** ⊘ give course more frequently than q6wk (cumulative toxicity); baseline PFTs recommended **Interactions:** ↑ Bleeding w/ ASA, anticoagulants; ↑ hepatic dysfunction w/ etoposide; ↑ myelosuppression w/ cimetidine; ↑ suppression of bone marrow w/ radiation or additional antineoplastics; ↓ effects of phenytoin, digoxin; ↓ pulmonary Fxn **Labs:** ↑ AST, alkaline phosphatase, bilirubin; monitor CBC, plts, LFTs, PFTs **NIPE:** ⊘ PRG, breast-feeding, exposure to infections, ASA products

Carteolol (Cartrol, Ocupress Ophthalmic)   **Uses:** *HTN,* ↑ intraocular pressure, chronic open-angle glaucoma* **Action:** Blocks β-adrenergic receptors (β$_1$, β$_2$), mild ISA **Dose:** PO 2.5–5 mg/d; ophth 1 gt in eye(s) bid; ↓ in renal impairment **Caution:** [C (1st tri); D (2nd & 3rd tri), ?/–] Cardiac failure, asthma **Contra:** Sinus bradycardia; heart block >1st degree; bronchospasm **Supplied:** Tabs 2.5, 5 mg; ophth soln 1% **SE:** Drowsiness, sexual dysfunction, bradycardia, edema, CHF; *ocular:* conjunctival hyperemia, anisocoria, keratitis, eye pain **Notes:** Not shown to be of value in CHF **Interactions:** ↑ Effects w/ amiodarone, adenosine, barbiturates, CCBs, digoxin, dipyridamole, fluoxetine, rifampin, tacrine, nitrates, EtOH; ↑ α-adrenergic effects w/ amphetamines, cocaine, ephedrine, epinephrine, phenylephrine; ↑ effects of theophylline; ↓ effects w/ antacids, NSAIDs, thyroid drugs, clonidine; ↓ effects of hypoglycemics, theophylline, dopamine **Labs:** ↑ BUN, uric acid, K$^+$, serum lipoprotein, triglycerides, glucose, ANA titers **NIPE:** Ophthalmic drug may cause photophobia & risk of burning; may ↑ cold sensitivity, mental confusion

Carvedilol (Coreg)   **Uses:** *HTN, CHF, MI* **Action:** Blocks adrenergic receptors, β$_1$, β$_2$, α **Dose:** *HTN:* 6.25–12.5 mg bid. *CHF:* 3.125–25 mg bid; take w/ food to minimize hypotension **Caution:** [C (1st tri); D (2nd & 3rd tri), ?/–] Bradycardia, asthma, diabetes **Contra:** Decompensated cardiac failure, 2nd-/3rd-degree heart block, SSS, severe hepatic impairment **Supplied:** Tabs 3.125, 6.25, 12.5, 25 mg **SE:** Dizziness, fatigue, hyperglycemia, bradycardia, edema, hypercholesterolemia **Notes:** ⊘ DC abruptly; **Interactions:** ↑ Effects w/ cimetidine, clonidine, MAOIs, reserpine, verapamil, fluoxetine, paroxetine; ↑ effects of digoxin, hypoglycemics, cyclosporine, CCBs; ↓ effects w/ rifampin, NSAIDs; **Labs:** ↑ LFTs, K$^+$, triglycerides, uric acid, BUN, creatinine, alkaline phosphatase; ↓ HDL **NIPE:** Food slows absorption, may cause dry eyes w/ contact lenses

Caspofungin (Cancidas)   **Uses:** *Invasive aspergillosis refractory/intolerant to standard therapy, esophageal candidiasis* **Action:** An echinocandin; inhibits fungal cell wall synthesis; highest activity in regions of active cell growth **Dose:** 70 mg IV load day 1, 50 mg/d IV; slow inf; ↓ dose in hepatic impairment **Caution:** [C, ?/–] ⊘ use w/ cyclosporine; not studied as initial therapy **Contra:** Hypersensitivity to any component **Supplied:** IV inf **SE:** Fever, HA, N/V, thrombophlebitis at site, ↑ LFTs **Notes:** Monitor during inf; limited experience beyond 2 wk of therapy **Interactions:** ↑ Effects w/ cyclosporine; ↓ effects w/ carbamazepine, dexamethasone, efavirenz, nelfinavir, nevirapine, phenytoin, rifampin; ↓ effect of tacrolimus **Labs:** ↑ LFTs, serum alkaline phosphatase, eosinophils, PT, urine protein & RBCs; ↓ K⁺, albumin, WBCs, Hgb, Hct, plts, neutrophils; **NIPE:** Infuse slowly over 1 h & ⊗ mix w/ other drugs

Cefaclor (Ceclor) Uses: *Rx bacterial infections of the upper & lower resp tract, skin, bone, urinary tract, abdomen, & gynecologic system* **Action:** 2nd-gen cephalosporin; inhibits cell wall synthesis. *Spectrum:* More gram(−)? activity than 1st-gen cephalosporins; effective against gram(+) including *S. aureus*; good gram(−) coverage against *H. influenzae* **Dose:** *Adults.* 250–500 mg PO tid; XR 375–500 mg bid. *Peds.* 20–40 mg/kg/d PO ÷ 8–12h; ↓ renal impairment **Caution:** [B, +] **Contra:** Allergy to cephalosporins **Supplied:** Caps 250, 500 mg; XR tabs 375, 500 mg; susp 125, 187, 250, 375 mg/5 mL **SE:** Diarrhea, rash, eosinophilia, ↑ transaminases **Interactions:** ↑ Bleeding w/ anticoagulants; ↑ nephrotoxicity w/ aminoglycosides, loop diuretics; ↑ effects w/ probenecid; ↓ effects w/ antacids, chloramphenicol **Labs:** + Direct Coombs' test; ↑ LFTs, alkaline phosphatase, bilirubin, LDH, BUN, creatinine; false + of serum or UCr, false + urine glucose **NIPE:** Food w/ ER tabs ↑ absorption, monitor for superinfection, ⊘ breast-feeding

Cefadroxil (Duricef, Ultracef) Uses: *Rx infections involving skin, bone, upper & lower resp tract, & urinary tract* **Action:** 1st-gen cephalosporin; inhibits cell wall synthesis. *Spectrum:* Good gram(+) coverage, including group A β-hemolytic *Streptococcus, Staphylococcus;* gram(−) coverage against *E. coli, Proteus, Klebsiella* **Dose:** *Adults.* 1–2 g/d PO, 2 ÷ doses *Peds.* 30 mg/kg/d ÷ bid; ↓ dose in renal impairment **Caution:** [B, +] **Contra:** Hypersensitivity to cephalosporins **Supplied:** Caps 500 mg; tabs 1 g; susp 125, 250, 500 mg/5 mL **SE:** Diarrhea, N/V, rash, eosinophilia, ↑ transaminases **Interactions:** ↑ Bleeding w/ anticoagulants; ↑ nephrotoxicity w/ aminoglycosides, loop diuretics; ↑ effects w/ probenecid; ↓ effects w/ antacids, chloramphenicol **Labs:** + Direct Coombs' test; ↑ LFTs, alkaline phosphatase, bilirubin, LDH, BUN, creatinine; false + of serum or UCr, false + urine glucose **NIPE:** Food w/ ER tabs ↑ absorption, monitor for superinfection, ⊘ breast-feeding; give w/o regard to food

Cefazolin (Ancef, Kefzol) Uses: *Rx infections of skin, bone, upper & lower resp tract, & urinary tract* **Action:** 1st-gen cephalosporin; inhibits cell wall synthesis. *Spectrum:* Good coverage against gram(+) bacilli & cocci, *Streptococcus, Staphylococcus* (except *Enterococcus*); some gram(−) coverage (*E. coli, Proteus, Klebsiella* **Dose:** *Adults.* 1–2 g IV q8h *Peds.* 25–100 mg/kg/d IV ÷ q6–8h; ↓ in renal impairment **Caution:**[B, +] **Contra:** Hypersensitivity to cephalosporins **Supplied:** Inj **SE:** Diarrhea, rash, eosinophilia, elevated transaminases, pain at inj site **Notes:** Widely used for surgical prophylaxis **Interactions:** ↑ Bleeding w/ anticoagulants; ↑ nephrotoxicity w/ aminoglycosides, loop diuretics; ↑ effects w/

probenecid; ↓ effects w/ antacids, chloramphenicol **Labs:** + Direct Coombs' test; ↑ LFTs, alkaline phosphatase, bilirubin, LDH, BUN, creatinine; false + of serum or UCr, false + urine glucose **NIPE:** Food w/ ER tabs ↑ absorption, monitor for superinfection, ◯ breast-feeding; monitor renal Fxn, I&O

Cefdinir (Omnicef) **Uses:** *Rx infections of the resp tract, skin, bone, & urinary tract* **Action:** 3rd-gen cephalosporin; inhibits cell wall synthesis *Spectrum:* Active in vitro against a wide range of gram(+) & gram(−) organisms; more active than cefaclor & cephalexin against *Streptococcus, Staphylococcus*; active against some anaerobes **Dose:** *Adults.* 300 mg PO bid or 600 mg/d PO. *Peds.* 7 mg/kg PO bid or 14 mg/kg/d PO; ↓ in renal impairment **Caution:** [B, +] In penicillin-sensitive Pts; serum sickness-like Rxns have been reported **Contra:** Hypersentivity to cephalosporins **Supplied:** Caps 300 mg; susp 125 mg/5 mL **SE:** Anaphylaxis, diarrhea, rare pseudomembranous colitis **Interactions:** ↑ Bleeding w/ anticoagulants; ↑ nephrotoxicity w/ aminoglycosides, loop diuretics; ↓ effects w/ probenecid; ↓ effects w/ antacids, chloramphenicol; ↓ effects w/ Fe suppls **Labs:** + Direct Coombs' test; ↑ LFTs, alkaline phosphatase, bilirubin, LDH, BUN, creatinine; false + of serum or UCr, false + urine glucose **NIPE:** Food w/ ER tabs ↑ absorption, monitor for superinfection, ◯ breast-feeding; stools may initially turn red in color, sucrose in suspension

Cefditoren (Spectracef) **Uses:** *Acute exacerbations of chronic bronchitis, pharyngitis, tonsillitis; skin infections* **Action:** 3rd-gen cephalosporin; inhibits cell wall synthesis. *Spectrum:* Good gram(+) activity against *Streptococcus* & *Staphylococcus* infections; gram(−) *H. influenzae* & *M. catarrhalis* **Dose:** *Adults & Peds >12 y. Skin:* 200 mg PO bid × 10 days. *Chronic bronchitis, pharyngitis, tonsillitis:* 400 mg PO bid × 10 days; ◯ antacids w/in 2 h; take w/ meals; adjust dose in renal impairment **Caution:** [B, ?] Renal or hepatic impairment **Contra:** Hypersensitivity to cephalosporins/penicillins, milk protein, or carnitine deficiency **Supplied:** 200-mg tabs **SE:** HA, N/V/D, colitis, nephrotoxicity, hepatic dysfunction, Stevens–Johnson syndrome, toxic epidermal necrolysis, hypersensitivity Rxns **Notes:** Causes renal excretion of carnitine **Interactions:** ↑ Bleeding w/ anticoagulants; ↑ nephrotoxicity w/ aminoglycosides, loop diuretics; ↑ effects w/ probenecid; ↓ effects w/ antacids, chloramphenicol **Labs:** + Direct Coombs' test; ↑ LFTs, alkaline phosphatase, bilirubin, LDH, BUN, creatinine; false + of serum or UCr, false + urine glucose **NIPE:** Food w/ ER tabs ↑ absorption, monitor for superinfection, ◯ breast-feeding, sensitive to milk protein; monitor for Sz activity

Cefepime (Maxipime) **Uses:** *UTI, pneumonia, febrile neutropenia, skin/soft tissue infections* **Action:** 4th-gen cephalosporin; inhibits cell wall synthesis. *Spectrum:* S. pneumoniae, S. aureus, K. pneumoniae, E. coli, P. aeruginosa, & Enterobacter sp **Dose:** *Adults.* 1–2 g IV q12h. *Peds.* 50 mg/kg q8h for febrile neutropenia; 50 mg/kg bid for skin/soft tissue infections; ↓ dose in renal impairment **Caution:** [B, +] **Contra:** Hypersensitivity to cephalosporins **Supplied:** Inj

500 mg, 1, 2 g **SE:** Rash, pruritus, N/V/D, fever, HA, + direct Coombs' test w/out hemolysis **Notes:** Administered as IM or IV **Interactions:** ↑ Bleeding w/ anticoagulants; ↑ nephrotoxicity w/ aminoglycosides, loop diuretics; ↓ effects w/ probenecid; ↓ effects w/ antacids, chloramphenicol; ↓ effects of oral contraceptives **Labs:** + Direct Coombs' test; ↑ LFTs, alkaline phosphatase, bilirubin, LDH, BUN, creatinine; false + of serum or UCr, false + urine glucose **NIPE:** Food w/ ER tabs ↑ absorption, monitor for superinfection, ⊘ breast-feeding or use EtOH w/ drug or w/in 3 d of taking drug

Cefixime (Suprax) **Uses:** *Rx infections of the resp tract, skin, bone, & urinary tract* **Action:** 3rd-gen cephalosporin; inhibits cell wall synthesis. *Spectrum: S. pneumoniae, S. pyogenes, H. influenzae,* & enterobacteria. **Dose: Adults.** 400 mg PO qd–bid. *Peds.* 8 mg/kg/d PO ÷ daily–bid; ↓ dose in renal impairment **Caution:** [B, +] **Contra:** Hypersensitivity to cephalosporins **Supplied:** Tabs 200, 400 mg; susp 100 mg/5 mL **SE:** N/V/D, flatulence, & abdominal pain **Notes:** Monitor renal & hepatic Fxn; use susp for otitis media **Interactions:** ↑ Bleeding w/ anticoagulants; ↑ nephrotoxicity w/ aminoglycosides, loop diuretics; ↓ effects w/ probenecid; ↓ effects w/ antacids, chloramphenicol ; ↓ effects of oral contraceptives **Labs:** + Direct Coombs' test; ↑ LFTs, alkaline phosphatase, bilirubin, LDH, BUN, creatinine; false + of serum or UCr, false + urine glucose **NIPE:** Food w/ ER tabs ↑ absorption, monitor for superinfection, ⊘ breast-feeding

Cefmetazole (Zefazone) **Uses:** *Rx infections of the upper & lower resp tract, skin, bone, urinary tract, abdomen, & gynecologic system* **Action:** 2nd-gen cephalosporin; inhibits cell wall synthesis. *Spectrum:* Gram(+) against *S. aureus;* gram(−) activity & some anaerobic activity; use in mixed aerobic–anaerobic infections where *Bacteroides fragilis* likely **Dose: Adults.** 2 g IV q6–12h; ↓ in renal impairment **Caution:** [B, +] **Contra:** Hypersensitivity to cephalosporins **Supplied:** Inj 1, 2 g **SE:** Eosinophilia, leukopenia, N/V/D, ↑ LFTs, bleeding risk, rash, pseudomembranous colitis, disulfram Rxn **Notes:** Safety not established in children **Interactions:** ↑ Bleeding w/ anticoagulants; ↑ nephrotoxicity w/ aminoglycosides, loop diuretics; ↓ effects w/ probenecid; ↓ effects w/ antacids, chloramphenicol **Labs:** + Direct Coombs' test; ↑ LFTs, alkaline phosphatase, bilirubin, LDH, BUN, creatinine; false + of serum or UCr, false + urine glucose **NIPE:** Food w/ ER tabs ↑ absorption, monitor for superinfection, ⊘ breast-feeding or use EtOH w/ drug or w/in 3 d of taking drug

Cefonicid (Monocid) **Uses:** *Rx bacterial infections (resp tract, skin, bone & joint, urinary tract, gynecologic, sepsis)* **Action:** 2nd-gen cephalosporin; inhibits bacterial cell wall synthesis. *Spectrum:* Gram(+) including MSSA & many streptococci; gram(−) bacilli including *E. coli, Klebsiella, P. mirabilis, H. influenzae,* & *Moraxella* **Dose:** 0.5–2 g/24 h IM/IV; ↓ in renal impairment **Caution:** [B, +] **Contra:** Hypersensitivity to cephalosporins **Supplied:** Powder for inj 500 mg, 1 g, 10 g **SE:** Diarrhea, rash, ↑ plts, eosinophilia, ↑ transaminases **Interactions:** ↑

Bleeding w/ anticoagulants; ↑ nephrotoxicity w/ aminoglycosides, loop diuretics; ↑ effects w/ probenecid; ↓ effects w/ antacids, chloramphenicol **Labs:** + Direct Coombs' test; ↑ LFTs, alkaline phosphatase, bilirubin, LDH, BUN, creatinine; false + of serum or UCr, false + urine glucose **NIPE:** Food w/ ER tabs ↑ absorption, monitor for superinfection. ⊘ breast-feeding

Cefoperazone (Cefobid) **Uses:** *Rx infections of the resp, skin, urinary tract, sepsis* **Action:** 3rd-gen cephalosporin; inhibits bacterial cell wall synthesis. *Spectrum:* Gram(–) (eg, *E. coli, Klebsiella*); variable against *Streptococcus* & *Staphylococcus* sp; active *P. aeruginosa* but < ceftazidime **Dose: Adults.** 2–4 g/d IM/IV ÷ q 8–12h (12 g/d max). **Peds.** (not approved) 100–150 mg/kg/d IM/IV ÷ bid–tid (12 g/d max); ↓ in renal/hepatic impairment **Caution:**[B, +] May ↑ risk of bleeding **Contra:** Hypersensitivity to cephalosporins **Supplied:** Powder for inj 1, 2 g **SE:** Diarrhea, rash, eosinophilia, ↑ LFTs, hypoprothrombinemia, & bleeding (due to MTT side chain) **Notes:** May interfere w/ warfarin **Interactions:** ↑ Bleeding w/ anticoagulants; ↑ nephrotoxicity w/ aminoglycosides, loop diuretics; ↑ effects w/ probenecid; ↓ effects w/ antacids, chloramphenicol **Labs:** + Direct Coombs' test; ↑ LFTs, alkaline phosphatase, bilirubin, LDH, BUN, creatinine; false + of serum or UCr, false + urine glucose **NIPE:** Food w/ ER tabs ↑ absorption, monitor for superinfection. ⊘ breast-feeding or use EtOH w/ drug or w/in 3 d of taking drug

Cefotaxime (Claforan) **Uses:** *Rx infections of resp tract, skin, bone, urinary tract, meningitis, sepsis* **Action:** 3rd-gen cephalosporin; inhibits cell wall synthesis. *Spectrum:* Most gram(–) (not *Pseudomonas*), some gram(+) cocci (not *Enterococcus*); many penicillin-resistant pneumococci **Dose: Adults.** 1–2 g IV q4–12h. **Peds.** 50–200 mg/kg/d IV ÷ q 4–12h; ↓ dose renal/hepatic impairment **Caution:** [B, +] Arrhythmia associated w/ rapid inj; caution in colitis **Contra:** Hypersensitivity to cephalosporins **Supplied:** Powder for inj 500 mg, 1, 2, 10 g **SE:** Diarrhea, rash, pruritus, colitis, eosinophilia, ↑ transaminases **Interactions:** ↑ Bleeding w/ anticoagulants; ↑ nephrotoxicity w/ aminoglycosides, loop diuretics; ↑ effects w/ probenecid; ↓ effects w/ antacids, chloramphenicol **Labs:** + Direct Coombs' test; ↑ LFTs, alkaline phosphatase, bilirubin, LDH, BUN, creatinine; false + of serum or UCr, false + urine glucose **NIPE:** Food w/ ER tabs ↑ absorption, monitor for superinfection. ⊘ breast-feeding or use EtOH w/ drug or wi/n 3 d of taking drug

Cefotetan (Cefotan) **Uses:** *Rx infections of the upper & lower resp tract, skin, bone, urinary tract, abdomen, & gynecologic system* **Action:** 2nd-gen cephalosporin; inhibits cell wall synthesis. *Spectrum:* Less active against gram(+); anaerobes including *B. fragilis*; gram(–), including *E. coli, Klebsiella,* & *Proteus* **Dose: Adults.** 1–2 g IV q12h. **Peds.** 20–40 mg/kg/d IV ÷ q12h; ↓ in renal impairment **Caution:** [B, +] May ↑ bleeding risk; in those Hx of penicillin allergies **Contra:** Hypersensitivity to cephalosporins **Supplied:** Powder for inj 1, 2, 10 g **SE:** Diarrhea, rash, eosinophilia, ↑ transaminases, hypoprothrombinemia, & bleeding (due to MTT side chain) **Notes:** Caution w/ other nephrotoxic drugs; may interfere w/ warfarin **Interactions:** ↑ Bleeding w/ anticoagulants; ↑ nephrotoxicity w/ aminoglycosides, loop diuretics; ↑ effects w/ probenecid; ↓ effects w/ antacids, chloramphenicol **Labs:** + Direct Coombs' test; ↑ LFTs, alkaline phosphatase, bilirubin, LDH, BUN, creatinine; false + of serum or UCr, false + urine glucose **NIPE:** Food w/ ER tabs ↑ absorption, monitor for superinfection, ⊘ breast-feeding or use EtOH w/ drug or w/in 3 d of taking drug

Cefoxitin (Mefoxin)
Uses: *Rx infections of the upper & lower resp tract, skin, bone, urinary tract, abdomen, & gynecologic system* **Action:** 2nd-gen cephalosporin; inhibits cell wall synthesis. *Spectrum:* Good gram(−) against enteric bacilli (ie, *E. coli, Klebsiella, & Proteus*); anaerobic activity against *B. fragilis* **Dose:** *Adults.* 1–2 mg IV q6–8h. *Peds.* 80–160 mg/kg/d ÷ q4–6h; ↓ in renal impairment **Caution:** [B, +] **Contra:** Hypersensitivity to cephalosporins **Supplied:** Powder for inj 1, 2, 10 g **SE:** Diarrhea, rash, eosinophilia, ↑ transaminases **Interactions:** ↑ Bleeding w/ anticoagulants; ↑ nephrotoxicity w/ aminoglycosides, loop diuretics; ↑ effects w/ probenecid; ↓ effects w/ antacids, chloramphenicol **Labs:** + Direct Coombs' test; ↑ LFTs, alkaline phosphatase, bilirubin, LDH, BUN, creatinine; false + of serum or UCr, false + urine glucose **NIPE:** Food w/ ER tabs ↑ absorption, monitor for superinfection, ⊘ breast-feeding

Cefpodoxime (Vantin)
Uses: *Rx resp, skin, & urinary tract infections* **Action:** 3rd-gen cephalosporin; inhibits cell wall synthesis. *Spectrum: S. pneumoniae* or non-β-lactamase-producing *H. influenzae*; acute uncomplicated *N. gonorrhoeae*; some uncomplicated gram(−)(*E. coli, Klebsiella, Proteus*) **Dose:** *Adults.* 200–400 mg PO q12h. *Peds.* 10 mg/kg/d PO ÷ bid; ↓ dose in renal impairment, take w/ food **Caution:** [B, +] **Contra:** Hypersensitivity to cephalosporins **Supplied:** Tabs 100, 200 mg; susp 50, 100 mg/5 mL **SE:** Diarrhea, rash, HA, eosinophilia, elevated transaminases **Notes:** Drug interactions w/ agents that ↑ gastric pH **Interactions:** ↑ Bleeding w/ anticoagulants; ↑ nephrotoxicity w/ aminoglycosides, loop diuretics; ↑ effects w/ probenecid; ↓ effects w/ antacids, chloramphenicol **Labs:** + Direct Coombs' test; ↑ LFTs, alkaline phosphatase, bilirubin, LDH, BUN, creatinine; false + of serum or UCr, false + urine glucose **NIPE:** Food w/ ER tabs ↑ absorption, monitor for superinfection, ⊘ breast-feeding. See Cefaclor. **Additional Interactions:** ↑ Effects if taken w/ food

Cefprozil (Cefzil)
Uses: *Rx resp tract, skin, & urinary tract infections* **Action:** 2nd-gen cephalosporin; inhibits cell wall synthesis. *Spectrum:* Active against MSSA, strep, & gram(−) bacilli (*E. coli, Klebsiella, P. mirabilis, H. influenzae, Moraxella*) **Dose:** *Adults.* 250–500 mg PO daily–bid. *Peds.* 7.5–15 mg/kg/d PO ÷ bid; ↓ dose in renal impairment **Caution:** [B, +] **Contra:** Hypersensitivity to cephalosporins **Supplied:** Tabs 250, 500 mg; susp 125, 250 mg/5 mL **SE:** Diarrhea, dizziness, rash, eosinophilia, ↑ transaminases **Notes:** Use higher doses for otitis & pneumonia **Interactions:** ↑ Bleeding w/ anticoagulants; ↑ nephrotoxicity w/ aminoglycosides, loop diuretics; ↑ effects w/ probenecid; ↓ effects w/ antacids,

chloramphenicol **Labs:** + Direct Coombs' test; ↑ LFTs, alkaline phosphatase, bilirubin, LDH, BUN, creatinine; false + of serum or UCr, false + urine glucose **NIPE:** Food w/ ER tabs ↑ absorption, monitor for superinfection, ⊘ breast-feeding

Ceftazidime (Fortaz, Ceptaz, Tazidime, Tazicef) Uses: *Rx resp tract, skin, bone, urinary tract infections, meningitis, & septicemia* **Action:** 3rd-gen cephalosporin; inhibits cell wall synthesis. *Spectrum: P. aeruginosa* sp, good gram(−)activity **Dose: Adults.** 500–2 g IV q8–12h. **Peds.** 30–50 mg/kg/dose IV q8h; ↓ dose in renal impairment **Caution:** [B, +] **Contra:** Hypersensitivity to cephalosporins **Supplied:** Powder for inj 1, 2, 10 g **SE:** Diarrhea, rash, eosinophilia, ↑ transaminases **Interactions:** ↑ Bleeding w/ anticoagulants; ↑ nephrotoxicity w/ aminoglycosides, loop diuretics; ↑ effects w/ probenecid; ↓ effects w/ antacids, chloramphenicol **Labs:** ↓ Direct Coombs' test; ↑ LFTs, alkaline phosphatase, bilirubin, LDH, BUN, creatinine; false ↓ of serum or UCr, false + urine glucose **NIPE:** Food w/ ER tabs ↑ absorption, monitor for superinfection, ⊘ breast-feeding or use EtOH w/in 3 d of taking drug

Ceftibuten (Cedax) Uses: *Rx resp tract, skin, urinary tract infections & otitis media* **Action:** 3rd-gen cephalosporin; inhibits cell wall synthesis. *Spectrum: H. influenzae* & *M. catarrhalis*; weak against *S. pneumoniae* **Dose: Adults.** 400 mg/d PO. **Peds.** 9 mg/kg/d PO; ↓ dose in renal impairment; take on an empty stomach **Caution:** [B, +] **Contra:** Hypersensitivity to cephalosporins **Supplied:** Caps 400 mg; susp 90, 180 mg/5 mL **SE:** Diarrhea, rash, eosinophilia, ↑ transaminases **Interactions:** ↑ Bleeding w/ anticoagulants; ↑ nephrotoxicity w/ aminoglycosides, loop diuretics; ↑ effects w/ probenecid; ↓ effects w/ antacids, chloramphenicol **Labs:** + Direct Coombs' test; ↑ LFTs, alkaline phosphatase, bilirubin, LDH, BUN, creatinine; false + of serum or UCr, false + urine glucose **NIPE:** Food w/ ER tabs ↑ absorption, monitor for superinfection, ⊘ breast-feeding or use EtOH w/in 3 d of taking drug

Ceftizoxime (Cefizox) Uses: *Rx resp tract, skin, bone, & urinary tract infections, meningitis, & septicemia* **Action:** 3rd-gen cephalosporin; inhibits cell wall synthesis. *Spectrum:* Good against gram(−) bacilli (not *Pseudomonas*), some gram(+) cocci (not *Enterococcus*), & some anaerobes **Dose: Adults.** 1–2 g IV q8–12h. **Peds.** 150–200 mg/kg/d IV ÷ q6–8h; ↓ dose in renal impairment **Caution:** [B, +] **Contra:** Hypersensitivity to cephalosporins **Supplied:** Inj 500 mg, 1, 2, 10 g **SE:** Diarrhea, fever, rash, eosinophilia, thrombocytosis, ↑ transaminases **Interactions:** ↑ Bleeding w/ anticoagulants; ↑ nephrotoxicity w/ aminoglycosides, loop diuretics; ↑ effects w/ probenecid; ↓ effects w/ antacids, chloramphenicol **Labs:** + Direct Coombs' test; ↑ LFTs, alkaline phosphatase, bilirubin, LDH, BUN, creatinine; false + of serum or UCr, false + urine glucose **NIPE:** Food w/ ER tabs ↑ absorption, monitor for superinfection, ⊘ breast-feeding

Ceftriaxone (Rocephin) Uses: *Resp tract, skin, bone, urinary tract infections, meningitis, & septicemia; pneumonia* **Action:** 3rd-gen cephalosporin; inhibits cell wall synthesis. *Spectrum:* Moderate against gram(+); excellent against β-lactamase producers **Dose: *Adults.*** 1–2 g IV q12–24h. **Peds.** 50–100 mg/kg/d IV ÷ q12–24h; ↓ dose in renal impairment **Caution:** [B, +] **Contra:** Hypersensitivity to cephalosporins; hyperbilirubinemic neonates (displaces bilirubin from binding sites) **Supplied:** Powder for inj 250 mg, 500 mg, 1, 2 g **SE:** Diarrhea, rash, leukopenia, thrombocytosis, eosinophilia, ↑ transaminases **Interactions:** ↑ Bleeding w/ anticoagulants; ↑ nephrotoxicity w/ aminoglycosides, loop diuretics; ↑ effects w/ probenecid; ↓ effects w/ antacids, chloramphenicol **Labs:** + Direct Coombs' test; ↑ LFTs, alkaline phosphatase, bilirubin, LDH, BUN, creatinine; false + of serum or UCr, false + urine glucose **NIPE:** Food w/ ER tabs ↑ absorption, monitor for superinfection, ⊘ breast-feeding or use EtOH w/in 3 d of taking drug (NR) mix w/ other antimicrobials

Cefuroxime (Ceftin [PO], Zinacef [parenteral]) Uses: *Upper & lower resp tract, skin, bone, urinary tract, abdomen, & gynecologic infections* **Action:** 2nd-gen cephalosporin; inhibits cell wall synthesis *Spectrum:* Staphylococci, group B streptococci, *H. influenzae, E. coli, Enterobacter, Salmonella,* & *Klebsiella* **Dose: *Adults.*** 750 mg–1.5 g IV q8h or 250–500 mg PO bid. **Peds.** 100–150 mg/kg/d IV ÷ q8h or 20–30 mg/kg/d PO ÷ bid; ↓ dose in renal impairment; take w/ food **Caution:** [B, +] **Contra:** Hypersensitivity to cephalosporins **Supplied:** Tabs 125, 250, 500 mg; susp 125, 250 mg/5 mL; powder for inj 750 mg, 1.5, 7.5 g **SE:** Diarrhea, rash, eosinophilia, ↑ LFTs **Notes:** Cefuroxime axetil film-coated tablets & PO susp not bioequivalent; ⊘ substitute on a mg/mg basis; IV crosses blood–brain barrier **Interactions:** ↑ Bleeding w/ anticoagulants; ↑ nephrotoxicity w/ aminoglycosides, loop diuretics; ↑ effects w/ probenecid; ↓ effects w/ antacids, chloramphenicol **Labs:** + Direct Coombs' test; ↑ LFTs, alkaline phosphatase, bilirubin, LDH, BUN, creatinine; false + of serum or UCr, false + urine glucose **NIPE:** Food w/ ER tabs ↑ absorption, monitor for superinfection, ⊘ breast-feeding or use EtOH w/ drug or w/in 3 d of taking drug, food will ↓ GI distress & ↑ absorption, swallow tabs whole

Celecoxib (Celebrex) Uses: *Osteoarthritis & RA*; acute pain, primary dysmenorrhea; preventive in familial adenomatous polyposis **Action:** NSAID; inhibits the COX-2 pathway **Dose:** 100–200 mg/d or bid; ↓ in hepatic impairment; take w/ food/milk to lessen GI SE **Caution:** [C/D (3rd tri), ?] Caution in renal impairment **Contra:** Allergy to sulfonamides **Supplied:** Caps 100, 200 mg **SE:** GI upset, HTN, edema, renal failure, HA **Notes:** Watch for Sxs of GI bleeding; no effect on plt/bleeding time; can affect drugs metabolized by P-450 pathway **Interactions:** ↑ Effects w/ fluconazole; ↑ effects of Li; ↑ risks of GI upset &/or bleeding w/ ASA, NSAIDs, warfarin, EtOH; ↓ effects w/ Al- & Mg-containing antacids, ↓ effects of thiazide diuretics, loop diuretics, ACEIs **Labs:** ↑ LFTs, BUN, creatinine, CPK, alkaline phosphatase; monitor for hypercholesterolemia, hyperglycemia, hypokalemia, hypophosphatemia, albuminuria, hematuria **NIPE:** Take w/ food if GI distress

Cephalexin (Keflex, Keftab) Uses: *Skin, bone, upper/lower resp tract, & urinary tract infections* **Action:** 1st-gen cephalosporin; inhibits cell wall synthesis. *Spectrum:* Streptococcus, Staphylococcus, E. coli, Proteus, Klebsiella **Dose: *Adults.*** 250–500 mg PO qid. ***Peds.*** 25–100 mg/kg/d ÷ qid; ↓ dose in renal impairment; take on an empty stomach **Caution:** [B, +] **Contra:** Hypersensitivity to cephalosporins **Supplied:** Caps 250, 500 mg; tabs 250, 500, 1000 mg; susp 125, 250 mg/5 mL **SE:** Diarrhea, rash, eosinophilia, ↑ LFTs **Interactions:** ↑ Bleeding w/ anticoagulants; ↑ nephrotoxicity w/ aminoglycosides, loop diuretics; ↑ effects w/ probenecid; ↓ effects w/ antacids, chloramphenicol **Labs:** + Direct Coombs' test; ↑ LFTs, alkaline phosphatase, bilirubin, LDH, BUN, creatinine; false + of serum or UCr, false + urine glucose **NIPE:** Food w/ ER tabs ↑ absorption, monitor for superinfection, ⊘ breast-feeding

Cephradine (Velosef) **Uses:** *Rx resp, genitourinary, GI, skin, soft tissue, bone, & joint infections* **Action:** 1st-gen cephalosporin; inhibits cell wall synthesis. *Spectrum.* Gram(+) bacilli & cocci (not *Enterococcus*); some gram(–) bacilli (*E. coli, Proteus,* & *Klebsiella*) **Dose: *Adults.*** 250–500 mg q6–12h (8 g/d max). ***Peds >9 mo.*** 25–100 mg/kg/d ÷ bid–qid (4 g/d max); ↓ dose in renal impairment **Caution:** [B, +] **Contra:** Hypersensitivity to cephalosporins **Supplied:** Caps: 250, 500 mg; powder for susp 125, 250 mg/5 mL, injectable **SE:** Diarrhea, rash, eosinophilia, ↑ LFTs, N/V **Interactions:** ↑ Bleeding w/ anticoagulants; ↑ nephrotoxicity w/ aminoglycosides, loop diuretics; ↑ effects w/ probenecid; ↓ effects w/ antacids, chloramphenicol **Labs:** + Direct Coombs' test; ↑ LFTs, alkaline phosphatase, bilirubin, LDH, BUN, creatinine; false + of serum or UCr, false + urine glucose **NIPE:** Food w/ ER tabs ↑ absorption, monitor for superinfection, ⊘ breast-feeding or use EtOH w/ drug or w/in 3 d of taking drug, ⊘ take w/ any other antibiotic, take w/ food

Cetirizine (Zyrtec) **Uses:** *Allergic rhinitis & other allergic Sxs including urticaria* **Action:** Nonsedating antihistamine **Dose: *Adults & Children >6 y.*** 5–10 mg/d. ***Peds. 6–11 mo:*** 2.5 mg qd. *12–23 mo:* 2.5 mg qd–bid; ↓ dosage in renal/hepatic impairment **Caution:** [B, ?/–] Elderly & nursing mothers; doses >10 mg/d may cause drowsiness **Contra:** Hypersensitivity to cetirizine, hydroxyzine **Supplied:** Tabs 5, 10 mg; syrup 5 mg/5 mL **SE:** HA, drowsiness, xerostomia **Notes:** Can cause sedation **Interactions:** ↑ Effects w/ anticholinergics, CNS depressants, theophylline, EtOH **Labs:** May cause false – w/ allergy skin tests **NIPE:** ⊘ take w/ EtOH or CNS depressants

Charcoal, Activated (Supchar, Actidose, Liqui-Char) **Uses:** *Emergency Rx in poisoning by most drugs & chemicals* **Action:** Adsorbent detoxicant **Dose:** Give w/70% sorbitol (2 mL/kg); repeated use of sorbitol ⊘ *Adults. Acute intoxication:* 30–100 g/dose. *GI dialysis:* 20–50 g q6h for 1–2 d. ***Peds 1–12 y.*** *Acute intoxication:* 1–2 g/kg/dose. *GI dialysis:* 5–10 g/dose q4–8h **Caution:** [C, ?] May cause vomiting (hazardous in petroleum distillate & caustic ingestions); ⊘ mix w/ milk, ice cream, or sherbet **Contra:** Not effective for cyanide, mineral acids, caustic alkalis, organic solvents, Fe, EtOH, methanol poisoning, Li; ⊘ use sorbitol in Pts w/ fructose intolerance **Supplied:** Powder, liq, caps **SE:** Some liq dosage forms in sorbitol base (a cathartic); vomiting, diarrhea, black stools, constipation **Notes:** Charcoal w/ sorbitol is ⊘ in children < 1 y; monitor for hypokalemia & hypomagnesemia; protect the airway in lethargic or comatose Pts **Interactions:** ↓ Effects if taken w/ ice cream, milk, or sherbet; ↓ effects of digoxin & absorption of other oral meds, ↓ effects of syrup of ipecac **NIPE:** Most effective if given w/in 30 min of acute poisoning, only give to conscious patients

Chloral Hydrate (Aquachloral, Supprettes) [C-IV] Uses:

Short-term nocturnal & preoperative sedation **Action:** Sedative hypnotic; active metabolite trichloroethanol **Dose:** *Adults. Hypnotic:* 500 mg–1 g PO or PR 30 min hs or before procedure. *Sedative:* 250 mg PO or PR tid. **Peds.** *Hypnotic:* 20–50 mg/kg/24 h PO or PR 30 min hs or before procedure. *Sedative:* 5–15 mg/kg/dose q8h; ⊘ w/ CrCl <50 mL/min or severe hepatic impairment **Caution:** [C, +] Porphyria & neonates **Contra:** Hypersensitivity to components; severe renal, hepatic or cardiac Dz **Supplied:** Caps 500 mg; syrup 250, 500 mg/5 mL; supp 324, 500, 648 mg **SE:** GI irritation, drowsiness, ataxia, dizziness, nightmares, rash **Notes:** May accumulate; tolerance may develop >2 wk; taper dose; mix syrup in water or fruit juice; ⊘ EtOH & CNS depressants **Interactions:** ↑ Effects w/ antihistamines, barbiturates, paraldehyde, CNS depressants, opioid analgesics, EtOH; ↑ effects of anticoagulants **Labs:** False + of urine glucose, may interfere w/ tests for catecholamines and urinary 17-hydroxycorticosteroids **NIPE:** ⊘ Take w/ EtOH, CNS depressants; ⊘ chew or crush capsules

Chlorambucil (Leukeran) Uses:

CLL, Hodgkin's Dz, Waldenström's macroglobulinemia **Action:** Alkylating agent **Dose:** 0.1–0.2 mg/kg/d for 3–6 wk or 0.4 mg/kg/dose q2wk (refer to specific protocol) **Caution:** [D, ?] Sz disorder & bone marrow suppression; affects human fertility **Contra:** Previous resistance; hypersensitivity to alkylating agents **Supplied:** Tabs 2 mg **SE:** Myelosuppression, CNS stimulation, N/V, drug fever, skin rash, chromosomal damage that can result in secondary leukemias, alveolar dysplasia, pulmonary fibrosis, hepatotoxicity **Notes:** Monitor LFTs, CBC, leukocyte counts, plts, serum uric acid; reduce initial dosage if Pt has received radiation therapy **Interactions:** ↑ Bone marrow suppression w/ antineoplastic drugs and immunosuppressants; ↑ risk of bleeding w/ ASA, anticoagulants **Labs:** ↑ Urine and serum uric acid, ALT, alkaline phosphatase **NIPE:** ⊘ PRG, breast-feeding, infection; ↑ fluids to 2–3 L/d; monitor lab work periodically & CBC w/ differential weekly during drug use, may cause hair loss

Chlordiazepoxide (Librium, Mitran, Libritabs) [C-IV] Uses:

Anxiety, tension, EtOH withdrawal, & *preoperative apprehension* **Action:** Benzodiazepine; antianxiety agent **Dose:** *Adults. Mild anxiety:* 5–10 mg PO tid–qid or PRN. *Severe anxiety:* 25–50 mg IM, IV, or PO q6–8h or PRN. *EtOH withdrawal:* 50–100 mg IM or IV; repeat in 2–4 h if needed, up to 300 mg in 24 h; gradually taper daily dose. *Peds >6 y.* 0.5 mg/kg/24 h PO or IM ÷ q6–8h; ↓ dose in renal impairment, elderly **Caution:** [D, ?] Resp depression, CNS impairment, or a Hx of drug dependence; ⊗ in hepatic impairment **Contra:** Preexisting CNS depression **Supplied:** Caps 5, 10, 25 mg; tabs 10, 25 mg; inj 100 mg **SE:** Drowsiness, CP, rash, fatigue, memory impairment, xerostomia, weight gain **Notes:** Erratic IM absorption **Interactions:** ↑ Effects w/ antidepressants, antihistamines, anticonvulsants, barbiturates, general anesthetics, MAOIs, narcotics, phenothiazines cimetidine, disulfiram, fluconazole, itraconazole, ketoconazole, oral contraceptives, INH, metoprolol, propoxyphene, propranolol, valproic acid, EtOH, grapefruit juice, kava kava, valerian; ↑ effects of digoxin, phenytoin; ↓ effects w/ aminophylline, antacids, carbamazepine, theophylline, rifampin, rifabutin, tobacco; ↓ effects of levodopa **Labs:** ↑ LFTs, alkaline phosphatase, bilirubin, triglycerides; false ↑ urine 5-HIAA, urine 17-ketosteroids; false + urine PRG test; false ↓ urine 17 ketogenic steroids; ↓ HDL **NIPE:** ⊗ EtOH, PRG, breast-feeding; risk of photosensitivity—use sunscreen, orthostatic hypotension, tachycardia

Chlorothiazide (Diuril) Uses: *HTN, edema* Action: Thiazide diuretic

Dose: *Adults.* 500 mg–1 g PO qd–bid; 100–500 mg/d IV (for edema only). *Peds >6 mo.* 20–30 mg/kg/24 h PO ÷ bid; 4 mg/kg/d IV **Caution:** [D, +] ⊗ administer inj IM or SQ **Contra:** Cross-sensitivity to thiazides/sulfonamides, anuria **Supplied:** Tabs 250, 500 mg; susp 250 mg/5 mL; inj 500 mg/vial **SE:** ↓ K⁺, ↓ Na⁺, dizziness, hyperglycemia, hyperuricemia, hyperlipidemia, photosensitivity **Notes:** May be taken w/ food/milk; take early in the day to ⊗ nocturia; use sunblock; monitor electrolytes **Interactions:** ↑ Effects w/ ACEI, amphotericin B, corticosteroids; ↑ effects of diazoxide, Li, MRX; ↓ effects w/ colestipol, cholestyramine, NSAIDs; ↓ effects of hypoglycemics **Labs:** ↑ CPK, ammonia, amylase, Ca²⁺, Cl⁻, cholesterol, glucose, Mg²⁺, K⁺, Na⁺, uric acid **NIPE:** Monitor for gout, hyperglycemia, photosensitivity, I&O, weight

Chlorpheniramine (Chlor-Trimeton, others [OTC]) Uses: *Allergic Rxns; common cold* Action: Antihistamine Dose: Adults. 4 mg PO q4–6h

or 8–12 mg PO bid of SR **Peds.** 0.35 mg/kg/24 h PO ÷ q4–6h or 0.2 mg/kg/24 h SR **Caution:** [C, ?/–] bladder obstruction; narrow-angle glaucoma; hepatic insufficiency **Contra:** Hypersensitivity **Supplied:** Tabs 4 mg; chew tabs 2 mg; SR tabs 8, 12 mg; syrup 2 mg/5 mL; inj 10, 100 mg/mL **SE:** Anticholinergic SE & sedation common, postural hypotension, QT changes, extrapyramidal Rxns, photosensitivity **Interactions:** ↑ Effects w/ other CNS depressants, EtOH, opioids, sedatives, MAOIs, atropine, haloperidol, phenothiazines, quinidine, disopyramide; ↑ effects of epinephrine; ↓ effects of heparin, sulfonylureas **Labs:** False – w/ allergy testing **NIPE:** Stop drug 4 d prior to allergy testing, take w/ food if GI distress

Chlorpromazine (Thorazine) Uses: *Psychotic disorders, N/V,* apprehension, intractable hiccups Action: Phenothiazine antipsychotic; antiemetic

Dose: *Adults. Psychosis:* 10–25 mg PO or PR bid–tid (usual 30–800 mg/d in ÷ doses). *Severe Sxs:* 25 mg IM/IV initial; may repeat in 1–4 h; then 25–50 mg PO or PR tid. *Hiccups:* 25–50 mg PO bid–tid. *Children >6 mo. Psychosis & N/V:* 0.5–1 mg/kg/dose PO q4–6h or IM/IV q6–8h; ⊗ in severe hepatic impairment **Caution:**

[C, ?/–] Safety in children <6 mo not established; caution in known Szs, BM suppression **Contra:** Cross-sensitivity w/ other phenothiazines; ⊘ in narrow-angle glaucoma **Supplied:** Tabs 10, 25, 50, 100, 200 mg; SR caps 30, 75, 150 mg; syrup 10 mg/5 mL; conc 30, 100 mg/mL; supp 25, 100 mg; inj 25 mg/mL **SE:** Extrapyramidal SE & sedation; α-adrenergic blocking properties; ↓ BP; prolongs QT interval **Notes:** ⊘ Stop abruptly; dilute PO concentrate in 2–4 oz of liquid **Interactions:** ↑ Effects w/ amodiaquine, chloroquine, sulfadoxine–pyrimethamine, antidepressants, narcotic analgesics, propranolol, quinidine, BBs, MAOIs, TCAs, EtOH, kava kava; ↑ effects of anticholinergics, centrally acting antihypertensives, propranolol, valproic acid; ↓ effects w/ antacids, antidiarrheals, barbiturates, Li, tobacco; ↓ effects of anticonvulsants, guanethidine, levodopa, Li, warfarin **Labs:** False + for amylase, phenylketonuria, urine bilirubin, urine protein, uroporphyrins, urobilinogen, PRG test; ↑ plasma cholesterol **NIPE:** Risk of photosensitivity—use sunscreen & tardive dyskinesia, take w/ food if GI upset, may darken urine

Chlorpropamide (Diabinese) **Uses:** *Type 2 DM* **Action:** Sulfonylurea; ↑ release of insulin from pancreas; ↑ peripheral insulin sensitivity; ↓ hepatic glucose output **Dose:** 100–500 mg/d; take w/ food **Caution:** [C, ?/–] ⊘ use in CrCl < 50 mL/min; ↓ in hepatic impairment **Contra:** Cross-sensitivity w/ sulfonamides **Supplied:** Tabs 100, 250 mg **SE:** HA, dizziness, rash, photosensitivity, hypoglycemia, SIADH **Notes:** ⊘ EtOH (disulfiram-like Rxn) **Interactions:** ↑ Effects w/ ASA, NSAIDs, anticoagulants, BBs, chloramphenicol, guanethidine, insulin, MAOIs, phenytoin, probenecid, rifampin, sulfonamides, EtOH, juniper berries, ginseng, garlic, fenugreek, coriander, dandelion root, celery, bitter melon, ginkgo biloba; ↓ effects of anticoagulants, phenytoin, ASA, NSAIDs; ↓ effects w/ diazoxide, thiazide diuretics **Labs:** False ↑ serum Ca

Chlorthalidone (Hygroton, others) **Uses:** *HTN* **Action:** Thiazide diuretic **Dose:** *Adults.* 50–100 mg PO daily. *Peds.* (not approved) 2 mg/kg/dose PO 3×/wk or 1–2 mg/kg/d PO; ↓ in renal impairment **Caution:** [D, +] **Contra:** Cross-sensitivity w/ thiazides or sulfonamides; anuria **Supplied:** Tabs 15, 25, 50, 100 mg **SE:** ↓ K⁺, dizziness, photosensitivity, hyperglycemia, hyperuricemia, sexual dysfunction **Interactions:** ↑ Effects w/ ACEIs, diazoxide; ↑ effects of digoxin, Li, MRX; ↓ effects w/ cholestyramine, colestipol, NSAIDs; ↓ effects of hypoglycemics; ↓ K⁺ w/ amphotericin B, carbenoxolone, corticosteroids **Labs:** ↑ CPK, amylase, Ca²⁺, Cl⁻, cholesterol, glucose, uric acid; ↓ Cl⁻, Mg²⁺, K⁺, Na⁺ **NIPE:** May take w/ food, and milk, take early in day, use sunscreen

Chlorzoxazone (Paraflex, Parafon Forte DSC, others) **Uses:** *Adjunct to rest & physical therapy for the relief of discomfort associated w/ acute, painful musculoskeletal conditions* **Action:** Centrally acting skeletal muscle relaxant **Dose:** *Adults.* 250–500 mg PO tid–qid. *Peds.* 20 mg/kg/d in 3–4 ÷ doses **Caution:** [C, ?] ⊘ EtOH & CNS depressants **Contra:** Severe liver Dz **Supplied:** Tabs 250; caps 250, 500 mg **SE:** Drowsiness, tachycardia, dizziness, hepatotoxicity, angioedema **Interactions:** ↑ Effects w/ antihistamines, CNS depressants,

MAOIs, TCAs, opioids, EtOH, watercress **Labs:** Monitor LFTs **NIPE:** Urine may turn reddish purple or orange

Cholecalciferol [Vitamin D₃] (Delta D)   Uses: Dietary suppl to Rx vitamin D deficiency **Action:** Enhances intestinal Ca absorption **Dose:** 400–1000 IU/d PO **Caution:** [A (D doses above the RDA), +] **Contra:** Hypercalcemia, hypervitaminosis, hypersensitivity **Supplied:** Tabs 400, 1000 IU **SE:** Vitamin D toxicity (renal failure, HTN, psychosis) **Notes:** 1 mg of cholecalciferol = 40,000 IU of vitamin D activity

Cholestyramine (Questran, LoCHOLEST)   Uses: *Hypercholesterolemia; Rx pruritus associated w/ partial biliary obstruction; diarrhea associated w/ excess fecal bile acids* **Action:** Binds intestinal bile acids to form insoluble complexes **Dose: *Adults.*** Individualize: 4 g/d–bid (↑ to max 24 g/d & 6 doses/d). *Peds.* 240 mg/kg/d in 3 ÷ doses **Caution:** [C, ?] Constipation & phenylketonuria **Contra:** Complete biliary obstruction; hypolipoproteinemia types III, IV, V **Supplied:** 4 g of cholestyramine resin/9 g of powder; w/ aspartame: 4 g resin/5 g of powder **SE:** Constipation, abdominal pain, bloating, HA, rash **Notes:** OD may result in GI obstruction; mix 4 g of cholestyramine in 2–6 oz of noncarbonated beverage **Interactions:** ↓ Effects of acetaminophen, amiodarone, anticoagulants, ASA, cardiac glycosides, clindamycin, corticosteroids, diclofenac, fat-soluble vitamins, gemfibrozil, glipizide, Fe salts, MRX, methyldopa, nicotinic acid, penicillins, phenobarbital, phenytoin, propranolol, thiazide diuretics, tetracyclines, thyroid drugs, troglitazone, warfarin **Labs:** ↑ LFTs, PT, P, Cl, alkaline phosphatase; ↓ serum Ca²⁺, Na⁺, K⁺, cholesterol **NIPE:** ↑ fluids, take other drugs 1 h before or 6 h after

Ciclopirox (Loprox)   Uses: *Tinea pedis, tinea cruris, tinea corporis, cutaneous candidiasis, tinea versicolor* **Action:** Antifungal antibiotic **Dose: *Adults & Peds >10 y.*** Massage into affected area bid **Caution:** [B, ?] **Contra:** Component sensitivity **Supplied:** Cream; lotion 1% **SE:** Pruritus, local irritation, burning **Notes:** DC if irritation occurs; ⊘ occlusive dressings **Interactions:** None noted **NIPE:** Nail lacquer may take 6 mo to see improvement, cream/gel/lotion see improvement by 4 wk

Cidofovir (Vistide)   WARNING: Renal impairment is the major toxicity. Follow administration instructions **Uses:** *CMV retinitis in Pts w/ HIV* **Action:** Selective inhibition of viral DNA synthesis **Dose:** *Rx:* 5 mg/kg IV over 1 h once/wk for 2 wk; administered w/ probenecid. *Maint:* 5 mg/kg IV once/2 wk; administered w/ probenecid. *Probenecid:* 2 g PO 3 h prior to cidofovir, & then 1 g PO at 2 h & 8 h after cidofovir; ↓ in renal impairment **Caution:** [C, –] SCr >1.5 mg/dL or CrCl = 55 mL/min or urine protein >100 mg/dL; other nephrotoxic drugs **Contra:** Hypersensitivity to probenecid or sulfa **Supplied:** Inj 75 mg/mL **SE:** Renal toxicity, chills, fever, HA, N/V/D, thrombocytopenia, neutropenia **Notes:** Hydrate w/ NS prior to each inf **Interactions:** ↑ Nephrotoxicity w/ aminoglycosides, amphotericin B, foscarnet, IV pentamidine, NSAIDs, vancomycin; ↑ effects

w/ zidovudine **Labs:** ↑ SCr, BUN, alkaline phosphatase, LFTs, urine protein, WBCs; monitor for hematuria, glycosuria, hypocalcemia, hyperglycemia, hypokalemia, hyperlipidemia **NIPE:** Coadminister oral probenecid w/ each dose, possible hair loss

Cilostazol (Pletal)
Uses: *Reduce Sxs of intermittent claudication* **Action:** Phosphodiesterase III inhibitor; ↑s cAMP in plts & blood vessels, to inhibit plt aggregation & vasodilation **Dose:** 100 mg PO bid, ½ h before or 2 h after breakfast & dinner **Caution:** [C, +/–] ↓ dose when used w/ other drugs that inhibit CYP3A4 & CYP2C19 **Contra:** In CHF of any severity **Supplied:** Tabs 50, 100 mg **SE:** HA, palpitation, diarrhea **Interactions:** ↑ Effects with diltiazem, macrolides, omeprazole, fluconazole, itraconazole, ketoconazole, sertraline, grapefruit juice; ↑ effects of ASA; ↓ effects with cigarette smoking; **Labs:** ↑ BUN/creatinine, ↓ Hgb, Hct **NIPE:** Take on empty stomach; may take up to 12 wk to ↓ cramping pain; may cause dizziness

Cimetidine (Tagamet, Tagamet HB) [OTC]
Uses: *Duodenal ulcer; ulcer prophylaxis in hypersecretory states, eg, trauma, burns, surgery; & GERD* **Action:** H₂ receptor antagonist **Dose:** *Adults.* Active ulcer: 2400 mg/d IV cont inf or 300 mg IV q6h; 400 mg PO bid or 800 mg hs. *Maint:* 400 mg PO hs. *GERD:* 300–600 mg PO q6h; maint 800 mg PO hs. *Peds.* Infants: 10–20 mg/kg/24 h PO or IV ÷ q6–12h. *Children:* 20–40 mg/kg/24 h PO or IV ÷ q6h; ↑ dosing interval w/ renal insufficiency; ↓ dose in the elderly **Caution:** [B, +] Many drug interactions (P-450 system) **Contra:** Component sensitivity **Supplied:** Tabs 200, 300, 400, 800 mg; liq 300 mg/5 mL; inj 300 mg/2 mL **SE:** Dizziness, HA, agitation, thrombocytopenia, gynecomastia **Notes:** Take 1 h before or 2 h after antacids; ∅ excessive EtOH **Interactions:** ↑ Effects of benzodiazepines, disulfram, flecainide, INH, lidocaine, oral contraceptives, sulfonylureas, warfarin, theophylline, phenytoin, metronidazole, triamterene, procainamide, quinidine, propranolol, diazepam, nifedipine, TCAs, procainamide, tacrine, carbamazepine, valproic acid, xanthines; ↓ effects w/ antacids, tobacco; ↓ effects of digoxin, ketoconazole, cefpodoxime, indomethacin, tetracyclines **Labs:** ↑ Creatinine, LFTs, false + hemoccult **NIPE:** Take w/ meals, monitor for gynecomastia, breast pain, impotence

Cinacalcet (Sensipar)
Uses: *Secondary hyperparathyroidism in CRF; hypercalcemia in parathyroid carcinoma* **Action:** ↑ PTH by ↑ Ca-sensing receptor sensitivity **Dose:** *Secondary hyperparathyroidism:* 30 mg PO daily. *Parathyroid carcinoma:* 30 mg PO bid; titrate q2–4wk based on Ca & PTH levels; swallow whole; take w/ food **Caution:** [C, ?/–] Dose adjust w/ addition/deletion of CYP3A4 inhibitors **Supplied:** Tabs 30, 60, 90 mg **SE:** N/V/D, myalgia, dizziness, hypocalcemia **Notes:** Monitor Ca²⁺, PO₄⁻², PTH **Labs:** Monitor serum Ca and serum P **NIPE:** Must take drug with vitamin D and/or phosphate binders

Ciprofloxacin (Cipro)
Uses: *Rx lower resp tract, sinuses, skin & skin structure, bone/joints, & UTI infections including prostatitis* **Action:** Quinolone antibiotic; inhibits DNA gyrase. *Spectrum:* Broad-spectrum gram(+) & gram(–)

aerobics; little against streptococci; *Pseudomonas, E. coli, Bacteroides fragilis, Proteus mirabilis, Klebsiella pneumoniae, Campylobacter jejuni,* or *Shigella* **Dose: Adults.** 250–750 mg PO q12h; XR 500–1000 mg PO q24h; or 200–400 mg IV q12h; ↓ in renal impairment **Caution:** [C, ?/–] Children <18 y **Contra:** Component sensitivity **Supplied:** Tabs 100, 250, 500, 750 mg; Tabs XR 500, 1000 mg; susp 5 g/100 mL, 10 g/100 mL; inj 200, 400 mg **SE:** Restlessness, N/V/D, rash, ruptured tendons, ↑ LFTs **Notes:** ⊘ Antacids; reduce/restrict caffeine intake; interactions w/ theophylline, caffeine, sucralfate, warfarin, antacids **Interactions:** ↑ Effects w/ probenecid; ↑ effects of diazepam, theophylline, caffeine, metoprolol, propranolol, phenytoin, warfarin; ↓ effects w/ antacids, didanosine, Fe salts, Mg, sucralfate, Na bicarbonate, Zn **Labs:** ↑ LFTs, alkaline phosphatase, serum bilirubin, LDH, BUN, SCr, amylase, uric acid, K⁺, PT, triglycerides, cholesterol; ↓ Hmg, Hct; **NIPE:** ⊘ give to children <18 y, ↑ fluids to 2–3 L/d, may cause photosensitivity—use sunscreen

Ciprofloxacin, Ophthalmic (Ciloxan)
Uses: *Rx & prevention of ocular infections (conjunctivitis, blepharitis, corneal abrasions)* **Action:** Quinolone antibiotic; inhibits DNA gyrase **Dose:** 1–2 gtt in eye(s) q2h while awake for 2 d, then 1–2 gtt q4h while awake for 5 d **Caution:** [C, ?/–] **Contra:** Component sensitivity **Supplied:** Soln 3.5 mg/mL **SE:** Local irritation **Interactions:** None reported **NIPE:** Limited systemic absorption

Ciprofloxacin, Otic (Cipro HC Otic)
Uses: *Otitis externa* **Action:** Quinolone antibiotic; inhibits DNA gyrase **Dose:** *Adult & Peds >1 mo.* 1–2 gtt in ear(s) bid for 7 d **Caution:** [C, ?/–] **Contra:** Perforated tympanic membrane, viral infections of the external canal **Supplied:** Susp ciprofloxacin 0.2% & hydrocortisone 1% **SE:** HA, pruritus **NIPE:** W/ diabetics, first-choice therapy for otitis externa

Cisplatin (Platinol, Platinol AQ)
Uses: *Testicular, small-cell & non-small-cell lung, bladder, ovarian, breast, head & neck, & penile CAs; osteosarcoma; pediatric brain tumors* **Action:** DNA-binding; denatures double helix; intrastrand cross-linking, formation of DNA adducts **Dose:** 10–20 mg/m² for 5 d q3wk; 50–120 mg/m² q3–4wk; refer to specific protocols; ↓ dose in renal impairment **Caution:** [D, –] Cumulative renal toxicity may be severe; serum Mg²⁺, electrolytes, should be monitored before & w/in 48 h after cisplantin therapy **Contra:** Hypersensitivity to platinum-containing compounds; preexisting renal insufficiency, myelosuppression, hearing impairment **Supplied:** Inj 1 mg/mL **SE:** Allergic Rxns, N/V, nephrotoxicity (worse w/administration of other nephrotoxic drugs; minimize by NS inf & mannitol diuresis), high-frequency hearing loss in 30%, peripheral "stocking glove"-type neuropathy, cardiotoxicity (ST-, T-wave changes), ↓ Mg²⁺, mild myelosuppression, hepatotoxicity; renal impairment dose-related & cumulative **Notes:** Give taxanes before platinum derivatives **Interactions:** ↑ Effects of antineoplastic drugs and radiation therapy; ↑ ototoxicity w/ loop diuretics; ↑ nephrotoxicity w/ aminoglycosides, amphotericin B, vancomycin; ↓ effects w/ Na

thiosulfate; ↓ effects of phenytoin **Labs:** ↑ BUN, creatinine, serum bilirubin, AST; ↓ Ca^{2+}, Mg^{2+}, phosphate, Na^+, K^+ **NIPE:** Drug ineffective w/ Al needles or equipment, may cause infertility; ⊘ immunizations

Citalopram (Celexa) WARNING: Closely monitor for worsening depression or emergence of suicidality, particularly in pediatric Pts **Uses:** *Depression* **Action:** SSRI **Dose:** Initial 20 mg/d, may be ↑ to 40 mg/d; ↓ dose in elderly & hepatic/renal insufficiency **Caution:** [C, +/–] Hx of mania; Hx Szs & Pts at risk for suicide **Contra:** MOAI or w/in 14 d of MAOI use **Supplied:** Tabs 10, 20, 40 mg; Soln 10 mg/5 mL **SE:** Somnolence, insomnia, anxiety, xerostomia, diaphoresis; sexual dysfunction **Notes:** May cause hyponatremia/SIADH **Interactions:** ↑ Effects w/ azole antifungals, cimetidine, Li, macrolides, EtOH; ↑ effects of BBs, carbamazepine, warfarin; ↓ effects w/ carbamazepine; ↓ effects of phenytoin; may cause fatal Rxn w/ MAOIs **Labs:** ↑ LFTs, alkaline phosphatase **NIPE:** ⊘ PRG, breast-feeding, use barrier contraception

Cladribine (Leustatin) Uses: *HCL, CLL, NHLs, progressive MS* **Action:** Induces DNA strand breakage; interferes w/ DNA repair/synthesis; purine nucleoside analog **Dose:** 0.09–0.1 mg/kg/d cont IV inf for 1–7 d (refer to specific protocols) **Caution:** [D, ?/–] Observe for signs of neutropenia & infection **Contra:** Component sensitivity **Supplied:** Inj 1 mg/mL **SE:** Myelosuppression, T-lymphocyte suppression may be prolonged (26–34 wk), fever in 46% (possibly tumor lysis), infections (especially lung & IV sites), rash (50%), HA, fatigue **Notes:** Consider prophylactic allopurinol; **Interactions:** ↑ Risk of bleeding w/ anticoagulants, NSAIDs, salicylates, ↑ risk of nephrotoxicity w/ amphotericin B; **Labs:** Monitor CBC, LFTs, SCr; **NIPE:** ⊘ PRG, breast-feeding

Clarithromycin (Biaxin, Biaxin XL) Uses: *Upper/lower resp tract, skin/skin structure infections, H. pylori infections, & infections caused by nontuberculosis (atypical) *Mycobacterium;* prevention of MAC infections in HIV-infection* **Action:** Macrolide antibiotic; inhibits protein synthesis. *Spectrum: H. influenzae, M. catarrhalis, S. pneumoniae, Mycoplasma pneumoniae, H. pylori* **Dose:** *Adults.* 250–500 mg PO bid or 1000 mg (2 × 500 mg XR tab)/d. *Mycobacterium:* 500–1000 mg PO bid. *Peds >9 mo.* 7.5 mg/kg/dose PO bid; ↓ in renal/hepatic impairment **Caution:** [C, ?] Antibiotic-associated colitis; rare QT prolongation & ventricular arrhythmias, including torsades de pointes **Contra:** Hypersensitivity to macrolides; combo w/ ranitidine in Pts w/ Hx of porphyria or CrCl < 25 mL/min **Supplied:** Tabs 250, 500 mg; susp 125, 250 mg/5 mL; 500 mg XR tab **SE:** Prolongs QT interval, causes metallic taste, diarrhea, nausea, abdominal pain, HA, rash **Notes:** Multiple drug interactions, ↑s theophylline & carbamazepine levels; ⊘ refrigerate suspension **Interactions:** ↑ Effects w/ amprenavir, indinavir, nelfinavir, ritonavir; ↑ effects of atorvastatin, buspirone, clozapine, colchicine, diazepam, felodipine, itraconazole, lovastatin, simvastatin, methylprednisolone, theophylline, phenytoin, quinidine, digoxin, carbamazepine, triazolam, warfarin, ergotamine, alprazolam, valproic acid; ↓ effects w/ EtOH; ↓ effects of penicillin, zafirlukast **Labs:** ↑ Serum AST, ALT, GTT, alkaline phosphatase, LDH, total bilirubin, BUN, creatinine, PT: ↓ WBC **NIPE:** May take w/ food

Clemastine Fumarate (Tavist, Tavist-1) [OTC] Uses: *Allergic rhinitis & Sxs of urticaria* Action: Antihistamine Dose: Adults & Peds >12 y.

1.34 mg bid–2.68 mg tid; max 8.04 mg/d *<12 y*: 0.4 mg PO bid **Caution:** [C, M] Bladder neck obstruction, symptomatic BPH **Contra:** Narrow-angle glaucoma **Supplied:** Tabs 1.34, 2.68 mg; syrup 0.67 mg/5 mL **SE:** Drowsiness, dyscoordination, epigastric distress **Notes:** ⊘ EtOH **Interactions:** ↑ Effects w/ CNS depressants, MAOIs, EtOH: ↓ effects of heparin, sulfonylureas

Clindamycin (Cleocin, Cleocin-T) Uses: *Rx aerobic & anaerobic infections; topical for severe acne & vaginal infections* Action: Bacteriostatic; interferes w/ protein synthesis. *Spectrum:* Streptococci, pneumococci, staphylococci, & gram(+) & gram(–) anaerobes; no activity against gram(–) aerobes & bacterial vaginosis **Dose:** *Adults*. *PO:* 150–450 mg PO q6–8h. *Intravenous:* 300–600 mg IV q6h or 900 mg IV q8h. *Vaginal:* 1 applicatorful hs for 7 d. *Topical:* Apply 1% gel, lotion, or soln bid. **Peds.** *Neonates:* (⊘ use; contains benzyl EtOH) 10–15 mg/kg/24 h ÷ q8–12h. *Children >1 mo:* 10–30 mg/kg/24 h ÷ q6–8h, to a max of 1.8 g/d PO or 4.8 g/d IV. *Topical:* Apply 1%, gel, lotion, or soln bid; ↓ in severe hepatic impairment **Caution:** [B, +] Can cause fatal colitis **Contra:** Previous pseudomembranous colitis **Supplied:** Caps 75, 150, 300 mg; susp 75 mg/5 mL; inj 300 mg/2 mL; vaginal cream 2% **SE:** Diarrhea may be pseudomembranous colitis caused by *C. difficile*, rash, ↑ LFTs **Notes:** DC drug if significant diarrhea. **Interactions:** ↑ Effects of neuromuscular blockage w/ tubocurarine, pancuronium; ↓ effects w/ erythromycin, kaolin, foods w/ sodium cyclamate **Labs:** Monitor CBC, LFTs, BUN, creatinine; false ↑ serum theophylline **NIPE:** ⊘ Intercourse, tampons, douches while using vaginal cream; take oral meds w/ 8 oz water

Clofazimine (Lamprene) Uses: *Leprosy & combination therapy for MAC in AIDS* Action: Bactericidal; inhibits DNA synthesis. *Spectrum:* Multibacillary dapsone-sensitive leprosy; erythema nodosum leprosum; *Mycobacterium avium-intracellulare* **Dose:** *Adults*. 100–300 mg PO daily. **Peds.** 1 mg/kg/d in combo w/ dapsone & rifampin; take w/ meals **Caution:** [C, +/–] In Pts w/ GI problems; use dosages >100 mg/d for as short a duration as possible **Contra:** Hypersensitivity to any component **Supplied:** Caps 50 mg **SE:** Pink to brownish-black discoloration of the skin & conjunctiva, dry skin, GI intolerance **Notes:** Orphan drug for the Rx of dapsone-resistant leprosy; monitor for GI complaints. **Interactions:** ↑ Effects w/ INH, food, ↓ effect w/ dapsone **Labs:** ↑ Effects of AST, serum bilirubin, albumin, glucose, ESR **NIPE:** Take w/ food

Clonazepam (Klonopin) [C-IV] Uses: *Lennox–Gastaut syndrome, akinetic & myoclonic Szs, absence Szs, panic attacks,* restless legs syndrome, neuralgia, parkinsonian dysarthria, bipolar disorder **Action:** Benzodiazepine; anticonvulsant **Dose:** *Adults*. 1.5 mg/d PO in 3 ÷ doses; ↑ by 0.5–1 mg/d q3d PRN up to 20 mg/d. **Peds.** 0.01–0.03 mg/kg/24 h PO ÷ tid; ↑ to 0.1–0.2 mg/kg/24 h–tid; ⊘

abrupt withdrawal **Caution:** [D, M] Elderly Pts, resp Dz, CNS depression, severe hepatic impairment, narrow-angle glaucoma **Contra:** Severe liver Dz, acute narrow-angle glaucoma **Supplied:** Tabs 0.5, 1, 2 mg **SE:** CNS side effects, including drowsiness, dizziness, ataxia, memory impairment **Notes:** Can cause retrograde amnesia; CYP3A4 substrate **Interactions:** ↑ Effects w/ anticonvulsants, antihistamines, cimetidine, ciprofloxacin, clarithromycin, clozapine, CNS depressants, diltiazem, disulfiram, digoxin, erythromycin, fluconazole, fluoxetine, INH, itraconazole, ketoconazole, labetalol, levodopa, metoprolol, opioids, ritonavir, valproic acid, verapmil, EtOH, kava kava, valerian; ↑ effects of phenytoin; ↓ effects w/ barbiturates, carbamazepine, phenytoin, rifampin, rifabutin; ↓ effects of levodopa **NIPE:** ⊘ DC abruptly

Clonidine, Oral (Catapres) Uses: *HTN*; opioid, EtOH, & tobacco withdrawal **Action:** Centrally acting α-adrenergic stimulant **Dose:** *Adults.* 0.1 mg PO bid adjust daily by 0.1- to 0.2-mg increments (max 2.4 mg/d). *Peds.* 5–10 μg/kg/d ÷ q8–12h (max 0.9 mg/d); ↓ dose in renal impairment **Caution:** [C, +/–] ⊘ w/ BBs; withdraw slowly **Contra:** Component sensitivity **Supplied:** Tabs 0.1, 0.2, 0.3 mg **SE:** Rebound HTN w/ abrupt cessation of doses >0.2 mg bid; drowsiness, orthostatic hypotension, xerostomia, constipation, bradycardia, dizziness **Notes:** More effective for HTN if combined w/ diuretics

Clonidine, Transdermal (Catapres TTS) Uses: *HTN* Action: Centrally acting α-adrenergic stimulant **Dose:** Apply 1 patch q7d to hairless area (upper arm/torso); titrate to effect; ↓ in severe renal impairment; ⊘ DC abruptly (rebound HTN) **Caution:** [C, +/–] ⊘ w/ BBs, withdraw slowly **Contra:** Component sensitivity **Supplied:** TTS-1, TTS-2, TTS-3 (delivers 0.1, 0.2, 0.3 mg, respectively, of clonidine/d for 1 wk) **SE:** Drowsiness, orthostatic hypotension, xerostomia, constipation, bradycardia **Notes:** Doses >2 TTS usually not associated w/ ↑ efficacy; steady state in 2–3 d **Interactions:** ↑ Effects w/ BBs, neuroleptics, nitroprusside, EtOH; ↑ effects of barbiturates; ↓ effects w/ MAOIs, TCAs, tolazoline, antidepressants, prazosin, capsicum; ↓ effects of levodopa **Labs:** ↑ Glucose, phosphatase, CPK **NIPE:** Tolerance develops w/ long-term use

Clonidine, Transdermal (Catapres TTS) Uses: HTN Action: Centrally acting α-adrenergic stimulant **Dose:** Apply 1 patch q7–10d to hairless area (upper arm/torso); titrate to effect; ↓ in severe renal impairment. ⊘ DC abruptly (rebound HTN) **Caution:** [C, +/–] **Contra:** ⊘ w/ BBs **Supplied:** TTS-1, TTS-2, TTS-3 (delivers 0.1, 0.2, 0.3 mg, respectively, of clonidine/d for 1 wk) **Notes** Doses >2 TTS-3 usually not associated w/ ↑ efficacy; steady state in 3 d **SE:** Drowsiness, orthostatic hypotension, xerostomia, constipation, bradycardia. See Clonidine. **NIPE:** Rotate transdermal site weekly

Clopidogrel (Plavix) Uses: *Reduction of atherosclerotic events* Action: Inhibits plt aggregation **Dose:** 75 mg/d **Caution:** [B, ?] Active bleeding; TTP; liver Dz **Contra:** Active pathologic bleeding; intracranial bleeding **Supplied:** Tabs 75 mg **SE:** Prolongs bleeding time, GI intolerance, HA, dizziness, rash, thrombocy-

topenia, leukopenia **Notes:** Use w/ caution in persons at risk of bleeding from trauma & other causes; plt aggregation returns to baseline ≈5 d after DC; plt transfusion reverses effects acutely; 300 mg PO × 1 dose can be used to load Pts **Interactions:** ↑ Risk of GI bleed w/ ASA, NSAIDs, heparin, warfarin, feverfew, garlic, ginger, ginkgo biloba; ↑ effects of phenytoin, tamoxifen, tolbutamide **Labs:** ↑ LFTs; ↓ plts, neutrophils **NIPE:** DC drug 1 wk prior to surgery

Clorazepate (Tranxene) [C-IV]
Uses: *Acute anxiety disorders, acute EtOH withdrawal Sxs, adjunctive therapy in partial Szs* **Action:** Benzodiazepine; antianxicty agent **Dose:** *Adults.* 15–60 mg/d PO single or ÷ doses. *Elderly & debilitated Pts:* Start at 7.5–15 mg/d in ÷ doses. *EtOH withdrawal:* Day 1: Initially, 30 mg; then 30–60 mg in ÷ doses; Day 2: 45–90 mg in ÷ doses; Day 3: 22.5–45 mg in ÷ doses; Day 4: 15–30 mg in ÷ doses. *Peds.* 3.75–7.5 mg/dose bid to 60 mg/d max ÷ bid–tid **Caution:** [D, ?/–] ↓ for <9 y of age; caution in elderly & w/ Hx depression **Contra:** Narrow angle glaucoma **Supplied:** Tabs 3.75, 7.5, 15 mg; Tabs-SD (once-daily) 11.25, 22.5 mg **SE:** CNS depressant effects (drowsiness, dizziness, ataxia, memory impairment), hypotension **Notes:** Monitor Pts w/ renal/hepatic impairment (drug may accumulate); may cause dependence **Interactions:** ↑ Effects w/ antidepressants, antihistamines, barbiturates, MAOIs, narcotics, phenothiazines, cimetidine, disulfiram, EtOH; ↓ effects of levodopa; ↓ effects w/ ginkgo, tobacco **Labs:** ↓ Hct, abnormal LFTs, BUN, creatinine **NIPE:** ⊘ DC abruptly

Clotrimazole (Lotrimin, Mycelex) [OTC]
Uses: *Candidiasis & tinea infections* **Action:** Antifungal; alters cell wall permeability. *Spectrum:* Oropharyngeal candidiasis, dermatophytoses, superficial mycoses, cutaneous candidasis, & vulvovaginal candidiasis **Dose:** *PO: Prophylaxis:* One troche dissolved in mouth TID *Rx:* One troche dissolved in mouth 5 ×/d for 14 d. *Vaginal 1% Cream:* 1 applicatorful hs for 7 d. *2% Cream:* 1 applicatorful hs for 3 d *Tabs:* 100 mg vaginally hs for 7 d or 200 mg (2 tabs) vaginally hs for 3 d or 500-mg tabs vaginally hs once. *Topical:* Apply bid for 10–14 d **Caution:** [B, (C if PO), ?] Not for systemic fungal infection; safety in children <3 y not established **Contra:** Hypersensitivity to any component **Supplied:** 1% cream; soln; lotion; troche 10 mg; vaginal tabs 100, 500 mg; vaginal cream 1%, 2% **SE:** *Topical:* Local irritation; *PO:* N/V, ↑ LFTs **Notes:** PO prophylaxis used for immunosuppressed Pts **Interactions:** ↑ Effects of cyclosporine, tacrolimus; ↓ effects of spermicides

Clotrimazole & Betamethasone (Lotrisone)
Uses: *Fungal skin infections* **Action:** Imidazole antifungal & anti-inflammatory. *Spectrum:* Tinea pedis, cruris, & corpora **Dose:** *Pts ≥17 y.* Apply & massage into area bid for 2–4 wk **Caution:** [C, ?] Varicella infection **Contra:** Children <12 y **Supplied:** Cream 15, 45 g; lotion 30 mL **SE:** Local irritation, rash **Notes:** ⊘ use for diaper dermatitis or under occlusive dressings

Clozapine (Clozaril)
WARNING: Myocarditis, agranulocytosis, Szs, & orthostatic hypotension have been associated w/ clozapine **Uses:** *Refractory severe schizophrenia*; childhood psychosis **Action:** Tricyclic "atypical" antipsy-

chotic **Dose:** 25 mg daily–bid initial; ↑ to 300–450 mg/d over 2 wk. Maintain at the lowest dose possible; ⊘ DC abruptly **Caution:** [B, +/–] Monitor for psychosis & cholinergic rebound **Contra:** Uncontrolled epilepsy; comatose state; WBC count ≤3500 cells/mm³ before Rx or <3000 cells/mm³ during Rx **Supplied:** Tabs 25, 100 mg **SE:** Tachycardia, drowsiness, weight gain, constipation, urinary incontinence, rash, Szs, CNS stimulation **Notes:** Benign, self-limiting temperature elevations may occur during the 1st 3 wk of Rx, weekly CBC mandatory for 1st 6 mo, then qowk **Interactions:** ↑ Effects w/ clarithromycin, cimetidine, erythromycin, fluoxetine, paroxetine, quinidine, sertraline; ↑ depressant effects w/ CNS depressants, EtOH; ↑ effects of digoxin, warfarin; ↓ effects w/ carbamazepine, phenytoin, primidone, phenobarbital, valproic acid, St. John's wort, nutmeg, caffeine; ↓ effects of phenytoin **Labs:** Monitor WBCs **NIPE:** ↑ Risk of developing agranulocytosis

Cocaine [C-II] **Uses:** *Topical anesthetic for mucous membranes* **Action:** Narcotic analgesic, local vasoconstrictor **Dose:** Apply lowest amount of topical soln that provides relief; 1 mg/kg max **Caution:** [C, ?] **Contra:** PRG **Supplied:** Topical soln & viscous preps 4, 10%; powder, soluble tabs (135 mg) for soln **SE:** CNS stimulation, nervousness, loss of taste/smell, chronic rhinitis **Notes:** Use only on mucous membranes of the PO, laryngeal, & nasal cavities; ⊘ use on extensive areas of broken skin **Interactions:** ↑ Effects w/ MAOIs, ↑ risk of HTN & arrhythmias w/ epinephrine

Codeine [C-II] **Uses:** *Mild/moderate pain; symptomatic relief of cough* **Action:** Narcotic analgesic; depresses cough reflex **Dose:** *Adults.* Analgesic: 15–60 mg PO or IM qid PRN. *Antitussive:* 10–20 mg PO q4h PRN; max 120 mg/d. *Peds.* Analgesic: 0.5–1 mg/kg/dose PO q4–6h PRN. *Antitussive:* 1–1.5 mg/kg/24 h PO ÷ q4h; max 30 mg/24 h; ↓ in renal/hepatic impairment **Caution:** [C, (D if prolonged use or high doses at term), +] **Contra:** Component sensitivity **Supplied:** Tabs 15, 30, 60 mg; soln 15 mg/5 mL; inj 30, 60 mg/mL **SE:** Drowsiness, constipation **Notes:** Usually combined w/ APAP for pain or w/ agents (eg, terpin hydrate) as an antitussive; 120 mg IM = 10 mg IM morphine **Interactions:** ↑ CNS depression w/ CNS depressants, antidepressants, MAOIs, TCAs, barbiturates, benzodiazepines, muscle relaxants, phenothiazines, cimetidine, antihistamines, sedatives, EtOH; ↑ effects of digitoxin, phenytoin, rifampin; ↓ effects w/ nalbuphine, pentazocine, tobacco **Labs:** False ↑ amylase, lipase, ↑ urine morphine

Colchicine **Uses:** *Acute gouty arthritis & prevention of recurrences; familial Mediterranean fever*; primary biliary cirrhosis **Action:** Inhibits migration of leukocytes; ↓ production of lactic acid by leukocytes **Dose:** *Initially:* 0.5–1.2 mg PO, then 0.5–0.6 mg q1–2h until relief or GI SE develop (max 8 mg/d); ⊘ repeat for 3 d. *IV:* 1–3 mg, then 0.5 mg q6h until relief (max 4 mg/d); ⊘ repeat for 7 d. *Prophylaxis:* PO: 0.5–0.6 mg/d or 3–4 d/wk; ↓ renal impairment; caution in elderly **Caution:** [D, +] Severe local irritation can occur following SQ/IM **Contra:** Serious renal, GI, hepatic, or cardiac disorders; blood dyscrasias **Supplied:** Tabs 0.5,

0.6 mg; inj 1 mg/2 mL **SE:** N/V/D, abdominal pain, bone marrow suppression, hepatotoxicity **Notes:** Colchicine 1–2 mg IV w/in 24–48 h of an acute attack diagnostic/therapeutic in monoarticular arthritis **Interactions:** ↑ GI effects w/ NSAIDs; ↑ effects of sympathomimetics, CNS depressants, bone marrow depressants, radiation therapy; ↓ effects of vitamin B $_{12}$ **Labs:** Monitor CBC, BUN, creatinine; false + urine Hgb & RBCs **NIPE:** ⊘ EtOH

Colesevelam (Welchol) **Uses:** *Reduction of LDL & total cholesterol alone or in combination w/ an HMG-CoA reductase inhibitor* **Action:** Bile acid sequestrant **Dose:** 3 tabs PO bid w/ meals **Caution:** [B, ?] Severe GI motility disorders; safety & efficacy not established in peds **Contra:** Bowl obstruction **Supplied:** Tabs 625 mg **SE:** Constipation, dyspepsia, myalgia, weakness **Notes:** May decrease absorption of fat-soluble vitamins **Interactions:** ↓ Effects of verapamil **Labs:** Monitor lipids **NIPE:** Take w/ food and liquid

Colestipol (Colestid) **Uses:** *Adjunct to ↓ serum cholesterol in primary hypercholesterolemia* **Action:** Binds intestinal bile acids to form an insoluble complex **Dose:** Granules: 5–30 g/d ÷ 2–4 doses; tabs: 2–16 g/d daily–bid **Caution:** [C, ?] ⊘ w/ high triglycerides, GI dysfunction **Contra:** Bowl obstruction **Supplied:** Tabs 1 g; granules 5, 300, 500 g **SE:** Constipation, abdominal pain, bloating, HA **Notes:** ⊘ Use dry powder; mix w/ beverages, soups, cereals, etc; may decrease absorption of other medications; may decrease absorption of fat-soluble vitamins **Interactions:** ↓ Absorption of numerous drugs especially anticoagulants, cardiac glycosides, digitoxin, digoxin, phenobarbital, penicillin G, tetracycline, thiazide diuretics, thyroid drugs **Labs:** ↓ Serum cholesterol, ↑ PT **NIPE:** Take other meds 1 h before or 4 h after colestipol

Colfosceril Palmitate (Exosurf Neonatal) **Uses:** *Prophylaxis & Rx for RDS in infants* **Action:** Synthetic lung surfactant **Dose:** 5 mL/kg/dose through ET tube as soon after birth as possible & again at 12 & 24 h **Caution:** [?, ?] Pulmonary hemorrhaging **Supplied:** Inj 108 mg **SE:** Pulmonary hemorrhage possible in infants weighing <700 g at birth; mucous plugging **Notes:** Monitor pulmonary compliance & oxygenation carefully; monitor ECG **Interactions:** None noted

Cortisone See Steroids, Tables 4 and 5 (pages 271 & 272)

Cromolyn Sodium (Intal, NasalCrom, Opticrom) **Uses:** *Adjunct to the Rx of asthma; prevent exercise-induced asthma; allergic rhinitis; ophth allergic manifestations*; food allergy **Action:** Antiasthmatic; mast cell stabilizer **Dose:** *Adults & Children >12 y.* Inhal: 20 mg (as powder in caps) inhaled qid or met-dose inhaler 2 puffs qid. *PO:* 200 mg qid 15–20 min ac, up to 400 mg qid. *Nasal instillation:* Spray once in each nostril 2–6×/d. *Ophth:* 1–2 gtt in each eye 4–6×/d. *Peds.* Inhal: 2 puffs qid of met-dose inhaler. *PO: Infants <2 y:* (⊘) 20 mg/kg/d in 4 ÷ doses. *2–12 y:* 100 mg qid ac **Caution:** [B, ?] **Contra:** Acute asthmatic attacks **Supplied:** PO conc 100 mg/5 mL; soln for neb 20 mg/2 mL; met-dose inhaler; nasal soln 40 mg/mL; ophth soln 4% **SE:** Unpleasant taste, hoarseness, coughing **Notes:** No benefit in acute Rx; 2–4 wk for maximal effect in perennial allergic disorders **Interactions:** None noted **Labs:** Monitor pulmonary Fxn tests

Cyanocobalamin [Vitamin B₁₂]

Uses: *Pernicious anemia & other vitamin B₁₂ deficiency states; ↑d requirements due to PRG; thyrotoxicosis; liver or kidney Dz* **Action:** Dietary suppl of vitamin B₁₂ **Dose:** *Adults.* 100 μg IM or SQ qd for 5–10 d, then 100 μg IM 2×/wk for 1 mo, then 100 μg IM monthly. *Peds.* 100 μg/d IM or SQ for 5–10 d. then 30–50 μg IM q4wk **Caution:** [A (C if dose exceeds RDA), +] **Contra:** Hypersensitivity to Co; hereditary optic nerve atrophy; Leber's Dz **Supplied:** Tabs 50, 100, 250, 500, 1000 μg; inj 100, 1000 μg/mL; gel 500 μg/0.1 mL **SE:** Itching, diarrhea, HA, anxiety **Notes:** PO absorption erratic, altered by many drugs & ⊘; for use w/ hyperalimentation **Interactions:** ↓ Effects w/ aminosalicylic acid, chloramphenicol, cholestyramine, cimetidine, colchicines, neomycin, amino salicylate, EtOH **Labs:** Antibiotics, MRX, pyrimethamine invalidate blood assays of vitamin B₁₂ and folic acid

Cyclobenzaprine (Flexeril)

Uses: *Relief of muscle spasm* **Action:** Centrally acting skeletal muscle relaxant; reduces tonic somatic motor activity **Dose:** 10 mg PO 2–4×/d (2–3 wk max) **Caution:** [B. ?] Shares the toxic potential of the TCAs; urinary hesitancy or angle-closure glaucoma **Contra:** ⊘ Use concomitantly or w/in 14 days of MAOIs; hyperthyroidism; HF; arrhythmias **Supplied:** Tabs 10 mg **SE:** Sedation & anticholinergic side effects **Notes:** May inhibit mental alertness or physical coordination **Interactions:** ↑ Effects of CNS depression w/ CNS depressants, TCAs, barbiturates, EtOH; ↑ risk of HTN & convulsions w/ MAOIs **NIPE:** ↑ Fluids & fiber for constipation

Cyclopentolate (Cyclogyl)

Uses: *Diagnostic procedures requiring cycloplegia & mydriasis* **Action:** Cycloplegic & mydriatic agent (can last up to 24 h) **Dose:** 1 gt then another in 5 min **Caution:** [C. ?] **Contra:** Narrow-angle glaucoma **Supplied:** Soln. 0.5, 1, 2% **SE:** Blurred vision, ↑ sensitivity to light, tachycardia, restlessness **Interactions:** ↓ Effects of carbachol, cholinesterase inhibitors, pilocarpine **NIPE:** Burning sensation when instilled

Cyclophosphamide (Cytoxan, Neosar)

Uses: *Hodgkin's & NHLs; multiple myeloma; small-cell lung, breast, & ovarian CAs; mycosis fungoides; neuroblastoma; retinoblastoma; acute leukemias; & allogeneic & ABMT in high doses; severe rheumatologic disorders* **Action:** Converted to acrolein & phosphoramide mustard, the active alkylating moieties **Dose:** 500–1500 mg/m² as a single dose at 2–4-wk intervals; 1.8 g/m² to 160 mg/kg (or ≈12 g/m² in a 75-kg individual) in the BMT setting (refer to specific protocols); adjust in renal/hepatic impairment **Caution:** [D, ?] In bone marrow suppression **Contra:** Component sensitivity **Supplied:** Tabs 25, 50 mg; inj 100 mg **SE:** Myelosuppression (leukopenia & thrombocytopenia); hemorrhagic cystitis, SIADH, alopecia, anorexia; N/V; hepatotoxicity & rarely interstitial pneumonitis; irreversible testicular atrophy possible; cardiotoxicity rare; 2nd malignancies (bladder CA & acute leukemias);

cumulative risk 3.5% at 8 y, 10.7% at 12 y **Notes:** Hemorrhagic cystitis prophylaxis: continuous bladder irrigation & mesna uroprotection; encourage adequate hydration **Interactions:** ↑ Effects w/ allopurinol, cimetidine, phenobarbital, rifampin; ↑ effects of succinylcholine, warfarin; ↓ effects of digoxin **Labs:** May inhibit + Rxns to skin tests for PPD, risk of false + Pap smear results **NIPE:** May cause sterility, hair loss, ⊘ PRG, breast-feeding, immunizations

Cyclosporine (Sandimmune, Neoral)

Uses: *Organ rejection in kidney, liver, heart, & BMT w/ steroids; RA; psoriasis;* CA Rx; BMT **Action:** Immunosuppressant; reversible inhibition of immunocompetent lymphocytes **Dose:** **Adults & Peds.** PO: 15 mg/ kg/d 12 h pretransplant; after 2 wk, taper by 5 mg/wk to 5–10 mg/kg/d. *IV:* If NPO, give ⅓ PO dose IV; ↓ in renal/hepatic impairment **Caution:** [C, ?] Dose-related risk of nephrotoxicity/hepatotoxicity; live, attenuated vaccines may be less effective **Contra:** Abnormal renal Fxn; uncontrolled HTN **Supplied:** Caps 25, 50, 100 mg; PO soln 100 mg/mL; inj 50 mg/mL **SE:** May ↑ BUN & creatinine & mimic transplant rejection; HTN; HA; hirsutism **Notes:** Administer in glass containers; many drug interactions; Neoral & Sandimmune not interchangeable; interaction w/ St. John's wort. **Interactions:** ↑ Effects w/ azole antifungals, allopurinol, amiodarone, anabolic steroids, CCBs, cimetidine, chloroquine, clarithromycin, clonidine, diltiazem, macrolides, metoclopramide, nicardipine, NSAIDs, oral contraceptives, ticlopidine, grapefruit juice; ↑ nephrotoxicity w/ aminoglycosides, amphotericin B, acyclovir, colchicine, enalapril, ranitidine, sulfonamides; ↑ risk digoxin toxicity; ↑ risk of hyperkalemia w/ diuretics, ACEIs; ↓ effects w/ barbiturates, carbamazepine, INH, nafcillin, pyrazinamide, phenytoin, rifampin, sulfonamides, St. John's wort, alfalfa sprouts, astragalus, echinacea, licorice; ↓ effects immunizations **Labs:** ↑ SCr, BUN, total bilirubin, K⁺, alkaline phosphatase, lipids **NIPE:** Monitor for hyperglycemia, hyperkalemia, hyperuricemia, risk of photosensitivity—use sunscreen

Cyproheptadine (Periactin)

Uses: *Allergic Rxns; itching* **Action:** Phenothiazine antihistamine; serotonin antagonist **Dose:** **Adults.** 4–20 mg PO ÷ q8h; max 0.5 mg/kg/d. **Peds.** *2–6 y:* 2 mg bid–tid (max 12 mg/24 h). *7–14 y:* 4 mg bid–tid; ↓ dose in hepatic impairment **Caution:** [B, ?] Symptomatic BPH **Contra:** Neonates or <2 y; narrow-angle glaucoma; bladder neck obstruction; acute asthma; GI obstruction **Supplied:** Tabs 4 mg; syrup 2 mg/5 mL **SE:** Anticholinergic, drowsiness, **Notes:** May stimulate appetite **Interactions:** ↑ Effects w/ CNS depressants, MAOIs, EtOH; ↓ effects of epinephrine, fluoxetine **Labs:** False – skin testing; false + urine TCA assay; ↑ serum amylase, prolactin; ↓ FBS **NIPE:** ↑ Risk photosensitivity—use sunscreen, take w/ food if GI distress

Cytarabine [ARA-C] (Cytosar-U)

Uses: *Acute leukemias, CML, NHL; IT administration for leukemic meningitis or prophylaxis* **Action:** Antimetabolite; interferes w/ DNA synthesis **Dose:** 100–150 mg/m²/d for 5–10 d (low dose); 3 g/m² q12h for 8–12 doses (high dose); 1 mg/kg 1–2/wk (SQ maintenance regimens); 5–70 mg/m² up to 3/wk IT (refer to specific protocols); ↓ in renal/hepatic impairment **Caution:** [D, ?] In marked bone marrow suppression, ↓ dosage by ↓ the number of days of administration **Contra:** Component sensitivity **Supplied:** Inj 100, 500 mg, 1, 2, g **SE:** Myelosuppression, N/V/D, stomatitis, flu-like syndrome, rash on palms/soles, hepatic dysfunction, cerebellar dysfunction, noncardiogenic pulmonary edema, neuropathy **Notes:** Of little use in solid tumors; toxicity of high-dose regimens (conjunctivitis) ameliorated by corticosteroid ophth soln **Interactions:** ↑ Effects w/ alkylating drugs and radiation therapy; ↓ effects of digoxin, gentamicin, MRX, flucytosine **Labs:** ↑ Uric acid, monitor CBC, BUN, creatinine, LFTs **NIPE:** ⊘ EtOH, NSAIDs, ASA, PRG, breast-feeding, immunizations

Cytarabine Liposome (DepoCyt)
Uses: *Lymphomatous meningitis* **Action:** Antimetabolite; interferes w/ DNA synthesis **Dose:** 50 mg IT q14d for 5 doses, then 50 mg IT q28d for 4 doses; use dexamethasone prophylaxis **Caution:** [D, ?] May cause neurotoxicity; blockage to CSF flow may ↑ the risk of neurotoxicity; use in peds not established **Contra:** Active meningeal infection **Supplied:** IT inj 50 mg/5 mL **SE:** Neck pain/rigidity, HA, confusion, somnolence, fever, back pain, N/V, edema, neutropenia, thrombocytopenia, anemia **Notes:** Cytarabine liposomes are similar in microscopic appearance to WBCs; care must be taken in interpreting CSF examinations **Interactions:** None noted, perhaps because of limited systemic exposure **Labs:** May interfere w/ CSF interpretation **NIPE:** ⊘ PRG, use contraception

Cytomegalovirus Immune Globulin [CMV-IG IV] (CytoGam)
Uses: *Attenuation of primary CMV Dz associated w/ transplantation* **Action:** Exogenous IgG antibodies to CMV **Dose:** 150 mg/kg/dose w/in 72 h of transplant, for 16 wk posttransplant; see insert for dosing schedule **Caution:** [C, ?] Anaphylactic Rxns; renal dysfunction **Contra:** Hypersensitivity to immunoglobulins; immunoglobulin A deficiency **Supplied:** Inj 50 mg/mL **SE:** Flushing, N/V, muscle cramps, wheezing, HA, fever **Notes:** IV use only; administer by separate line; ⊘ shake **Interactions:** ↓ Effects of live virus vaccines **NIPE:** Admin immunizations at least 3 mo after CMV-IG

Dacarbazine (DTIC)
Uses: *Melanoma, Hodgkin's Dz, sarcoma* **Action:** Alkylating agent; antimetabolite as a purine precursor; inhibits protein synthesis, RNA, & especially DNA **Dose:** 2–4.5 mg/kg/d for 10 consecutive d or 250 mg/m²/d for 5 d (refer to specific protocols); ↓ in renal impairment **Caution:** [C, ?] In bone marrow suppression; renal/hepatic impairment **Contra:** Component sensitivity **Supplied:** Inj 100, 200, 500 mg **SE:** Myelosuppression, severe N/V, hepatotoxicity, flu-like syndrome, ↓ BP, photosensitivity, alopecia, facial flushing, facial paresthesias, urticaria, phlebitis at inj site **Notes:** ⊘ extravasation **Interactions:** ↑ Effects w/ amphotericin B, anticoagulants, ASA, bone-marrow suppressants; ↑ effects of phenobarbital, phenytoin **Labs:** ↑ AST, ALT **NIPE:** Risk of photosensitivity—use sunscreen, hair loss, infection

Daclizumab (Zenapax)
Uses: *Prevent acute organ rejection* **Action:** IL-2 receptor antagonist **Dose:** 1 mg/kg/dose IV; 1st dose pretransplant, then 4

doses 14 d apart posttransplant **Caution:** [C, ?] **Contra:** Component sensitivity **Supplied:** Inj 5 mg/mL **SE:** Hyperglycemia, edema, HTN, hypotension, constipation, HA, dizziness, anxiety, nephrotoxicity, pulmonary edema, pain **Notes:** Administer w/in 4 h of prep **Interactions:** ⊘ Echinacea **NIPE:** ⊘ Immunizations, infections, ↑ fluid intake

Dactinomycin (Cosmegen) **Uses:** *Choriocarcinoma, Wilms' tumor, Kaposi's sarcoma, Ewing's sarcoma, rhabdomyosarcoma, testicular CA* **Action:** DNA intercalating agent **Dose:** 0.5 mg/d for 5 d; 2 mg/wk for 3 consecutive wk; 15 μg/kg or 0.45 mg/m²/d (max 0.5 mg) for 5 d q3–8wk in pediatric sarcoma (refer to specific protocols); ↓ in renal impairment **Caution:** [C, ?] **Contra:** Use w/ concurrent or recent chickenpox or herpes zoster; ⊘ in infants <6 mo **Supplied:** Inj 0.5 mg **SE:** Myelo- & immunosuppression, severe N/V, alopecia, acne, hyperpigmentation, radiation recall phenomenon, tissue damage w/ extravasation, hepatotoxicity **Interactions:** ↑ Effects bone marrow suppressants, radiation therapy; ↓ effects of vitamin K **Labs:** ↑ Uric acid; monitor CBC w/ differential & plts, LFTs, BUN, creatinine **NIPE:** ⊘ PRG, breast-feeding; risk of irreversible infertility, reversible hair loss, ↓ fluids to 2–3 L/d

Dalteparin (Fragmin) **Uses:** *Unstable angina, non-Q-wave MI, prevention of ischemic complications due to clot formation in Pts on concurrent ASA, prevention & Rx of DVT following surgery* **Action:** LMW heparin **Dose:** *Angina/MI:* 120 IU/kg (max 10,000 IU) SQ q12h w/ ASA. *DVT prophylaxis:* 2500–5000 IU SC 1–2 h preop, then qd for 5–10 d. *Systemic anticoagulation:* 200 IU/kg/d SQ or 100 IU/kg bid SQ; use w/ caution in renal/hepatic impairment **Caution:** [B, ?] Active hemorrhage, cerebrovascular Dz, cerebral aneurysm, severe uncontrolled HTN **Contra:** HIT; hypersensitivity to pork products; **Supplied:** Inj 2500 IU (16 mg/0.2 mL), 5000 IU (32 mg/0.2 mL), 10,000 IU (64 mg/mL) **SE:** Bleeding, pain at inj site, thrombocytopenia **Notes:** Predictable antithrombotic effects eliminate need for laboratory monitoring; not for IM or IV use **Interactions:** ↑ Bleeding w/ oral anticoagulants, plt inhibitors, penicillins, cephalosporins, garlic, ginger, ginkgo biloba, ginseng, chamomile, vitamin E **Labs:** ↑ AST, ALT, monitor CBC and plts **NIPE:** ⊘ Give PO or IM; give deep SC

Danaparoid (Orgaron) **Uses:** *Prophylaxis of DVT to prevent PE, in hip replacement surgery* **Action:** Antithrombotic; inhibits factor Xa & IIa **Dose:** 750 anti-Xa units bid SQ 1–4 h preop & starting no sooner than 2 h postop; ↓ dose in severe renal impairment **Caution:** [B, ?/–] **Contra:** Active major bleeding, hemophilia, ITP, type II thrombocytopenia w/ a + antiplt antibody test **Supplied:** Amps & prefilled syringes 0.6 mL (750 anti-Xa units) **SE:** Bleeding, fever, inj site pain, ↑d risk of epidural & spinal hematoma in Pts receiving epidural/spinal anesthesia **Notes:** aPTT monitoring not necessary

Dantrolene (Dantrium) **Uses:** *Rx clinical spasticity due to upper motor neuron disorders, eg, spinal cord injuries, strokes, CP, MS; Rx malignant hyperthermia* **Action:** Skeletal muscle relaxant **Dose:** *Adults.* Spasticity: Initially, 25

mg PO qd; ↑ to effect by 25 mg to a max dose of 100 mg PO qid PRN. **Peds.** Initially, 0.5 mg/kg/dose bid; ↑ by 0.5 mg/kg to effect to a max dose of 3 mg/kg/dose qid PRN. **Adults & Peds.** Malignant hyperthermia: Rx: Continuous rapid IV push, start at 1 mg/kg until Sxs subside or 10 mg/kg is reached. *Postcrisis follow-up:* 4–8 mg/kg/d in 3–4 ÷ doses for 1–3 d to prevent recurrence **Caution:**[C, ?] ↓ Cardiac Fxn or pulmonary Fxn **Contra:** Active hepatic Dz; should not be used where spasticity is used to maintain posture or balance **Supplied:** Caps 25, 50, 100 mg; powder for inj 20 mg/vial **SE:** Hepatotoxicity w/↑ LFTs, drowsiness, dizziness, rash, muscle weakness, pleural effusion w/ pericarditis, diarrhea, blurred vision, hepatitis **Notes:** Monitor transaminases; ⊘ sunlight/ EtOH /CNS depressants **Interactions:** ↑ effects w/ CNS depressants, antihistamines, opioids, EtOH; ↑ risk of hepatotoxicity w/ estrogens; ↑ risk of CV collapse & ventricular fib w/ CCBs; ↓ plasma protein binding w/ clofibrate, warfarin **Labs:** ↑ AST, ALT, alkaline phosphatase, LDH, BUN, total serum bilirubin **NIPE:** ↑ Risk of photosensitivity—use sunscreen

Dapsone (Avlosulfon)
Uses: *Rx & prevent PCP; toxoplasmosis prophylaxis; leprosy* **Action:** Unknown; bactericidal **Dose:** **Adults.** PCP prophylaxis 50–100 mg/d PO; Rx PCP 100 mg/d PO w/ TMP 15–20 mg/kg/d for 21 d. **Peds.** Prophylaxis of PCP 1–2 mg/kg/24 h PO qd; max 100 mg/d **Caution:** [C, +] G6PD deficiency; severe anemia **Contra:** Component sensitivity **Supplied:** Tabs 25, 100 mg **SE:** Hemolysis, methemoglobinemia, agranulocytosis, rash, cholestatic jaundice **Notes:** Absorption ↑ by an acidic environment; w/ leprosy, combine w/ rifampin & other agents **Interactions:** ↑ Effects w/ probenecid, trimethoprim; ↓ effects w/ activated charcoal, rifampin **Labs:** Monitor CBC, LFTs **NIPE:** ↑ Risk of photosensitivity—use sunscreen

Darbepoetin Alfa (Aranesp)
Uses: *Anemia associated w/ CRF* **Action:** Stimulates erythropoiesis, recombinant variant of erythropoietin **Dose:** 0.45 µg/kg single IV or SQ qwk; titrate dose, ⊘ exceed target Hgb of 12 g/dL; see insert if converting from Epogen **Caution:** [C, ?] May ↑ risk of CV &/or neurologic SE in renal failure; HTN; Hx of Szs **Contra:** Uncontrolled hypertension, allergy to components **Supplied:** 25, 40, 60, 100 µg/mL, in polysorbate or albumin excipient **SE:** May ↑ risk of cardiac events, CP, hypo-/hypertension, N/V/D, myalgia, arthralgia, dizziness, edema, fatigue, fever, ↑ risk infection **Notes:** Longer ½-life than Epogen; follow weekly CBC until stable **Interactions:** None noted **Labs:** Monitor CBC w/ differential & plts, BUN, creatinine, serum P, K⁺, Fe stores **NIPE:** Monitor BP & for Sz activity, shaking vial inactivates drug

Daunorubicin (Daunomycin, Cerubidine)
WARNING: Cardiac Fxn should be monitored due to potential risk for cardiac toxicity & CHF **Uses:** Acute leukemias **Action:** DNA intercalating agent; inhibits topoisomerase II; generates oxygen free radicals **Dose:** 45–60 mg/m²/d for 3 consecutive d; 25 mg/m²/wk (refer to specific protocols); ↓ dose in renal/hepatic impairment **Caution:** [D, ?] **Contra:** Component sensitivity **Supplied:** Inj 20 mg **SE:** Myelosup-

pression, mucositis, N/V, alopecia, radiation recall phenomenon, hepatotoxicity (hyperbilirubinemia), tissue necrosis on extravascular extravasation, & cardiotoxicity (1–2% CHF risk w/ 550 mg/m^2 cumulative dose) **Notes:** Prevent cardiotoxicity w/ dexrazoxane; administer allopurinol prior to initiating Rx to prevent hyperuricemia **Interactions:** ↑ Risk of cardiotoxicity w/ cyclophosphamide; ↑ myelosuppression w/ antineoplastic agents; ↓ response to live virus vaccines **Labs:** ↑ Serum alkaline phosphatase, bilirubin, AST, monitor uric acid, CBC, LFTs **NIPE:** ⊘ ASA, NSAIDs, EtOH, PRG, breast-feeding, immunizations; risk of hair loss

Delavirdine (Rescriptor) **Uses:** *HIV infection* **Action:** Nonnucleoside RT inhibitor **Dose:** 400 mg PO tid **Caution:** [C, ?] CDC recommends HIV-infected mothers not breast-feed due to risk of HIV transmission to infant; use caution in renal/hepatic impairment **Contra:** Concomitant use w/ drugs highly dependent on CYP 3A for clearance (ie, alprazolam, ergot alkaloids, midazolam, pimozide, triazolam) **Supplied:** Tabs 100 mg **SE:** HA, fatigue, rash, ↑ serum transaminases, N/V/D **Notes:** ⊘ Antacids; inhibits cytochrome P-450 enzymes; numerous drug interactions; monitor LFTs **Interactions:** ↑ Effects w/ fluoxetine; (up) benzodiazepines, cisapride, clarithromycin, dapsone, ergotamins, indinavir, lovastatin, midazolam, nifedipine, quinidine, ritonavir, simvastatin, terfenadine, triazolam, warfarin; ↓ effects w/ antacids, barbiturates, carbamazepine, cimetidine, famotidine, lansoprazole, nizatidine, phenobarbital, phenytoin, ranitidine, rifabutin, rifampin; ↓ effects of didanosine **Labs:** ↑ AST, ALT, ↓ neutrophil counts **NIPE:** Take w/o regard to food

Demeclocycline (Declomycin) **Uses:** SIADH **Action:** Antibiotic, antagonizes action of ADH on renal tubules **Dose:** 300–600 mg PO q12h on an empty stomach; ↓ in renal failure; ⊘ antacids **Caution:** [D, +] ⊘ in hepatic/renal dysfunction & children **Contra:** Hypersensitivity to tetracyclines **Supplied:** Tabs 150, 300 mg **SE:** Diarrhea, abdominal cramps, photosensitivity, DI **Notes:** ⊘ prolonged exposure to sunlight **Interactions:** Effects of digoxin, anticoagulants; ↓ effects w/ antacids, Bi salts, Fe, Na bicarbonate, barbiturates, carbamazepine, hydantoins, food; ↓ effects of oral contraceptives, penicillin **Labs:** False – urine glucose; monitor CBC, LFTs, BUN, creatinine **NIPE:** Risk of photosensitivity—use sunscreen

Desipramine (Norpramin) **Uses:** *Endogenous depression,* chronic pain, & peripheral neuropathy **Action:** TCA; ↑s synaptic conc of serotonin or norepinephrine in CNS **Dose:** 25–200 mg/d single or ÷ doses; usually a single hs dose (max 300 mg/d) **Caution:** [C, ?/–] Caution in CV Dz, Sz disorder, hypothyroidism **Contra:** Use of MAOIs w/in 14 d; during recovery phase of MI **Supplied:** Tabs 10, 25, 50, 75, 100, 150 mg; caps 25, 50 mg **SE:** Anticholinergic (blurred vision, urinary retention, xerostomia); orthostatic hypotension; prolongs QT interval, arrhythmias **Notes:** Numerous drug interactions; may cause urine to turn blue-green; ⊘ sunlight **Interactions:** ↑ Effects w/ cimetidine, diltiazem, fluoxetine, indinavir, MAOIs, paroxetine, propoxyphene, quinidine, ritonavir ranitidine, EtOH, grapefruit juice; ↑ effects of Li, sulfonylureas; ↓ effects w/ barbiturates, carbamazepine rifampin, tobacco **NIPE:** Full effect of drug may take 4 wk, risk of photosensitivity—use sunscreen

Desloratadine (Clarinex) Uses: *Symptoms of seasonal & perennial allergic rhinitis; chronic idiopathic urticaria* Action: Active metabolite of Claritin, H_1-antihistamine, blocks inflammatory mediators Dose: *Adults & Peds >12 y.* 5 mg PO qd; in hepatic/renal impairment 5 mg PO qod Caution: [C, ?/–] RediTabs contain phenylalanine; safety not established for <12 y Supplied: Tabs & RediTabs (rapid dissolving) 5 mg SE: Hypersensitivity Rxns, anaphylaxis somnolence, HA, dizziness, fatigue, pharyngitis, xerostomia, nausea, dyspepsia, myalgia Labs: ↑ LFTs, bilirubin NIPE: Take w/o regard to food

Desmopressin (DDAVP, Stimate) Uses: *DI (intranasal & parenteral); bleeding due to uremia, hemophilia A, & type I von Willebrand's Dz (parenteral), nocturnal enuresis* Action: Synthetic analog of vasopressin, a naturally occurring human ADH; ↑ factor VIII Dose: *DI: Intranasal: Adults.* 0.1–0.4 mL (10–40 µg/d in 1–4 ÷ doses. *Peds 3 mo–12 y.* 0.05–0.3 mL/d in 1 or 2 doses. *Parenteral: Adults.* 0.5–1 mL (2–4 µg/d in 2 ÷ doses; if converting from nasal to parenteral, use $\frac{1}{10}$ nasal dose. *PO: Adults.* 0.05 mg bid; ↑ to max of 1.2 mg. *Hemophilia A & von Willebrand's Dz (type I): Adults & Peds >10 kg.* 0.3 µg/kg in 50 mL NS, inf over 15–30 min. *Peds <10 kg.* As above w/ dilution to 10 mL w/ NS. *Nocturnal enuresis: Peds >6 y.* 20 µg intranasally hs Caution: [B, M] ⊘ overhydration Contra: Hemophilia B; severe classic von Willebrand's Dz; Pts w/ factor VIII antibodies Supplied: Tabs 0.1, 0.2 mg; inj 4 µg/mL; nasal soln 0.1, 1.5 mg/mL SE: Facial flushing, HA, dizziness, vulval pain, nasal congestion, pain at inj site, hyponatremia, water intoxication Notes: In very young & old Pts, ↓ fluid intake to ⊘ water intoxication & hyponatremia Interactions: ↑ Antidiuretic effects w/ carbamazepine, chlorpropamide, clofibrate; ↑ effects of vasopressors; ↓ antidiuretic effects w/ demeclocycline, Li, norepinephrine NIPE: Monitor I&O, ⊘ EtOH, overhydration

Dexamethasone, Nasal (Dexacort Phosphate Turbinaire) Uses: *Chronic nasal inflammation or allergic rhinitis* Action: Antiinflammatory corticosteroid Dose: *Adult & Peds >12 y.* 2 sprays/nostril bid–tid, max 12 sprays/d. *Peds 6–12 y.* 1–2 sprays/nostril bid, max 8 sprays/d Caution: [C, ?] Contra: Untreated infection Supplied: Aerosol, 84 µg/activation SE: Local irritation NIPE: Use decongestant nose gtt 1st if nasal congestion

Dexamethasone, Ophthalmic (AK-Dex Ophthalmic, Decadron Ophthalmic) Uses: *Inflammatory or allergic conjunctivitis* Action: Antiinflammatory corticosteroid Dose: Instill 1–2 gtt tid–qid Caution: [C, ?/–] Contra: Active untreated bacterial, viral, & fungal eye infections Supplied: Susp & soln 0.1%; oint 0.05% SE: Long-term use associated w/ cataract formation NIPE: Eval intraocular pressure and lens if prolonged use

Dexamethasone Systemic, Topical (Decadron) See Steroids, Systemic, page 223, & Table 4, page 271, & Steroids, Topical, Table 5, page 272

Interactions: ↑ Effects w/ cyclosporine, estrogens, oral contraceptives, macrolides; ↑ effects of cyclosporine; ↓ effects w/ aminoglutethimide, antacids, barbiturates, carbamazepine, cholestyramine, colestipol, phenytoin, phenobarbital, rifampin; ↓ effects of anticoagulants, hypoglycemics, INH, toxoids, salicylates, vaccines **Labs:** False – allergy skin tests **NIPE:** ⊘ Vaccines, breast-feeding, use on broken skin

Dexpanthenol (Ilopan-Choline PO, Ilopan)
Uses: *Minimize paralytic ileus, Rx postop distention* **Action:** Cholinergic agent **Dose:** *Adults. Relief of gas:* 2–3 tabs PO tid. *Prevent postop ileus:* 250–500 mg IM stat, repeat in 2 h, then q6h PRN. *Ileus:* 500 mg IM stat, repeat in 2 h, followed by doses q6h, PRN **Caution:** [C, ?] **Contra:** Hemophilia, mechanical obstruction **Supplied:** Inj; tabs 50 mg; cream **SE:** GI cramps

Dexrazoxane (Zincard)
Uses: *Prevent anthracycline-induced cardiomyopathy* **Action:** Chelates heavy metals; binds intracellular Fe & prevents anthracycline-induced free radicals **Dose:** 10:1 ratio dexrazoxane:doxorubicin 30 min prior to each dose **Caution:** [C, ?] **Contra:** Component sensitivity **Supplied:** Inj 10 mg/mL **SE:** Myelosuppression (especially leukopenia), fever, infection, stomatitis, alopecia, N/V/D; mild ↑ transaminase, pain at inj site **Interactions:** ↑ Length of muscle relaxation w/ succinylcholine

Dextran 40 (Rheomacrodex)
Uses: *Shock, prophylaxis of DVT & thromboembolism, adjunct in peripheral vascular surgery* **Action:** Expands plasma volume; ↓ blood viscosity **Dose:** *Shock:* 10 mL/kg inf rapidly; 20 mL/kg max in the 1st 24 h; beyond 24 h 10 mL/kg max; DC after 5 d. *Prophylaxis of DVT & thromboembolism:* 10 mL/kg IV day of surgery, then 500 mL/d IV for 2–3 d, then 500 mL IV q2–3d based on risk for up to 2 wk **Caution:** [C, ?] Inf Rxns; Pts receiving corticosteroids **Contra:** Major hemostatic defects of all types; cardiac decompensation; renal Dz w/ severe oliguria/anuria **Supplied:** 10% dextran 40 in 0.9% NaCl or 5% dextrose **SE:** Hypersensitivity/anaphylactoid Rxn (observe closely during 1st min of inf), arthralgia, cutaneous Rxns, hypotension, fever **Notes:** Monitor Cr & electrolytes; Pts should be well hydrated **Interactions:** ↑ Bleeding times w/ antiplt agents or anticoagulants **Labs:** False ↑ serum glucose, urinary protein, bilirubin assays, & total protein assays **NIPE:** Draw blood before administration of drug, Pt should be well hydrated prior to inf

Dextromethorphan (Mediquell, Benylin DM, PediaCare 1, others) [OTC]
Uses: *Controlling nonproductive cough* **Action:** Depresses the cough center in the medulla **Dose:** *Adults.* 10–30 mg PO q4h PRN (max 120 mg/24 h). *Peds. 7 mo–1 y:* 2–4 mg q6–8h. *2–6 y:* 2.5–7.5 mg q4–8h (max 30 mg/24 h). *7–12 y:* 5–10 mg q4–8h (max 60 mg/24/h) **Caution:** [C, ?/–] Not for persistent or chronic cough **Supplied:** Caps 30 mg; lozenges 2.5, 5, 7.5, 15 mg; syrup 15 mg/15 mL, 10 mg/5 mL; liq 10 mg/15 mL, 3.5, 7.5, 15 mg/5 mL; sustained-action liq 30 mg/5 mL **SE:** GI disturbances **Notes:** May be found in combination OTC products w/ guaifenesin **Interactions:** ↑ Effects w/ amiodarone,

fluoxetin, quinidine, terbinafine; ↑ risk of serotonin syndrome w/ sibutramine, MAOIs; ↑ CNS depression w/ antihistamines, antidepressants, sedative, opioids, EtOH **NIPE:** ↑ Fluids, humidity to environment, stop MAOIs for 2 wk before administering drug

Dezocine (Dalgan) **Uses:** *Moderate to severe pain* **Action:** Narcotic agonist–antagonist **Dose:** 5–20 mg IM or 2.5–10 mg IV q2–4h PRN; ↓ in renal impairment **Caution:** [C, ?] **Contra:** Pts <18 y **Supplied:** Inj 5, 10, 15 mg/mL **SE:** Sedation, dizziness, vertigo, N/V, inj site Rxn **Notes:** Withdrawal possible in Pts dependent on narcotics **Interactions:** ↑ Effects w/ CNS depressants, ⊘ MAOIs **NIPE:** ↑ Resp depression greatest 1st h after admin

Diazepam (Valium) [C-IV] **Uses:** *Anxiety, EtOH withdrawal, muscle spasm, status epilepticus, panic disorders, amnesia, preoperative sedation* **Action:** Benzodiazepine **Dose:** *Adults.* Status epilepticus: 5–10 mg q10–20min to 30 mg max in 8-h period. *Anxiety, muscle spasm:* 2–10 mg PO bid–qid or IM/IV q3–4h PRN. *Preop:* 5–10 mg PO or IM 20–30 min or IV just prior to procedure. *EtOH withdrawal:* Initial 2–5 mg IV, then 5–10 mg q5–10min, 100 mg in 1 h max. May require up to 1000 mg in 24-h period for severe withdrawal. Titrate to agitation; ⊘ excessive sedation; may lead to aspiration or resp arrest. *Peds.* Status epilepticus: <5 y: 0.05–0.3 mg/kg/dose IV q15–30min up to a max of 5 mg. >5 y: Give up to max of 10 mg. *Sedation, muscle relaxation:* 0.04–0.3 mg/kg/dose q2–4h IM or IV to max of 0.6 mg/kg in 8 h, or 0.12–0.8 mg/kg/24 h PO ÷ tid–qid; ↓ in hepatic impairment; ⊘ abrupt withdrawal **Caution:** [D, ?/–] **Contra:** Coma, CNS depression, resp depression, narrow-angle glaucoma, severe uncontrolled pain, PRG **Supplied:** Tabs 2, 5, 10 mg; soln 1, 5 mg/mL; inj 5 mg/mL; rectal gel 5 mg/mL **SE:** Sedation, amnesia, bradycardia, hypotension, rash, decreased resp rate **Notes:** ⊘ exceed 5 mg/min IV in adults or 1–2 mg/min in peds because resp arrest possible; IM absorption erratic **Interactions:** ↑ Effects w/ antihistamines, azole antifungals, BBs, CNS depressants, cimetidine, ciprofloxin, disulfiram, INH, oral contraceptives, omeprazole, phenytoin, valproic acid, verapamil, EtOH, kava kava, valerian; ↑ effects of digoxin, diuretics; ↓ effects w/ barbiturates, carbamazepine, theophylline, ranitidine, tobacco; ↓ effects of haloperidol, levodopa **Labs:** False – urine glucose; monitor LFTs, BUN, creatinine, CBC w/ long-term drug use **NIPE:** Risk ↑ Sz activity

Diazoxide (Hyperstat, Proglycem) **Uses:** *Hypoglycemia due to hyperinsulinism (Proglycem); hypertensive crisis (Hyperstat)* **Action:** Inhibits pancreatic insulin release; antihypertensive **Dose:** *Hypertensive crisis:* 1–3 mg/kg IV (150 mg max in a single inj); repeat in 5–15 min until BP controlled; repeat every 4–24 h; monitor BP closely. *Hypoglycemia:* **Adults & Peds.** 3–8 mg/kg/24 h PO ÷ q8–12h. **Neonates.** 8–15 mg/kg/24 h ÷ in 3 equal doses; maint 8–10 mg/kg/24 h PO in 2–3 equal doses **Caution:** [C, ?] ↓ effect w/ phenytoin; ↑ effect w/ diuretics, warfarin **Contra:** Hypersensitivity to thiazides or other sulfonamide-containing products; HTN associated w/ aortic coarctation, AV shunt, or pheochromocytoma

Supplied: Inj 15 mg/mL; caps 50 mg; PO susp 50 mg/mL **SE:** Hyperglycemia, hypotension, dizziness, Na & water retention, N/V, weakness **Notes:** Can give false – insulin response to glucagons; treat extravasation w/ warm compress **Interactions:** ↑ Effects w/ carboplatin, cisplatin, diuretics, phenothiazines; ↑ effects of anticoagulants; ↓ effects w/ sulfonylureas; ↓ effects of phenytoin, sulfonylureas; **Labs:** ↑ Serum uric acid, AST, alkaline phosphatase, false – response to glucagon **NIPE:** Daily weights, ↑ reversible body hair growth

Dibucaine (Nupercainal) Uses: *Hemorrhoids & minor skin conditions* **Action:** Topical anesthetic **Dose:** Insert PR w/ applicator bid & after each bowel movement; apply sparingly to skin **Caution:** [C, ?] **Contra:** Component sensitivity **Supplied:** 1% oint w/ rectal applicator; 0.5% cream **SE:** Local irritation, rash **Interactions:** None noted

Diclofenac (Cataflam, Voltaren) Uses: *Arthritis & pain* **Action:** NSAID **Dose:** 50–75 mg PO bid; w/ food or milk **Caution:** [B (D 3rd tri or near delivery), ?] CHF, HTN, renal/hepatic dysfunction, & Hx PUD **Contra:** Hypersensitivity to NSAIDs or ASA; porphyria **Supplied:** Tabs 50 mg; tabs DR 25, 50, 75, 100 mg; XR tabs 100 mg; ophthalmic soln 0.1% **SE:** Abdominal cramps, heartburn, GI ulceration, rash, interstitial nephritis **Notes:** Watch for GI bleed **Interactions:** ↑ Risk of bleeding w/ feverfew, garlic, ginger, ginkgo biloba; ↑ effects of digoxin, MRX, cyclosporine, Li, insulin, sulfonylureas, K-sparing diuretics, warfarin; ↓ effects w/ ASA; ↓ effects of thiazide diuretics, furosemide, BBs **Labs:** ↑ LFTs, serum glucose & cortisol, ↓ serum uric acid; **NIPE:** Risk of photosensitivity—use sunscreen, monitor LFTs, CBC, BUN, creatinine, take w/ food, ⊘ crush tablets

Dicloxacillin (Dynapen, Dycill) Uses: *Rx of pneumonia, skin & soft tissue infections, & osteomyelitis caused by penicillinase-producing staphylococci* **Action:** Bactericidal; inhibits cell wall synthesis. *Spectrum: S. aureus & Streptococcus* **Dose:** *Adults.* 250–500 mg qid *Peds <40 kg.* 12.5–25 mg/kg/d ÷ qid; take on empty stomach **Caution:** [B, ?] **Contra:** Component or PCN sensitivity **Supplied:** Caps 125, 250, 500 mg; soln 62.5 mg/5 mL **SE:** Diarrhea, nausea, abdominal pain **Notes:** Monitor PTT if Pt concurrently on warfarin **Interactions:** ↑ Effects w/ disulfiram, probenecid; ↑ effects of MRX, ↓ effects w/ macrolides, tetracyclines, food; ↓ effects of oral contraceptives, warfarin **Labs:** False ↑ nafcillin level, urine & serum proteins, uric acid **NIPE:** Take w/ water

Dicyclomine (Bentyl) Uses: *Functional IBSs* **Action:** Smooth muscle relaxant **Dose:** *Adults.* 20 mg PO qid; ↑ to max dose of 160 mg/d or 20 mg IM q6h *Peds.* Infants >6 mo: 5 mg/dose tid–qid. *Children:* 10 mg/dose tid–qid **Caution:** [B, –] **Contra:** Infants < 6 mo, narrow-angle glaucoma, MyG, severe UC, obstructive uropathy **Supplied:** Caps 10, 20 mg; tabs 20 mg; syrup 10 mg/5 mL; inj 10 mg/mL **SE:** Anticholinergic side effects may limit dose **Notes:** Take 30–60 min before meal; **Interactions:** ↑ Anticholinergic effects w/ anticholinergics, antihistamines, amantadine, MAOIs, TCAs, phenothiazides; ↑ effects of atenolol, digoxin;

↓ effects w/ antacids; ↓ effects of haloperidol, ketoconazole, levodopa, phenothiazines **NIPE**: ⊘ EtOH, CNS depressant; adequate hydration

Didanosine [ddI] (Videx)
WARNING: Hypersensitivity manifested as fever, rash, fatigue, GI/resp Sxs reported; stop drug immediately & ⊘ rechallenge; lactic acidosis & hepatomegaly/steatosis reported **Uses**: *HIV infection in zidovudine-intolerant Pts* **Action**: Nucleoside antiretroviral agent **Dose**: *Adults*. >60 kg: 400 mg/d PO or 200 mg PO bid. <60 kg: 250 mg/d PO or 125 mg PO bid; adults should take 2 tabs/administration. *Peds*. Dose by following table; ↓ in renal impairment:

BSA (m²)	Tablets (mg)	Powder (mg)
1.1–1.4	100 bid	125 bid
0.8–1	75 bid	94 bid
0.5–0.7	50 bid	62 bid
<0.4	25 bid	31 bid

Caution: [B, –] CDC recommends HIV-infected mothers not breast-feed due to risk of transmission of HIV to their infant **Contra**: Component sensitivity **Supplied**: Chew tabs 25, 50, 100, 150, 200 mg; powder packets 100, 167, 250, 375 mg; powder for soln 2, 4 g **SE**: Pancreatitis, peripheral neuropathy, diarrhea, HA **Notes**: ⊘ Take w/ meals; thoroughly chew tablets, ⊘ mix w/ fruit juice or other acidic beverages; reconstitute powder w/ water **Interactions**: ↑ Effects w/ allopurinol, ganciclovir; ↓ effects w/ methadone, food; ↑ risk of pancreatitis w/ thiazide diuretics, IV pentamidine, EtOH; ↓ effects of azole antifungals, dapsone, delavirdine, ganciclovir, indinavir, quinolones, ranitidine, tetracyclines **Labs**: ↑ LFTs, uric acid, amylase, lipase, triglycerides **NIPE**: May cause hyperglycemia, take w/o food, chew or crush tabs

Diflunisal (Dolobid)
Uses: *Mild to moderate pain; osteoarthritis* **Action**: NSAID **Dose**: *Pain*: 500 mg PO bid. *Osteoarthritis*: 500–1500 mg PO in 2–3 ÷ doses; ↓ in renal impairment, take w/ food/milk **Caution**: [C (D 3rd tri or near delivery), ?] CHF, HTN, renal/hepatic dysfunction, & Hx PUD. **Contra**: Hypersensitivity to NSAIDs or ASA, active GI bleed **Supplied**: Tabs 250, 500 mg **SE**: May prolong bleeding time; HA, abdominal cramps, heartburn, GI ulceration, rash, interstitial nephritis, fluid retention **Interactions**: ↑ Effects w/ probenecid; ↑ effects of acetaminophen, anticoagulants, digoxin, HCTZ, indomethacin, Li, MRX, phenytoin, sulfonamides, sulfonylureas; ↓ effects w/ antacids, ASA; ↓ effects of furosemide **Labs**: ↑ Salicylate levels, PT, ↓ uric acid, T₃, T₄; **NIPE**: Take w/ food, ⊘ chew or crush tabs

Digoxin (Lanoxin, Lanoxicaps)
Uses: *CHF, AF & flutter, & PAT* **Action**: + Inotrope; ↑ AV node refractory period **Dose**: *Adults*. PO digitalization:

0.5–0.75 mg PO, then 0.25 mg PO q6–8h to total 1–1.5 mg. *IV or IM digitaliza-tion:* 0.25–0.5 mg IM or IV, then 0.25 mg q4–6h to total ≈1 mg. *Daily maint:* 0.125–0.5 mg/d PO, IM, or IV (average daily dose 0.125–0.25 mg). *Peds.* Preterm infants: Digitalization: 30 µg/kg PO or 25 µg/kg IV; give ½ of dose initially, then ¼ of dose at 8–12-h intervals for 2 doses. *Maint:* 5–7.5 µg/kg/24 h PO or 4–6 µg/kg/24 h IV ÷ q12h. *Term infants:* Digitalization: 25–35 µg/kg PO or 20–30 µg/kg IV; give ½ the dose initially, then ¼ of the dose at 8–12 h. *Maint:* 6–10 µg/kg/24 h PO or 5–8 µg/kg/24 h IV ÷ q12h. *1 mo–2 y: Digitalization:* 35–60 µg/kg PO or 30–50 µg/kg IV; give ½ the dose initially, then ¼ dose at 8–12-h intervals for 2 doses. *Maint:* 10–15 µg/kg/24 h PO or 7.5–15 µg/kg/24 h IV ÷ q12h. *2–10 y: Digitaliza-tion:* 30–40 µg/kg PO or 25 µg/kg IV; give ½ dose initially, then ¼ of the dose at 8–12-h intervals for 2 doses. *Maint:* 8–10 µg/kg/24 h PO or 6–8 µg/kg/24 h IV ÷ q12h. *7–10 y:* Same as for adults; ↓ in renal impairment, follow serum levels **Cau-tion:** [C, +] **Contra** AV block; idiopathic hypertrophic subaortic stenosis; constric-tive pericarditis **Supplied:** Caps 0.05, 0.1, 0.2 mg; tabs 0.125, 0.25, 0.5 mg; elixir 0.05 mg/mL; inj 0.1, 0.25 mg/mL **SE:** Can cause heart block; ↓ K⁺ potentiates tox-icity; N/V, HA, fatigue, visual disturbances (yellow-green halos around lights), car-diac arrhythmias **Notes:** Multiple drug interactions; IM inj painful, has erratic absorption & should not be used; see Drug Levels, Table 2, page 265. **Interac-tions:** ↑ Effects w/ alprazolam, amiodarone, azole antifungals, BBs, carvedilol, cy-closporine, corticosteroids, diltiazem, diuretics, erythromycin, NSAIDs, quinidine, spironolactone, tetracyclines, verapamil, goldenseal, hawthorn, licorice, quinine, Siberian ginseng; ↓ effects w/ charcoal, cholestyramine, cisapride, neomycin, ri-fampin, sucralfate, thyroid hormones, psyllium, St. John's wort **Labs:** ↓ PT, moni-tor serum electrolytes, LFTs, BUN, creatinine **NIPE:** Different bioavailability in various brands

Digoxin Immune Fab (Digibind)

Uses: *Life-threatening digoxin in-toxication* **Action:** Antigen-binding fragments bind & inactivate digoxin **Dose:** *Adults & Peds.* Based on serum level & Pt's weight; see charts provided w/ the drug **Caution:** [C, ?] **Contra:** Hypersensitivity to sheep products **Supplied:** Inj 38 mg/vial **SE:** Worsening of cardiac output or CHF, hypokalemia, facial swelling, & redness **Notes:** Each vial binds ≈ 0.6 mg of digoxin; in renal failure may require re-dosing in several days because of breakdown of the immune complex **Interac-tions:** ↓ Effects of cardiac glycosides **NIPE:** Will take up to 1 wk for accurate serum digoxin levels after use of Digibind

Diltiazem (Cardizem, Cardizem CD, Cardizem SR, Cartia XT, Dilacor XR, Diltia XT, Tiamate, Tiazac)

Uses: *Angina, prevention of reinfarction, HTN, AF or flutter, & PAT* **Action:** CCB **Dose:** *PO:* Initially, 30 mg PO qid; ↑ to 180–360 mg/d in 3–4 ÷ doses PRN. *SR:* 60–120 mg PO bid; ↑ to 360 mg/d max. *CD or XR:* 120–360 mg/d (max 480 mg/d). *IV:* 0.25 mg/kg IV bolus over 2 min; may repeat in 15 min at 0.35 mg/kg; may begin inf of 5–15 mg/h **Caution:** [C, +] ↑ effect w/ amiodarone, cimetidine, fentanyl, Li, cyclosporine, digoxin, BBss, cisapride, theophylline **Contra:** SSS, AV block, hypotension, AMI, pulmonary congestion **Supplied:** *Cardizem CD:* Caps 120, 180, 240, 300, 360 mg; *Cardizem SR:* caps 60, 90, 120 mg; *Cardizem:* Tabs 30, 60, 90, 120 mg; *Cartia XT:* Caps 120, 180, 240, 300 mg; *Dilacor XR:* Caps 180, 240 mg; *Diltia XT:* Caps 120, 180, 240 mg; *Tiazac:* Caps 120, 180, 240, 300, 360, 420 mg; *Tiamate (XR):* Tabs 120, 180, 240 mg; inj 5 mg/mL **SE:** Gingival hyperplasia, bradycardia, AV block, ECG abnormalities, peripheral edema, dizziness, HA **Notes:** Cardizem CD, Dilacor XR, & Tiazac not interchangeable **Interactions:** ↑ Effects w/ α-blockers, azole antifungals, BBs, erythromycin, H₂ receptor antagonists, nitroprusside, quinidine, EtOH, grapefruit juice; ↑ effects of carbamazepine, cyclosporine, digitalis glycosides, quinidine, phenytoin, prazosin, theophylline, TCAs; ↓ effects w/ NSAIDs, phenobarbital, rifampin **Labs:** False ↑ urine ketones, ↑ LFTs, BUN, creatinine **NIPE:** ⊘ Chew or crush SR or ER preps, risk of photosensitivity—use sunscreen

Dimenhydrinate (Dramamine, others) Uses: *Prevention & Rx of N/V, dizziness, or vertigo of motion sickness* Action: Antiemetic Dose: *Adults.* 50–100 mg PO q4–6h, max 400 mg/d; 50 mg IM/IV PRN. *Peds.* 5 mg/kg/24 h PO or IV ÷ qid (max 300 mg/d) Caution: [B, ?] Contra: Component sensitivity Supplied: tab 50 mg; chew tabs 50 mg; liq 12.5 mg/4 mL, 12.5 mg/5 mL, 15.62 mg/5 mL; inj 50 mg/mL SE: Anticholinergic side effects Interactions: ↑ Effects w/ CNS depressants, antihistamines, opioids, quinidine, MAOIs, TCAs, EtOH Labs: False ↓ allergy skin tests NIPE: ⊘ Drug 72 h prior to allergy skin testing, take before motion sickness occurs

Dimethyl Sulfoxide [DMSO] (Rimso 50) Uses: *Interstitial cystitis* Action: Unknown Dose: Intravesical, 50 mL, retain for 15 min; repeat q2wk until relief Caution: [C, ?] Contra: Component sensitivity Supplied: 50% soln in 50 mL SE: Cystitis, eosinophilia, GI, & taste disturbance Interactions: ↓ Effects of sulindac Labs: Monitor CBC, LFTs, BUN, creatinine levels NIPE: ↑ Taste & smell of garlic

Dinoprostone (Cervidil Vaginal Insert, Prepidil Vaginal Gel) Uses: *Induce labor; terminate PRG (12–28 wk); evacuate uterus in missed abortion or fetal death* Action: prostaglandin, changes consistency, dilatation, & effacement of the cervix; induces uterine contraction Dose: *Gel:* 0.5 mg; if no cervical/uterine response, repeat 0.5 mg q6h (max 24-h dose 1.5 mg). *Vaginal insert:* 1 insert (10 mg = 0.3 mg dinoprostone/h over 12 h); remove w/ onset of labor or 12 h after insertion. *Vaginal supp:* 20 mg repeated every 3–5 h; adjust PRN supp: 1 high in vagina, repeat at 3–5-h intervals until abortion (240 mg max) Caution: [X, ?] Contra: Ruptured membranes, hypersensitivity to prostaglandins, placenta previa or unexplained vaginal bleeding during PRG, when oxytocic drugs contraindicated or if prolonged uterine contractions are inappropriate (Hx C-section or major uterine surgery, presence of cephalopelvic disproportion, etc) Supplied *Gel, endocervical:* 0.5 mg in 3-g syringes (each package contains a 10-mm & 20-mm shielded catheter); *vaginal gel:* 0.5 mg/3 g; *vaginal supp:* 20 mg; vagi-

nal insert, CR: 0.3 mg/h **SE:** N/V/D, dizziness, flushing, headache, fever **Interactions:** ↑ Effects of oxytocics; ↓ effects w/ large amts EtOH **NIPE:** Pt supine after insertion of supp or gel up to ½ h

Diphenhydramine (Benadryl) [OTC]
Uses: *Rx & prevent allergic Rxns, motion sickness, potentiate narcotics, sedation, cough suppression, & Rx of extrapyramidal Rxns* **Action:** Antihistamine, antiemetic **Dose:** *Adults.* 25–50 mg PO, IV, or IM bid–tid. *Peds.* 5 mg/kg/24 h PO or IM ÷ q6h (max 300 mg/d); ↑ dosing interval in moderate/severe renal failure **Caution:** [B, –] **Contra:** ⊘ Use in acute asthma release **Supplied:** Tabs & caps 25, 50 mg; chew tabs 12.5 mg; elixir 12.5 mg/5 mL; syrup 12.5 mg/5 mL; liq 6.25 mg/5 mL, 12.5 mg/5 mL; inj 50 mg/mL **SE:** Anticholinergic side effects (xerostomia, urinary retention, sedation) **Interactions:** ↑ Effects w/ CNS depressants, antihistamines, opioids, MAOIs, TCAs, EtOH; ↑ effects of metoprolol **Labs:** ↓ Response to allergy skin testing **NIPE:** ↑ Risk of photosensitivity—use sunscreen

Diphenoxylate + Atropine (Lomotil) [C-V]
Uses: *Diarrhea* **Action:** Constipating meperidine congener, reduces GI motility **Dose:** *Initial,* 5 mg PO tid–qid until under control, then 2.5–5.0 mg PO bid. *Peds >2 y:* 0.3–0.4 mg/kg/24 h (of diphenoxylate) bid–qid **Caution:** [C, +] **Contra:** Obstructive jaundice, diarrhea due to bacterial infection; children <2 y **Supplied:** Tabs 2.5 mg of diphenoxylate/0.025 mg of atropine; liq 2.5 mg diphenoxylate/0.025 mg atropine/5 mL **SE:** Drowsiness, dizziness, xerostomia, blurred vision, urinary retention, constipation **Interactions:** ↑ Effects w/ CNS depressants, opioids, EtOH, ↑ risk HTN crisis w/ MAOIs **NIPE:** ↓ Effectiveness w/ diarrhea caused by antibiotics

Diphtheria, Tetanus Toxoids, & Acellular pertussis adsorbed, Hepatitis B (recombinant), & Inactivated Poliovirus Vaccine [IPV] combined (Pediarix)
Uses: *Vaccine against diphtheria, tetanus, pertussis, HBV, polio(types 1, 2, 3) as a three-dose primary series in infants & children <7, born to HBsAg-negative mothers* **Actions:** Active immunization **Dose:** Infants 3 0.5-mL doses IM, at 6–8-wk intervals, start at 2 mo; child given 1 dose of hep B vaccine, same; child previously vaccinated w/ one or more doses IPV, use to complete series **Caution:** [C, N/A] **Contra:** If HbsAG+ mother, adults, children >7 y, immunosuppressed, hypersensitivity to yeast, neomycin, or polymyxin B, Hx allergy to any component of the vaccine, encephalopathy, or progressive neurologic disorders; caution in bleeding disorders. **Supplied:** Single-dose vials 0.5 mL **SE:** Drowsiness, restlessness, fever, fussiness, ↓ appetite, nodule redness, pain, & swelling at inj site **Notes:** Give IM only **Interactions:** ↓ Effects w/ immunosuppressants

Dipivefrin (Propine)
Uses: *Open-angle glaucoma* **Action:** α-Adrenergic agonist **Dose:** 1 gt into eye q12h **Caution:** [B, ?] **Contra:** Closed-angle glaucoma **Supplied:** 0.1% soln **SE:** HA, local irritation, blurred vision, photophobia, hypertension **Interactions:** ↑ Effects w/ BBs, ophthalmic anhydrase inhibitors, osmotic

drugs, sympathomimetics, ↑ risk of cardiac arrhythmias w/ digoxin, TCAs **NIPE:** Discard discolored solutions

Dipyridamole (Persantine) Uses: *Prevent postop thromboembolic disorders, often in combination w/ ASA or warfarin (eg, CABG, vascular graft); w/ warfarin after artificial heart valve; chronic angina; w/ ASA to prevent coronary artery thrombosis; dipyridamole IV used in place of exercise stress test for CAD* **Action:** Antiplt activity; coronary vasodilator **Dose:** *Adults.* 75–100 mg PO tid–qid; stress test 0.14 mg/kg/min (max 60 mg over 4 min). *Peds >12 y.* 3–6 mg/kg/d divided tid **Caution:** [B, ?/–] Caution w/ other drugs that affect coagulation **Contra:** Component sensitivity **Supplied:** Tabs 25, 50, 75 mg; inj 5 mg/mL **SE:** HA, hypotension, nausea, abdominal distress, flushing rash, dyspnea **Notes:** IV use can worsen angina **Interactions:** ↑ Effects w/ anticoagulants, heparin, evening primrose oil, feverfew, garlic, ginger, ginkgo biloba, ginseng, grapeseed extract; ↑ effects of adenosine; ↑ bradycardia w/ BBs; ↓ effects w/ aminophylline **NIPE:** ⊘ EtOH or tobacco because of vasoconstriction effects; + effects may take several mo

Dipyridamole & Aspirin (Aggrenox) Uses: *↓ Reinfarction after MI; prevent occlusion after CABG; ↓ risk of stroke* **Action:** ↓ Plt aggregation (both agents) **Dose:** 1 cap PO bid **Caution:** [C, ?] **Contra:** Ulcers, bleeding diathesis **Supplied:** Dipyridamole (XR) 200 mg/ASA 25 mg **SE:** ASA component: allergic Rxns, skin Rxns, ulcers/GI bleed, bronchospasm; dipyridamole component: dizziness, HA, rash **Notes:** Swallow capsule whole

Dirithromycin (Dynabac) Uses: *Bronchitis, community-acquired pneumonia, & skin & skin structure infections* **Action:** Macrolide antibiotic. *Spectrum: M. catarrhalis, Streptococcus pneumoniae, Legionella, H. influenzae, S. pyogenes, Staphylococcus aureus* **Dose:** 500 mg/d PO; take w/ food **Caution:** [C, M] **Contra:** Use w/ pimozide **Supplied:** Tabs 250 mg **SE:** Abdominal discomfort, HA, rash, hyperkalemia **Notes:** Swallow whole **Interactions:** ↑ Effects w/ antacids, H$_2$ antagonists, food; ↑ effects of theophylline; ↓ effects of penicillins **NIPE:** Take w/ food, ⊘ crush or chew

Disopyramide (Norpace, NAPamide) Uses: *Suppression & prevention of VT* **Action:** Class 1A antiarrhythmic **Dose:** *Adults.* 400–800 mg/d ÷ q6h for regular & q12h for SR. *Peds.* <1 y: 10–30 mg/kg/24 h PO (÷ qid). *1–4 y:* 10–20 mg/kg/24 h PO (÷ qid). *4–12 y:* 10–15 mg/kg/24 h PO (÷ qid). *12–18 y:* 6–15 mg/kg/24 h PO (÷ qid); ↓ in renal/hepatic impairment **Caution:** [C, +] **Contra:** AV block, cardiogenic shock **Supplied:** Caps 100, 150 mg; SR caps 100, 150 mg **SE:** Anticholinergic side effects; negative inotropic properties may induce CHF **Notes:** See Drug Levels, Table 2, page 265. **Interactions:** ↑ Effects w/ cimetidine, clarithromycin, erythromycin, quinidine; ↑ effects of digoxin, hypoglycemics, insulin, warfarin; ↑ risk of arrhythmias w/ pimozide; ↓ effects w/ barbiturates, phenytoin, phenobarbital, rifampin **Labs:** ↑ LFTs, lipids, BUN, creatinine; ↓ serum glucose, Hmg, Hct **NIPE:** Risk of photosensitivity—use sunscreen, daily weights

Dobutamine (Dobutrex) Uses: *Short-term use in cardiac decompensation secondary to depressed contractility* **Action:** + inotropic agent **Dose:** *Adults & Peds.* Cont IV inf of 2.5–15 µg/kg/min; rarely, 40 µg/kg/min may be required; titrate to response **Caution:** [C, ?] **Contra:** Sensitivity to sulfites, idiopathic hypertrophic subaortic stenosis **Supplied:** Inj 250 mg/20 mL **SE:** Chest pain, HTN, dyspnea **Notes:** Monitor PWP & cardiac output if possible; check ECG for ↑ heart rate, ectopic activity; follow BP **Interactions:** ↑ Effects w/ furazolidone, methyldopa, MAOIs, TCAs; ↓ effects w/ BBs, NaHCO$_3$; ↓ effects of guanethidine **Labs:** ↓ K; **NIPE:** Eval for adequate hydration; monitor I&O, cardiac output, ECG, BP during inf

Docetaxel (Taxotere) Uses: *Breast (anthracycline-resistant), ovarian, lung cancers, & CAP* **Action:** Antimitotic agent; promotes microtubular aggregation; semisynthetic taxoid **Dose:** 100 mg/m^2 over 1 h IV q3wk (refer to specific protocols); start dexamethasone 8 mg bid prior to docetaxel & continue for 3–4 d; ↓ dose w/ ↑ bilirubin levels **Caution:** [D, –] **Contra:** Component sensitivity **Supplied:** Inj 20, 40, 80 mg/mL **SE:** Myelosuppression, neuropathy, N/V, alopecia, fluid retention syndrome; cumulative doses of 300–400 mg/m^2 w/o steroid prep & posttreatment & 600–800 mg/m^2 w/ steroid prep; hypersensitivity Rxns possible, but rare w/ steroid prep **Interactions:** ↑ Effects w/ cyclosporine, ketoconazole, erythromycin, terfenidine **Labs:** ↑ AST, ALT, alkaline phosphatase **NIPE:** ↑ Fluids to 2–3 L/d, ↑ risk of hair loss, ↑ susceptibility to infection, urine may become reddish-brown

Docusate Calcium (Surfak)/Docusate Potassium (Dialose)/ Docusate Sodium (DOS, Colace) Uses: *Constipation; adjunct to painful anorectal conditions (hemorrhoids)* **Action:** Stool softener **Dose:** *Adults.* 50–500 mg PO ÷ daily–qid. *Peds.* Infants–3 y: 10–40 mg/24 h ÷ daily–qid. *3–6 y:* 20–60 mg/24 h ÷ daily–qid. *6–12 y:* 40–150 mg/24 h ÷ daily–qid **Caution:**[C, ?] **Contra:** Concomitant use of mineral oil; intestinal obstruction, acute abdominal pain, N/V **Supplied:** *Ca:* Caps 50, 240 mg. *K:* Caps 100, 240 mg. *Na:* Caps 50, 100 mg; syrup 50, 60 mg/15 mL; liq 150 mg/15 mL; soln 50 mg/mL **SE:** No significant side effects, rare abdominal cramping, diarrhea; no laxative action **Notes:** Take w/ full glass of water; ⊘ use >1 wk **Interactions:** ↑ Absorption of mineral oil **Labs:** ↓ K$^+$ Cl **NIPE:** Short-term use, take w/ juices or milk to mask bitter taste

Dofetilide (Tikosyn) WARNING: To minimize the risk of induced arrhythmia, Pts initiated or reinitiated on Tikosyn should be placed for a minimum of 3 d in a facility that can provide calculations of CrCl, continuous ECG monitoring, & cardiac resuscitation Uses: *Maintain normal sinus rhythm in AF/A flutter after conversion* **Action:** Type III antiarrhythmic **Dose:** 125–500 µg PO bid based on CrCl & QTc (see insert) **Caution:** [C, –] **Contra:** Baseline QTc is > 440 ms (500 ms w/ ventricular conduction abnormalities) or CrCl < 20 mL/min; concomitant use of verapamil, cimetidine, trimethoprim, or ketoconazole **Supplied:** Caps 125, 250, 500 µg **SE:** Ventricular arrhythmias, HA, CP, dizziness **Notes:** ⊘ w/ other drugs that prolong the QT interval; hold class I or III antiarrhythmics for at least 3 ½-lives prior to dofetilide; amiodarone level should be < 0.3 mg/L prior to dofetilide **Interactions:** ↑ Effects w/ amiloride, amiodarone, azole antifungals, cimetidine, diltiazem, macrolides, metformin, megestrol, nefazodone, norfloxacin, SSRIs, TCAs, triamterene, trimethoprim, verapamil, zafirlukast, quinine, grapefruit juice **NIPE:** Take w/o regard to food; monitor LFTs, BUN, creatinine

Dolasetron (Anzemet) **Uses:** *Prevent chemotherapy-associated N/V* **Action:** 5-HT$_3$ receptor antagonist **Dose:** *Adults & Peds.* IV: 1.8 mg/kg IV as single dose 30 min prior to chemotherapy. *Adults.* PO: 100 mg PO as a single dose 1 h prior to chemotherapy. *Peds.* PO: 1.8 mg/kg PO to max 100 mg as single dose **Caution:** [B, ?] **Contra:** Component sensitivity **Supplied:** Tabs 50, 100 mg; inj 20 mg/mL **SE:** Prolongs QT interval, HTN, HA, abdominal pain, urinary retention, transient ↑ LFTs **Interactions:** ↑ Effects w/ cimetidine; ↑ risk of arrhythmias w/ diuretics; ↓ effects w/ rifampin **Labs:** ↑ ALT, AST, alkaline phosphatase, PTT **NIPE:** Monitor LFTs, PTT, CBC, plts, & alkaline phosphatase w/ prolonged use

Dopamine (Intropin) **Uses:** *Short-term use in cardiac decompensation secondary to decreased contractility; ↑s organ perfusion (at low dose)* **Action:** + Inotropic agent w/ dose response: 2–10 µg/kg/min β-effects (↑ CO & renal perfusion); 10–20 µg/kg/min β-effects (peripheral vasoconstriction, pressor). >20 µg/kg/min peripheral & renal vasoconstriction **Dose:** *Adults & Peds.* 5 µg/kg/min by cont inf, ↑ increments of 5 µg/kg/min to 50 µg/kg/min max based on effect **Caution:** [C, ?] **Contra:** Pheochromocytoma, VF, sulfite sensitivity **Supplied:** Inj 40, 80, 160 mg/mL **SE:** Tachycardia, vasoconstriction, hypotension, HA, N/V, dyspnea **Notes:** Dosage >10 µg/kg/min may ↓ renal perfusion; monitor urinary output; monitor ECG for ↑ in heart rate, BP, & ectopic activity; monitor PCWP & cardiac output if possible **Interactions:** ↑ Effects w/ α-blockers, diuretics, ergot alkaloids, MAOIs, BBs, anesthetics, phenytoin; ↓ effects w/ guanethidine **Labs:** False ↑ urine catecholamines, urine amino acids; false ↓ SCr **NIPE:** Maintain adequate hydration

Dornase Alfa (Pulmozyme) **Uses:** *↓ Frequency of resp infections in CF* **Action:** Enzyme that selectively cleaves DNA **Dose:** Inhal 2.5 mg/d **Caution:** [B, ?] **Contra:** Hypersensitivity to Chinese hamster ovary cell products **Supplied:** Soln for inhal 1 mg/mL **SE:** Pharyngitis, voice alteration, CP, rash **Notes:** Use w/ recommended nebulizer **Interactions:** None noted **NIPE:** ⊘ Mix or dilute w/ other drugs

Dorzolamide (Trusopt) **Uses:** *Glaucoma* **Action:** Carbonic anhydrase inhibitor **Dose:** 1 gt in eye(s) tid **Caution:** [C, ?] **Contra:** Component sensitivity **Supplied:** 2% soln **SE:** Local irritation, bitter taste, superficial punctate keratitis, ocular allergic Rxn **Interactions:** ↑ Effects w/ oral carbonic anhydrase inhibitors, salicylates **NIPE:** ⊘ Wear soft contact lenses

Dorzolamide & Timolol (Cosopt) Uses: **Glaucoma** Action: Carbonic anhydrase inhibitor w/ β-adrenergic blocker Dose: 1 gt in eye(s) bid Caution: [C, ?] Contra: Component sensitivity Supplied: Soln dorzolamide 2% & timolol 0.5% SE: Local irritation, bitter taste, superficial punctate keratitis, ocular allergic Rxn

Doxazosin (Cardura) Uses: **HTN & symptomatic BPH** Action: $α_1$-Adrenergic blocker; relaxes bladder neck smooth muscle Dose: *HTN:* Initial 1 mg/d PO; may be ↑ to 16 mg/d PO. *BPH:* Initial 1 mg/d PO, may be ↑ to 8 mg/d PO Caution: [B, ?] Contra: Component sensitivity Supplied: Tabs 1, 2, 4, 8 mg SE: Dizziness, HA, drowsiness, sexual dysfunction, doses >4 mg ↑ likelihood of postural hypotension Notes: Take first dose hs; syncope may occur w/in 90 min of initial dose Interactions: ↑ effects w/ nitrates, antihypertensives, EtOH; ↓ effects w/ NSAIDs, butcher's broom; ↓ effects of clonidine NIPE: May be taken w/ food

Doxepin (Sinequan, Adapin) Uses: **Depression, anxiety, chronic pain** Action: TCA; ↑s the synaptic CNS concs of serotonin or norepinephrine Dose: 25–150 mg/d PO, usually hs but can be in ÷ doses; ↓ in hepatic impairment Caution: [C, ?/–] Contra: Narrow-angle glaucoma Supplied: Caps 10, 25, 50, 75, 100, 150 mg; PO conc 10 mg/mL SE: Anticholinergic side effects, hypotension, tachycardia, drowsiness, photosensitivity Interactions: ↑ Effects w/ fluoxetine, MAOIs, alcohol, CNS depressants, anticholinergics, cimetidine, oral contraceptives, propoxyphene, quinidine, EtOH, grapefruit juice; ↑ effects of carbamazepine, anticoagulants, amphetamines, thyroid drugs, sympathomimetics; ↓ effects w/ ascorbic acid, cholestyramine, tobacco; ↓ effects of bretylium, guanethidine, levodopa Labs: ↑ Serum bilirubin, alkaline phosphatase, glucose NIPE: Risk of photosensitivity—use sunscreen, urine may turn blue-green, may take 4–6 wk for full effect

Doxepin, Topical (Zonalon) Uses: **Short-term Rx pruritus (atopic dermatitis or lichen simplex chronicus)** Action: Antipruritic; H_1- & H_2-receptor antagonism Dose: Apply thin coating qid for max 8 d Caution: [C, ?/–] Contra: Component sensitivity Supplied: 5% cream SE: ↓ BP, tachycardia, drowsiness, photosensitivity Notes: Limit application area to ⊘ systemic toxicity

Doxorubicin (Adriamycin, Rubex) Uses: **Acute leukemias; Hodgkin's & NHLs; breast CA; soft tissue & osteosarcomas; Ewing's sarcoma; Wilms' tumor; neuroblastoma; bladder, ovarian, gastric, thyroid, & lung CAs** Action: Intercalates DNA; inhibits DNA topoisomerases I & II Dose: 60–75 mg/m^2 q3wk; ↓ cardiotoxicity w/ weekly (20 mg/m^2/wk) or cont inf (60–90 mg/m^2 over 96 h); refer to specific protocols Caution: [D, ?] Contra: Severe CHF, cardiomyopathy, preexisting myelosuppression, ↓ cardiac Fxn, Pts who received previous Rx w/ complete cumulative doses of doxorubicin, idarubicin, daunorubicin Supplied: Inj 10, 20, 50, 75, 200 mg SE: Myelosuppression, venous streaking & phlebitis, N/V/D, mucositis, radiation recall phenomenon, cardiomyopathy rare but dose-related; limit of 550 mg/m^2 cumulative dose (400 mg/m^2 if prior mediastinal irradiation) **Notes:** Dexrazoxane may limit cardiac toxicity; extravasation leads to tissue damage; discolors urine red/orange **Interactions:** ↑ Effects w/ streptozocin, verapamil, green tea; ↑ bone-marrow depression w/ antineoplastic drugs and radiation; ↓ effects w/ phenobarbital; ↓ effects of digoxin, phenytoin, live virus vaccines **Labs:** ↑ Urine and plasma uric acid levels **NIPE:** ⊘ PRG, use contraception at least 4 mo after drug Rx

Doxycycline (Vibramycin) **Uses:** *Broad-spectrum antibiotic activity* **Action:** Tetracycline; interferes w/ protein synthesis. *Spectrum: Rickettsia* sp, *Chlamydia,* & *M. pneumoniae* **Dose:** *Adults.* 100 mg PO q12h on 1st day, then 100 mg PO qd–bid or 100 mg IV q12h. *Peds >8y.* 5 mg/kg/24 h PO, to a max of 200 mg/d ÷ daily–bid **Supplied:** Tabs 50, 100 mg; caps 20, 50, 100 mg; syrup 50 mg/5 mL; susp 25 mg/5 mL; inj 100, 200 mg/vial **Caution:** [D, +] **Contra:** Children <8 y, severe hepatic dysfunction **SE:** Diarrhea, GI disturbance, photosensitivity **Notes:** Useful for chronic bronchitis; ↓ effect w/ antacids containing Al, Ca, Mg; tetracycline of choice in renal impairment **Interactions:** ↑ Effects of digoxin, warfarin; ↓ effects w/ antacids, Fe, barbiturates, carbamazepine, phenytoins, food; ↓ effects of penicillins **Labs:** False – urine glucose, false ↑ urine catecholamines; false ↓ urine urobilinogen **NIPE:** ↑ Risk of superinfection, ⊘ PRG, use barrier contraception

Dronabinol (Marinol) [C-II] **Uses:** *N/V associated w/ CA chemotherapy; appetite stimulation* **Action:** Antiemetic; inhibits the vomiting center in the medulla **Dose:** *Adults & Peds.* Antiemetic: 5–15 mg/m²/dose q4–6h PRN. *Adults.* Appetite stimulant: 2.5 mg PO before lunch & dinner **Caution:** [C, ?] **Contra:** Should not be used in Pts w/ Hx schizophrenia **Supplied:** Caps 2.5, 5, 10 mg **SE:** Drowsiness, dizziness, anxiety, mood change, hallucinations, depersonalization, orthostatic hypotension, tachycardia **Notes:** Principal psychoactive substance present in marijuana **Interactions:** ↑ Effects w/ anticholinergics, CNS depressants, EtOH; ↓ effects of theophylline **Labs:** ↓ FSH, LH, growth hormone, testosterone

Droperidol (Inapsine) **Uses:** *N/V; anesthetic premedication* **Action:** Tranquilizer, sedation, & antiemetic **Dose:** *Adults.* Nausea: 2.5–5 mg IV or IM q3–4h PRN. *Premed:* 2.5–10 mg IV, 30–60 min preop. *Peds.* Premed: 0.1–0.15 mg/kg/dose **Caution:** [C, ?] **Contra:** Component sensitivity **Supplied:** Inj 2.5 mg/mL **SE:** Drowsiness, moderate hypotension, occasional tachycardia & extrapyramidal Rxns, QT interval prolongation, arrhythmias **Notes:** Give IV push slowly over 2–5 min **Interactions:** ↑ Effects w/ CNS depressants, fentanyl, EtOH; ↑ hypotension w/ antihypertensives, nitrates

Drotrecogin Alfa (Xigris) **Uses:** *Reduce mortality in adults w/ severe sepsis (associated w/ acute organ dysfunction) at high risk of death (eg, as determined by APACHE II)* **Action:** Recombinant of human activated protein C; mechanism unknown **Dose:** 24 µg/kg/h for a total of 96 h **Caution:** [C, ?] **Contra:** Active bleeding, recent stroke or CNS surgery, head trauma, epidural catheter, CNS lesion at risk for herniation **Supplied:** 5-, 20-mg vials for reconstitution **SE:**

Bleeding most common SE **Notes:** For percutaneous procedures stop inf 2 h before the procedure & resume 1 h after; major surgery stop inf 2 h before surgery & resume 12 h after surgery in absence of bleeding **Interactions:** ↑ Risk of bleeding w/ plt inhibitors, anticoagulants **Labs:** ↑ aPTT **NIPE:** DC drug 2 h before invasive procedures

Dutasteride (Avodart) Uses: *Symptomatic BPH* Action: 5α-reductase inhibitor **Dose:** 0.5 mg PO qd **Caution:** [X, –] Caution in hepatic impairment, PRG women should ⊘ handling pills **Contra:** Women & children **Supplied:** Caps 0.5 mg **SE:** ↓ PSA levels, impotence, ↓ libido, gynecomastia **Notes:** ⊘ Donate blood until 6 mo after discontinuation of this drug **Interactions:** ↑ Effects w/ cimetidine, ciprofloxacin, diltiazem, ketoconazole, ritonavir, verapamil **Labs:** ↓ PSA levels **NIPE:** ⊘ Handling by PRG women, take w/o regard to food

Echothiophate Iodine (Phospholine Ophthalmic) Uses: *Glaucoma* Action: Cholinesterase inhibitor **Dose:** 1 gt eye(s) bid w/ one dose hs **Caution:** [C, ?] **Contra:** Active uveal inflammation or any inflammatory Dz of iris/ciliary body; glaucoma associated w/ iridocyclitis **Supplied:** Powder to reconstitute 1.5 mg/0.03%; 3 mg/ 0.06%; 6.25 mg/0.125%; 12.5 mg/0.25% **SE:** Local irritation, myopia, blurred vision, hypotension, bradycardia **Interactions:** ↑ Effects w/ cholinesterase inhibitors, pilocarpine, succinylcholine, carbamate or organophosphate insecticides; ↑ effects of cocaine; ↓ effects w/ anticholinergics, atropine, cyclopentolate, ophthalmic adrenocorticoids **NIPE:** ⊘ Drug 2 wk before surgery if succinylcholine is to be administered, keep drug refrigerated, monitor for lens opacities

Econazole (Spectazole) Uses: *Tinea, cutaneous *Candida*, & tinea versicolor infections* Action: Topical antifungal **Dose:** Apply to areas bid (daily for tinea versicolor) for 2–4 wk **Caution:** [C, ?] **Contra:** Component sensitivity **Supplied:** Topical cream 1% **SE:** Local irritation, pruritus, erythema **Notes:** Symptom/clinical improvement seen early in Rx, must carry out course of therapy to ⊘ recurrence **Interactions:** ↓ Effects w/ corticosteroids **NIPE:** Topical use only, ⊘ eye area

Edrophonium (Tensilon) Uses: *Diagnosis of MyG; acute MyG crisis; curare antagonist* Action: Anticholinesterase **Dose:** *Adults.* Test for MyG: 2 mg IV in 1 min; if tolerated, give 8 mg IV; + test is brief ↑ in strength. *Peds.* Test for MyG: Total dose 0.2 mg/kg; 0.04 mg/kg test dose; if no Rxn, give remainder in 1-mg increments to 10 mg max; ↓ in renal impairment **Caution:** [C, ?] **Contra:** GI or GU obstruction; hypersensitivity to sulfite **Supplied:** Inj 10 mg/mL **SE:** N/V/D, excessive salivation, stomach cramps, ↑ aminotransferases **Notes:** Can cause severe cholinergic effects; keep atropine available **Interactions:** ↑ Effects w/ tacrine; ↑ cardiac effects w/ digoxin; ↑ effects of neostigmine, pyridostigmine, succinylcholine, jaborandi tree, pill-bearing spurge; ↓ effects w/ corticosteroids, procainamide, quinidine **Labs:** ↑ AST, ALT, serum amylase **NIPE:** ↑ Risk uterine irritability & premature labor in PRG Pts near term

Efalizumab (Raptiva) **WARNING:** Associated w/ serious infections, malignancy, thrombocytopenia **Uses:** Chronic moderate to severe plaque psoriasis **Action:** Monoclonal antibody **Dose:** *Adults.* 0.7 mg/kg SQ conditioning dose, followed by 1 mg/kg/wk; single doses should not exceed 200 mg **Caution:** [C, +/–] **Contra:** Admin of most vaccines **Supplied:** 125-mg vial **SE:** First-dose Rxn, HA, worsening psoriasis, ↑ LFT, immunosuppressive-related Rxns (see warning) **Notes:** Minimize first-dose Rxn by administering conditioning dose; monitor plts monthly, then every 3 mo & Rx progresses; Pts may be trained in self-admin **Interactions:** ↑ Risk of infection & malignancy with immunosuppressive agents; ↓ immune response with live virus vaccines; **Labs:** ↑ Lymphocyte **NIPE:** Reconstituted soln may be stored for 8 h; monitor for bleeding gums & bruising

Efavirenz (Sustiva) **Uses:** *HIV infections* **Action:** Antiretroviral; non-nucleoside RTI **Dose:** 600 mg/d PO q hs. *Peds.* See insert; ⊘ high-fat meals **Caution:** [C, ?] CDC recommends HIV-infected mothers not breast-feed due to risk of transmission of HIV to infant **Contra:** Component sensitivity **Supplied:** Caps 50, 100, 200 mg **SE:** Somnolence, vivid dreams, dizziness, rash, N/V/D **Notes:** Monitor LFT, cholesterol **Interactions:** ↑ Effects w/ ritonavir; ↑ effects of CNS depressants, ergot derivatives, midazolam, ritonavir, simvastatin, triazolam, warfarin; ↓ effects w/ carbamazepine, phenobarbital, rifabutin, rifampin, saquinavir, St. John's wort; ↓ effects of amprenavir, carbamazepine, clarithromycin, indinavir, phenobarbital, saquinavir, warfarin; may alter effectiveness of oral contraceptive **Labs:** ↑ AST, ALT, amylase, total cholesterol, triglycerides; false + urine cannabinoid test **NIPE:** ⊘ High–fat foods, take w/o regard to food, use barrier contraception

Emedastine (Emadine) **Uses:** *Allergic conjunctivitis* **Action:** Antihistamine; selective H_1-antagonist **Dose:** 1 gt in eye(s) up to qid **Caution:** [B, ?] **Contra:** Hypersensitivity to ingredients (preservatives benzalkonium, tromethamine) **Supplied:** 0.05% soln **SE:** HA, blurred vision, burning/stinging, corneal infiltrates/staining, dry eyes, foreign body sensation, hyperemia, keratitis, tearing, pruritus, rhinitis, sinusitis, asthenia, bad taste, dermatitis, discomfort **Notes:** ⊘ Use contact lenses if eyes are red **NIPE:** ⊘ Wear soft contact lens for 15 min after use

Emtricitabine (Emtriva) **WARNING:** Class warning for lipodystrophy, lactic acidosis, & severe hepatomegaly **Uses:** HIV-1 infection **Action:** Nucleoside RT inhibitor (NRTI) **Dose:** 200 mg PO daily; ↓ dose for renal impairment. **Caution:** [B, –] **Contra:** Component sensitivity **Supplied:** 200 mg caps **SE:** HA, diarrhea, nausea, rash **Notes:** Rare hyperpigmentation of feet & hands; posttreatment exacerbation of hepatitis; first NRTI w/ once-daily dosing **Interactions:** None noted w/ additional NRTIs **NIPE:** Take w/o regard to food, causes redistribution and accumulation of body fat; take w/ other antiretrovirals; not a cure for HIV or prevention of opportunistic infections

Enalapril (Vasotec) **Uses:** *HTN, CHF, LVD.* DN **Action:** ACEI **Dose:** *Adults.* 2.5–40 mg/d PO; 1.25 mg IV q6h. *Peds.* 0.05–0.08 mg/kg/dose PO q12–24h; ↓ dose in renal impairment **Caution** [C (1st tri; D 2nd & 3rd tri), +] Use w/ NSAIDs, K suppls **Contra:** Bilateral renal artery stenosis, angioedema **Supplied:** Tabs 2.5, 5, 10, 20 mg; IV 1.25 mg/mL (1, 2 mL) **SE:** Symptomatic ↓ BP w/ initial dose (especially w/ concomitant diuretics), ↑ K⁺, nonproductive cough, angioedema **Notes:** Monitor Cr; DC diuretic for 2–3 d prior to initiation **Interactions:** ↑ Effects w/ loop diuretics; ↑ risk of cough w/ capsaicin; ↑ effects of α-blockers, insulin, Li; ↑ risk of hyperkalemia w/ K suppl, K-sparing diuretics, salt substitutes, trimethoprim; ↓ effects w/ ASA, NSAIDs, rifampin **Labs:** May cause ↑ serum K⁺, direct Coombs' test, false + urine acetone **NIPE:** Several weeks needed for full hypotensive effect

Enfuvirtide (Fuzeon) **WARNING:** Rarely causes hypersensitivity; never rechallenge Pt **Uses:** *Combination w/ antiretroviral agents for Rx of HIV-1 infection in Rx-experienced Pts w/ evidence of viral replication despite ongoing antiretroviral therapy* **Action:** Fusion inhibitor **Dose:** 90 mg (1 mL) SQ bid in upper arm, anterior thigh, or abdomen **Caution:** [B, –] **Contra:** Previous hypersensitivity to drug **Supplied:** 90 mg/mL on reconstitution; dispensed as Pt convenience kit w/ monthly supplies **SE:** Inj site Rxns (in nearly all Pts); pneumonia, diarrhea, nausea, fatigue, insomnia, peripheral neuropathy **Notes:** Rotate inj site; available only via restricted drug distribution system; must be immediately administered on reconstitution or refrigerated for up to 24 h prior to use **Interactions:** None noted w/ other antiretrovirals **NIPE:** Does not cure HIV; does not ↓ risk of transmission or prevent opportunistic infections; take w/o regard to food

Enoxaparin (Lovenox) **WARNING:** Recent or anticipated epidural/ spinal anesthesia ↑s risk of spinal/epidural hematoma w/ subsequent paralysis **Uses:** *Prevention & Rx of DVT; Rx PE; unstable angina & non-Q-wave MI* **Action:** LMW heparin **Dose:** *Adults.* Prevention: 30 mg SQ bid or 40 mg SQ q24h. *DVT/PE Rx:* 1 mg/kg SQ q12h or 1.5 mg/kg SQ q24h. *Angina:* 1 mg/kg SQ q12h. *Peds.* Prevention: 0.5 mg/kg SQ q12h. *DVT/PE Rx:* 1mg/kg SQ q12h; ↓ or ⊘ w/ severe renal impairment **Caution** [B, ?] ⊘ for thromboprophylaxis in prosthetic heart valves **Contra:** Active bleeding, HIT antibody + **Supplied:** Inj 10 mg/0.1 mL (30-, 40-, 60-, 80-, 100-, 120-, & 150-mg syringes) **SE:** Bleeding, hemorrhage, bruising, thrombocytopenia, pain/hematoma at inj site, ↑ AST/ALT **Notes:** Does not significantly affect bleeding time, plt Fxn, PT, or aPTT; monitor plts, bleeding; may monitor anti-factor Xa **Interactions:** ↑ Bleeding effects w/ ASA, anticoagulants, cephalosporins, NSAIDs, penicillin, chamomile, garlic, ginger, ginkgo biloba, feverfew, horse chestnut **Labs:** ↑ AST, ALT **NIPE:** No need to monitor aPTT, admin deep ⊘ IM

Entacapone (Comtan) **Uses:** *Parkinson's Dz* **Action:** Selective & reversible carboxymethyl transferase inhibitor **Dose:** 200 mg w/ each levodopa/carbidopa dose; max 1600 mg/d; ↓ levodopa/carbidopa dose by 25% if levodopa dose >800 mg **Caution:** [C, ?] Hepatic impairment **Contra:** Concurrent use w/ nonselective MAOI **Supplied:** Tabs 200 mg **SE:** Dyskinesia, hyperkinesia, nausea, dizziness, hallucinations, orthostatic hypotension, brown-orange urine, diarrhea **Notes:** Monitor LFT; **Interactions:** ↑ Effects w/ ampicillin, choramphenicol, cholestyramine, erythromycin, MAOIs, probenecid, rifampin; ↑ risk of arrhythmias & HTN w/ bitolterol, dopamine, dobutamine, epinephrine, isoetharine, methyldopa, norepinephrine **NIPE:** ⊘ DC abruptly, breast-feed

Ephedrine **Uses:** *Acute bronchospasm, bronchial asthma, nasal congestion,* ↓ BP, narcolepsy, enuresis, & MyG **Action:** Sympathomimetic; stimulates α- & β-receptors; bronchodilator **Dose:** *Adults.* 25–50 mg IM or IV q10min to a max of 150 mg/d or 25–50 mg PO q3–4h PRN. *Peds.* 0.2–0.3 mg/kg/dose IM/IV q4–6h PRN **Caution:** [C, ?/–] **Contra:** Cardiac arrhythmias; angle-closure glaucoma **Supplied:** Inj 50 mg/mL; caps 25 mg; nasal spray 0.25% **SE:** CNS stimulation (nervousness, anxiety, trembling), tachycardia, arrhythmia, HTN, xerostomia, painful urination **Notes:** Protect from light; monitor BP, HR, urinary output; can cause false + amphetamine EMIT; take last dose 4–6h before hs **Interactions:** ↑ Effects w/ acetazolamide, antacids, MAOIs, TCAs, urinary alkalinizers; ↑ effects of sympathomimetics; ↓ response w/ diuretics, methyldopa, reserpine, urinary acidifiers; ↓ effects of antihypertensives, BBs, dexamethasone, guanethidine **Labs:** False ↑ urine amino acids **NIPE:** ⊘ EtOH, store away from light/heat

Epinephrine (Adrenalin, Sus-Phrine, EpiPen, others) **Uses:** *Cardiac arrest, anaphylactic Rxn, bronchospasm, open-angle glaucoma* **Action:** β-adrenergic agonist, some α-effects **Dose:** *Adults.* ACLS: 0.5–1 mg (5–10 mL of 1:10,000) IV q 5 min to response. *Anaphylaxis:* 0.3–0.5 mL SQ of 1:1000 dilution, may repeat q5–15min to a max of 1 mg/dose & 5 mg/d. *Asthma:* 0.1–0.5 mL SQ of 1:1000 dilution, repeated at 20-min–4-h intervals or 1 inhal (met-dose) repeat in 1–2 min or susp 0.1–0.3 mL SQ for extended effect. *Peds.* ACLS: 1st dose 0.1 mL/kg IV of 1:10,000 dilution, then 0.1 mL/kg IV of 1:1000 dilution q3–5min to response. *Anaphylaxis:* 0.001mg/kg SQ q15min ×2 doses, then q4h PRN. *Asthma:* 0.01 mL/kg SQ of 1:1000 dilution q8–12h. **Caution:** [C, ?] ↓ bronchodilation w/ BBs **Contra:** Cardiac arrhythmias, angle-closure glaucoma **Supplied:** Inj 1:1000, 1:2000, 1:10,000, 1:100,000; susp for inj 1:200; aerosol 220 μg/spray; soln for inhal 1% **SE:** CV (tachycardia, HTN, vasoconstriction), CNS stimulation (nervousness, anxiety, trembling), ↓ renal blood flow **Notes:** Can give via ET tube if no central line (2–2.5 × IV dose) **Interactions:** ↑ HTN effects w/ α-blockers, BBs, ergot alkaloids, furazolidone, MAOIs; ↑ cardiac effects w/ antihistamines, cardiac glycosides, levodopa, thyroid hormones, TCAs; ↑ effects of sympathomimetics; ↓ effects of diuretics, guanethidine, hypoglycemics, methyldopa **Labs:** ↑ Serum bilirubin, glucose, & uric acid, urine catecholamines **NIPE:** ⊘ OTC inhalation drugs

Epirubicin (Ellence) **Uses:** *Adjuvant therapy w/ evidence of axillary node tumor involvement following resection of primary breast CA* **Actions:** An anthracycline cytotoxic agent **Dose:** Refer to specific protocols; ↓ dose w/ hepatic impairment. **Caution:** [D, –] **Contra:** Baseline neutrophil count < 1500 cells/mm³.

severe myocardial insufficiency, recent MI, severe arrhythmias, severe hepatic dysfunction, previous Rx w/ anthracyclines up to max cumulative dose **Supplied:** Inj 50 mg/25 mL, 200 mg/100 mL **SE:** Mucositis, N/V/D, alopecia, myelosuppression, cardiotoxicity, secondary AML, severe tissue necrosis if extravasation occurs **Interactions:** ↑ Effects with cimetidine; ↑ effects of cytotoxic drugs, radiation therapy; ↑ risk of HF with CCBs, trastuzumab; incompatible chemically with fluorouracil, heparin **Labs:** Monitor before & after treatment AST, total bilirubin, creatinine, CBC, LVEF **NIPE:** ⊘ Handle if PRG breast-feeding; urine reddish up to 2 d after treatment, use contraception during treatment, burning at inj site indicates infiltration, menstruation may cease permanently

Eplerenone (Inspra) **Uses:** *HTN* **Action:** Selective aldosterone antagonist **Dose:** **Adults:** 50 mg PO daily–bid, doses >100 mg/d no benefit w/ ↑ hyperkalemia; ↓ dose to 25 mg PO qd if giving w/ weak CYP3A4 inhibitors **Caution:** [B, +/–] Use of CYP3A4 inhibitors (ketoconazole, itraconazole, erythromycin, fluconazole, verapamil, saquinavir); monitor K^+ w/ ACEIs, ARBs, NSAIDs, K-sparing diuretics; grapefruit juice, St. John's wort **Contra:** K^+ >5.5 mEq/L; NIDDM w/ microalbuminuria; SCr >2 mg/dL (males), >1.8 mg/dL (females); CrCl <50 mL/min; concurrent K suppls/K-sparing diuretics **Supplied:** Tabs 25, 50, 100 mg **SE:** Hypertriglyceridemia, ↑ K^+, HA, dizziness, gynecomastia, hypercholesterolemia, diarrhea, orthostatic hypotension **Notes:** May take 4 wk to see full effect **Interactions:** ↑ Risk hyperkalemia w/ ACEIs; ↑ risk of toxic effects w/ azole antifungals, erythromycin, saquinavir, verapamil, ↑ effects of Li; ↓ effects w/ NSAIDs **NIPE:** ⊘ High-K foods, may cause reversible breast pain or enlargement w/ use

Epoetin Alfa [Erythropoietin, EPO] (Epogen, Procrit) **Uses:** *Anemia associated w/ CRF,* zidovudine Rx in HIV-infected Pts, CA chemotherapy; reduction in transfusions associated w/ surgery **Action:** Induces erythropoiesis **Dose:** **Adults & Peds.** 50–150 units/kg IV/SQ 3×/wk; adjust the dose q4–6wk PRN. *Surgery:* 300 units/kg/d × 10 d prior to surgery to 4 d after; decrease dose if Hct approaches 36%/Hgb, or ↑ >4 points in 2-wk period **Caution:** [C, +] **Contra:** Uncontrolled HTN **Supplied:** Inj 2000, 3000, 4000, 10,000, 20,000, 40,000 units/mL **SE:** HTN, HA, fatigue, fever, tachycardia, N/V **Notes:** Store in refrigerator; monitor baseline & posttreatment Hct/Hgb, BP, ferritin **Interactions:** None noted **Labs:** ↑ WBCs, plts **NIPE:** Monitor for access line clotting, ⊘ shake vial

Epoprostenol (Flolan) **Uses:** *Pulmonary HTN* **Action:** Dilates pulmonary & systemic arterial vascular beds; inhibits plt aggregation **Dose:** Initial 2 ng/kg/min; ↑ by 2 ng/kg/min q15min until dose-limiting SE (CP, dizziness, N/V, HA, hypotension, flushing); IV cont inf 4 ng/kg/min less than maximum-tolerated rate; adjustments based on response; see package insert guidelines **Caution:** [B, ?] ↑ toxicity w/diuretics, vasodilators, acetate in dialysis fluids, anticoagulants **Contra:** Chronic use in CHF 2nd-deg severe LVSD **Supplied:** Inj 0.5, 1.5 mg **SE:** Flushing, tachycardia, CHF, fever, chills, nervousness, HA, N/V/D, jaw pain, flu-like Sxs **Notes:** Abrupt DC can cause rebound pulmonary HTN; monitor bleeding if using other antiplt/anticoagulants; watch hypotensive effects w/ other vasodilators/diuretics **Interactions:** ↑ Risk of bleeding w/ anticoagulants, antiplts; ↑ effects of digoxin; ↓ BP w/ antihypertensives, diuretics, vasodilators **NIPE:** ⊘ Mix or administer w/ other drugs

Eprosartan (Teveten) **Uses:** *HTN,* DN, CHF **Action:** ARB **Dose:** 400–800 mg/d single dose or bid **Caution:** [C (1st tri); D (2nd & 3rd tri), –] Li, ↑ K+ w/ K-sparing diuretics/suppls/high-dose trimethoprim **Contra:** Bilateral renal artery stenosis, 1st-deg aldosteronism **Supplied:** Tabs 400, 600 mg **SE:** Fatigue, depression, hypertriglyceridemia, URI, UTI, abdominal pain, rhinitis/pharyngitis/cough **Interactions:** ↑ Risk of hyperkalemia w/ K-sparing diuretics, K suppls, trimethoprim; ↑ effects of Li **Labs:** ↑ ALT, AST, alkaline phosphatase, BUN, creatinine; ↓ Hmg **NIPE:** Monitor LFTs, CBC & differential, renal Fxn; ⊘ PRG, breast-feeding

Eptifibatide (Integrilin) **Uses:** *ACS, PCI* **Action:** Glycoprotein IIb/IIIa inhibitor **Dose:** 180 μg/kg IV bolus, then 2 μg/kg/min cont inf; ↓ dose in renal impairment (SCr >2 mg/dL, <4 mg/dL: 135 μg/kg bolus & 0.5 μg/kg/min inf) **Caution:** [B, ?] Monitor bleeding w/ other anticoagulants **Contra:** Other GPIIb/IIIa inhibitors, Hx abnormal bleeding, hemorrhagic stroke (w/in 30 d), severe HTN, major surgery (w/in 6 wk), plt count <100,000 cells/mm³, renal dialysis **Supplied:** Inj 0.75, 2 mg/mL **SE:** Bleeding, hypotension, inj site Rxn, thrombocytopenia **Notes:** Monitor bleeding, coags, plts, SCr, activated coagulation time (ACT) w/ prothrombin consumption index (maintain ACT between 200–300 s) **Interactions:** ↑ Bleeding w/ ASA, cephalosporins, clopidogrel, heparin, NSAIDs, thrombolytics, ticlopidine, warfarin, evening primrose oil, feverfew, garlic, ginger, ginkgo biloba, ginseng, grapeseed extract

Ertapenem (Invanz) **Uses:** *Complicated intraabdominal, acute pelvic, & skin infections, pyelonephritis, community-acquired pneumonia* **Action:** A carbapenem; β-lactam antibiotic, inhibits cell wall synthesis. *Spectrum:* Good gram(+/–) & anaerobic coverage, but not *Pseudomonas,* penicillin-resistant pneumococci, MRSA, *Enterococcus,* β-lactamase(+) *H. influenza, Mycoplasma, Chlamydia* **Dose:** *Adults.* 1 g IM/IV daily; 500 mg/d in CrCl <30 mL/min **Caution:** [C, ?/–] Probenecid ↓ renal clearance of ertapenem **Contra:** <18 y, penicillin allergy **Supplied:** Inj 1 g/vial **SE:** HA, N/V/D, inj site Rxns, thrombocytosis, ↑ LFTs **Notes:** Can give IM × 7 d, IV × 14 d; 137 mg Na⁺(6 mEg)/g ertapenem **Interactions:** ↑ Effects w/ probenecid; **Labs:** ↑ AST, ALT, serum alkaline phosphatase, bilirubin, glucose, creatinine, PT, RBCs, urine WBCs **NIPE:** Monitor for superinfection

Erythromycin (E-Mycin, E.E.S., Ery-Tab) **Uses:** *Bacterial infections; bowel decontamination*; GI motility; *acne vulgaris* **Action:** Bacteriostatic; interferes w/ protein synthesis. *Spectrum:* Group A streptococci (S. pyogenes), S. pneumoniae, N. meningitides, N. gonorrhea (in penicillin-allergic Pts), Legionella, M. pneumoniae **Dose:** *Adults.* Base 250–500 mg PO q6–12h or ethylsuccinate 400–800 mg q6–12h; 500 mg–1 g IV q6h. *Prokinetic:* 250 mg PO tid 30 mins ac. *Peds.* 30–50 mg/kg/d PO ÷ q6–8h or 20–40 mg/kg/d IV ÷ q6h, max 2 g/d **Caution:** [B, +] ↑ toxicity of carbamazepine, cyclosporine, digoxin, methylpred-nisolone, theophylline, felodipine, warfarin, simvastatin/lovastatin **Contra:** Hepatic impairment, preexisting liver Dz (estolate), use w/ pimozide **Supplied:** *Powder for inj as lactobionate:* 500 mg, 1 g. *Base:* Tabs 250, 333, 500 mg; caps 250 mg. *Estolate:* Susp 125, 250 mg/5 mL. *Stearate:* Tabs 250, 500 mg. *Ethylsuc-cinate:* Chew tabs 200 mg; tabs 400 mg; susp 200, 400 mg/5 mL **SE:** HA, abdominal pain, N/V/D; [QT prolongation, torsades de pointes, ventricular arrhythmias/tachycardias (rarely)]; cholestatic jaundice (estolate) **Notes:** 400 mg ethylsuccinate = 250 mg base/state/estolate; take w/ food to minimize GI upset; lactobionate salt contains benzyl EtOH (caution in neonates) **Interactions:** ↑ Effects w/ ampre-navir, indinavir, ritonavir, saquinavir, grapefruit juice; ↑ effects of alprazolam, ben-zodiazepines, buspirone, carbamazepine, clozapine, colchicines, cyclosporine, digoxin, felodipine, lovastatin, midazolam, quinidine, sildenafil, simvastatin, tacrolimus, theophylline, triazolam, valproic acid; ↑ QT w/ astemizole, cisapride; ↓ effects of penicillin, zafirlukast **Labs:** False ↑ AST, ALT, serum bilirubin, urine amino acids, false ↓ folate assay **NIPE:** Take w/ food if GI upset, monitor for su-perinfection & ototoxicity

Erythromycin & Benzoyl Peroxide (Benzamycin) Uses: Topical
Rx of *acne vulgaris* **Action:** Macrolide antibiotic w/ keratolytic **Dose:** Apply bid (AM & PM) **Caution:** [C, ?] **Contra:** Component sensitivity **Supplied:** Gel ery-thromycin 30 mg/benzoyl peroxide 50 mg/g **SE:** Local irritation, dryness

Erythromycin & Sulfisoxazole (Eryzole, Pediazole) Uses:
*Upper & lower resp tract; bacterial infections; otitis media in children due to *H. influenzae** infections in penicillin-allergic Pts **Action:** Macrolide antibiotic w/ sulfonamide **Dose:** Based on erythromycin content. *Adults.* 400 mg ery-thromycin/1200 mg sulfisoxazole PO q6h. *Peds.* >2 mo. 40–50 mg/kg/d ery-thromycin & 150 mg/kg/d sulfisoxazole PO ÷ q6h; max 2 g/d erythromycin or 6 g/d sulfisoxazole × 10 d; ↓ in renal impairment **Caution:** [C (D if given near term), +] PO anticoagulants, MRX, hypoglycemics, phenytoin, cyclosporine **Contra:** In-fants <2 mo **Supplied:** Susp erythromycin ethylsuccinate 200 mg/sulfisoxazole 600 mg/5 mL (100, 150, 200 mL) **SE:** GI disturbance **Additional Interactions:** ↑ Effects of sulfonamides w/ ASA, diuretics, NSAIDs, probenecid **Labs:** False + urine protein **NIPE:** ↑ Risk of photosensitivity—use sunscreen, ↑ fluid intake

Erythromycin, Ophthalmic (Ilotycin Ophthalmic) Uses: *Con-
junctival/corneal infections* **Action:** Macrolide antibiotic **Dose:** ½ in. bid **Caution:** [B, +] **Contra:** Hypersensitivity to erythromycin **Supplied:** 0.5% oint **SE:** Local irritation **NIPE:** May cause burning, stinging, blurred vision

Erythromycin, Topical (A/T/S, Eryderm, Erycette, T-Stat)
Uses: *Acne vulgaris* **Action:** Macrolide antibiotic **Dose:** Wash & dry area, apply

2% product over area bid **Caution:** [B, +] **Contra:** Component sensitivity **Supplied:** Soln 1.5%, 2%; gel 2%; impregnated pads & swabs 2% **SE:** Local irritation

Escitalopram (Lexapro) **WARNING:** Closely monitor for worsening depression or emergence of suicidality, particularly in pediatric Pts **Uses:** Depression, anxiety **Action:** SSRI **Dose:** *Adults.* 10–20 mg PO daily; 10 mg/d in elderly & hepatic impairment **Caution:** [C, +/–] ↑ Risk of serotonin syndrome w/ other SSRI, tramadol, linezolid, sumatriptan **Contra:** W/ or w/in 14 d of MAOI **Supplied:** Tabs 5, 10, 20 mg; soln 1 mg/mL **SE:** N/V/D, sweating, insomnia, dizziness, xerostomia, sexual dysfunction **Interactions:** ↑ Risk of serotonin syndrome w/ linezolid; ↑ risk of bleeding w/ anticoagulants, ASA, NSAIDs; may ↑ CNS effects w/ CNS depressants **NIPE:** ⊘ DC abruptly; may take up to 2–4 wk for full effects; take w/o regard to food

Esmolol (Brevibloc) **Uses:** *SVT & noncompensatory sinus tachycardia, AF/flutter* **Action:** β_1-Adrenergic blocker; class II antiarrhythmic **Dose:** *Adults & Peds.* Initiate Rx w/ 500 µg/kg load over 1 min, then 50 µg/kg/min × 4 min; if inadequate response, repeat the loading dose & maint inf of 100 µg/kg/min × 4 min; titrate by repeating load, then incremental ↑ in the maint dose of 50 µg/kg/min for 4 min until desired heart rate reached or hypotension; average dose 100 µg/kg/min **Caution:** [C (1st tri; D 2nd or 3rd tri), ?] **Contra:** Sinus bradycardia, heart block, uncompensated CHF, cardiogenic shock, hypotension **Supplied:** Inj 10, 250 mg/mL; premix inf 10 mg/mL **SE:** Hypotension (↓ or discontinuing inf reverses hypotension in 30 min); bradycardia, diaphoresis, dizziness, pain on inj **Notes:** Hemodynamic effects back to baseline w/in 20–30 min after DC inf **Interaction:** ↑ Effects w/ verapamil; ↑ effects of digoxin, antihypertensives, nitrates; ↑ HTN w/ amphetamines, cocaine, ephedrine, epinephrine, MAOIs, norepinephrine, phenylephrine, pseudoephedrine; ↓ effects of glucagons, insulin, hypoglycemics, theophylline; ↓ effects w/ NSAIDs, thyroid hormones **Labs:** ↑ Glucose, cholesterol **NIPE:** Monitor BS of Pts w/ DM

Esomeprazole (Nexium) **Uses:** *Short-term (4–8 wk) Rx of erosive esophagitis/GERD; Rx of H. pylori infection in combination w/ antibiotics* **Action:** Proton pump inhibitor, ↓ gastric acid production **Dose:** *Adults.* GERD/erosive gastritis: 20–40 mg/d PO × 4–8 wk; *Maint:* 20 mg/d PO. *H. pylori infection:* 40 mg/d PO, plus clarithromycin 500 mg PO bid & amoxicillin 1000 mg/bid for 10 d **Caution:** [B, ?/–] **Contra:** Component sensitivity **Supplied:** Caps 20, 40 mg **SE:** HA, diarrhea, abdominal pain **Notes:** ⊘ Chew; may open capsule & sprinkle on applesauce; take on empty stomach 1 h ac

Estazolam (ProSom) [C-IV] **Uses:** *Short-term management of insomnia* **Action:** Benzodiazepine **Dose:** 1–2 mg PO qhs PRN; ↓ in hepatic impairment/elderly/debilitated **Caution:** [X, –] ↑ effects w/ CNS depressants **Contra:** PRG **Supplied:** Tabs 1, 2 mg **SE:** Somnolence, weakness, palpitations **Notes:** May cause psychological/physical dependence; ⊘ abrupt DC after prolonged use **Inter-**

actions: ↑ Effects w/ amoxicillin, clarithromycin; ↑ effects of diazepam, phenytoin, warfarin; ↓ effects w/ food; ↓ effects of azole antifungals, digoxin **Labs:** ↑ LFTs, bilirubin, SCr, uric acid, TSH; ↓ Hgb, WBC, plts, K⁺, Na⁺, thyroxine **NIPE:** Take at least 1 h ac

Esterified Estrogens (Estratab, Menest) WARNING: ⊘ Use in the prevention of CV Dz

Uses: *Vasomotor Sxs or vulvar/vaginal atrophy associated w/ menopause*; female hypogonadism **Action:** Estrogen suppl **Dose:** *Menopause:* 0.3–1.25 mg/d, cyclically 3 wk on, 1 wk off. *Hypogonadism:* 2.5–7.5 mg/d PO × 20 d, off × 10 d **Caution:** [X, –] **Contra:** Genital bleeding of unknown cause, breast CA, estrogen-dependent tumors, thromboembolic disorders, thrombophlebitis, recent MI, PRG, severe hepatic Dz **Supplied:** Tabs 0.3, 0.625, 1.25, 2.5 mg **SE:** Nausea, HA, bloating, breast enlargement/tenderness, edema, venous thromboembolism, hypertriglyceridemia, gallbladder Dz **Notes:** Use at lowest dose for shortest time; refer to Women's Health Initiatives (WHI) data **Interactions:** ↑ Effects of corticosteroids, cyclosporine, TCAs, theophylline, caffeine, tobacco; ↓ effects w/ barbiturates, phenytoin, rifampin; ↓ effects of anticoagulants, hypoglycemics, insulin, tamoxifen **Labs:** ↑ Prothrombin & factors VII, VIII, IX, X, plt aggregability, thyroid-binding globulin, T₄, triglycerides; ↓ antithrombin III, folate **NIPE:** ⊘ PRG, breast-feeding

Esterified Estrogens + Methyltestosterone (Estratest, Estratest HS)

Uses: *Vasomotor Sxs*; postpartum breast engorgement **Action:** Estrogen & androgen suppl **Dose:** 1 tab/d × 3 wk, 1 wk off **Caution:** [X, –] **Contra:** Genital bleeding of unknown cause, breast CA, estrogen-dependent tumors, thromboembolic disorders, thrombophlebitis, recent MI, PRG **Supplied:** Tabs (estrogen/methyltestosterone) 0.625 mg/1.25 mg (hs), 1.25 mg/2.5 mg **SE:** Nausea, HA, bloating, breast enlargement/tenderness, edema, ↑ triglycerides, venous thromboembolism, gallbladder Dz **Notes:** Use at lowest dose for shortest time. See Esterified Estrogens, page 110. **Additional Interactions:** ↑ Effects of insulin; ↓ effects of oral anticoagulants

Estradiol (Estrace)

Uses: *Atrophic vaginitis, vasomotor Sxs associated w/ menopause, osteoporosis* **Action:** Estrogen suppl **Dose:** *PO:* 1–2 mg/d, adjust PRN to control Sxs. *Vaginal cream:* 2–4 g/d × 2 wk, then 1 g 1–3×/wk **Caution:** [X, –] **Contra:** Genital bleeding of unknown cause, breast CA, estrogen-dependent tumors, thromboembolic disorders, thrombophlebitis; recent MI; hepatic impairment **Supplied:** Tabs 0.5, 1, 2 mg; vaginal cream 0.1 mg/g **SE:** Nausea, HA, bloating, breast enlargement/tenderness, edema, ↑ triglycerides, venous thromboembolism, gallbladder Dz **Interactions:** ↑ Effects w/ grapefruit juice; ↑ effects of corticosteroids, cyclosporine, TCAs, theophylline, caffeine, tobacco; ↓ effects w/ barbiturates, carbamazepine, phenytoin, primidone, rifampin; ↓ effects of clofibrate, hypoglycemics, insulin, tamoxifen, warfarin **Labs:** ↑ Prothrombin & factors VII, VIII, IX, X, plt aggregability, thyroid-binding globulin, T₄, triglycerides; ↓ antithrombin III, folate **NIPE:** ⊘ PRG, breast-feeding

Estradiol Cypionate & Medroxyprogesterone Acetate (Lunelle) **Warning:** Cigarette smoking ↑ risk of serious CV side effects from contraceptives containing estrogen. This risk ↑ w/ age & w/ heavy smoking (> 15 cigarettes/d) & is quite marked in women > 35 y. Women who use Lunelle should be strongly advised not to smoke **Uses:** *Contraceptive* **Action:** Estrogen & progestin **Dose:** 0.5 mL IM (deltoid, ant thigh, buttock) monthly, ⊘ exceed 33 d **Caution:** [X, M] HTN, gallbladder Dz, ↑ lipids, migraines, sudden HA, valvular heart Dz w/ complications **Contra:** PRG, heavy smokers >35 y, DVT, PE, cerebro-/CV Dz, estrogen-dependent neoplasm, undiagnosed abnormal uterine bleeding, hepatic tumors, cholestatic jaundice **Supplied:** Estradiol cypionate (5 mg), medroxyprogesterone acetate (25 mg) single-dose vial or prefilled syringe (0.5 mL) **SE:** Arterial thromboembolism, HTN, cerebral hemorrhage, MI, amenorrhea, acne, breast tenderness **Notes:** Start w/in 5 d of menstruation. Eee Estradiol. **Additional Interactions:** ↓ Effects w/ aminoglutethimide

Estradiol, Transdermal (Estraderm, Climara, Vivelle) **Uses:** *Severe menopausal vasomotor Sxs; female hypogonadism* **Action:** Estrogen suppl **Dose:** 0.1 mg/d patch 1–2×/wk depending on product; adjust PRN to control Sxs **Caution:** [X, –] (See estradiol) **Contra:** PRG, undiagnosed genital bleeding, carcinoma of breast, estrogen-dependent tumors, Hx of thrombophlebitis, thrombosis, thromboembolic disorders associated w/ estrogen use **Supplied:** TD patches (deliver mg/24 h) 0.025, 0.0375, 0.05, 0.075, 0.1 **SE:** Nausea, bloating, breast enlargement/tenderness, edema, HA, hypertriglyceridemia, gallbladder Dz **Notes:** ⊘ Apply to breasts, place on trunk of body & rotate sites. See Estradiol. **Additional NIPE:** Rotate application sites

Estramustine Phosphate (Estracyt, Emcyt) **Uses:** *Advanced CAP* **Action:** Antimicrotubule agent; weak estrogenic & antiandrogenic activity **Dose:** 14 mg/kg/d in 3–4 ÷ doses; take on empty stomach, ⊘ take w/ milk/milk products **Caution:** [NA, not used in females] **Contra:** Active thrombophlebitis or thromboembolic disorders **Supplied:** Caps 140 mg **SE:** N/V, exacerbation of pre-existing CHF, thrombophlebitis, MI, PE, gynecomastia in 20–100% **Interactions:** ↓ Effects w/ antacids, Ca suppls, Ca-containing foods; ↓ effects of anticoagulants **NIPE:** Take on empty stomach, several wk may be needed for full effects, store in refrigerator

Estrogen, Conjugated (Premarin) **WARNING:** Should not be used for the prevention of CV Dz. The WHI reported ↑ risk of MI, stroke, breast CA, PE, & DVT when combined w/ methoxyprogesterone over 5 y of Rx; ↑ risk of endometrial CA **Uses:** *Moderate to severe menopausal vasomotor Sxs; atrophic vaginitis; palliative therapy of advanced prostatic carcinoma; prevention & Rx of estrogen deficiency-induced osteoporosis* **Action:** Hormonal replacement **Dose:** 0.3–1.25 mg/d PO cyclically; prostatic carcinoma requires 1.25–2.5 mg PO tid; **Caution:** [X, –] **Contra:** Severe hepatic impairment, genital bleeding of unknown cause, breast CA, estrogen-dependent tumors, thromboembolic disorders, thrombosis, thrombophlebitis, recent MI **Supplied:** Tabs 0.3, 0.625, 0.9, 1.25, 2.5 mg; inj 25 mg/mL **SE:** ↑ Risk of endometrial carcinoma, gallbladder Dz, thromboembolism, HA, & possibly breast CA; generic products not equivalent **Interactions:** ↑ Effects of corticosteroids, cyclosporine, TCAs, theophylline, tobacco; ↓ effects of anticoagulants, clofibrate; ↓ effects w/ barbiturates, carbamazepine, phenytoin, rifampin **Labs:** ↑ Prothrombin & factors VII, VIII, IX, X, plt aggregability, thyroid-binding globulin, T₄, triglycerides; ↓ antithrombin III, folate **NIPE:** ⊘ PRG, breast-feeding

Estrogen, Conjugated-Synthetic (Cenestin)   **Uses:** *Rx of moderate to severe vasomotor Sxs associated w/ menopause* **Action:** Hormonal replacement **Dose:** 0.625–1.25 mg PO qd **Caution:** [X, –] **Contra:** See estrogen, conjugated **Supplied:** Tabs 0.625, 0.9, 1.25 mg **SE:** Associated w/ an ↑ risk of endometrial CA, gallbladder Dz, thromboembolism, & possibly breast CA. See Estrogen, Conjugated, page 111

Estrogen, Conjugated + Medroxyprogesterone (Prempro, Premphase)   **WARNING:** Should not be used for the prevention of CV Dz; the WHI study reported ↑ risk of MI, stroke, breast CA, PE, & DVT over 5 y of Rx **Uses:** *Moderate to severe menopausal vasomotor Sxs; atrophic vaginits; prevention of postmenopausal osteoporosis* **Action:** Hormonal replacement **Dose:** Prempro 1 tab PO qd; Premphase 1 tab PO qd **Caution:** [X, –] **Contra:** Severe hepatic impairment, genital bleeding of unknown cause, breast CA, estrogen-dependent tumors, thromboembolic disorders, thrombosis, thrombophlebitis **Supplied:** (expressed as estrogen/medroxyprogesterone) Prempro: tabs 0.625/2.5, 0.625/5 mg; Premphase: tabs 0.625/0 (days 1–14) & 0.625/5 mg (days 15–28) **SE:** Gallbladder Dz, thromboembolism, HA, breast tenderness. See Estrogen, Conjugated. **Additional Interactions:** ↓ Effects w/ aminoglutethimide

Estrogen, Conjugated + Methylprogesterone (Premarin + Methylprogesterone)   **Uses:** *Menopausal vasomotor Sxs; osteoporosis* **Action:** Estrogen & androgen combination **Dose:** 1 tab/d **Caution:** [X, –] **Contra:** Severe hepatic impairment, genital bleeding of unknown cause, breast CA, estrogen-dependent tumors, thromboembolic disorders, thrombosis, thrombophlebitis **Supplied:** Tabs 0.625 mg estrogen, conjugated, & 2.5 or 5 mg of methylprogesterone **SE:** Nausea, bloating, breast enlargement/tenderness, edema, HA, hypertriglyceridemia, gallbladder Dz. See Estrogen, Conjugated, page 111

Estrogen, Conjugated + Methyltestosterone (Premarin + Methyltestosterone)   **Uses:** *Moderate to severe menopausal vasomotor Sxs*; postpartum breast engorgement **Action:** Estrogen & androgen combination **Dose:** 1 tab/d × 3 wk, then 1 wk off **Caution:** [X, –] **Contra:** Severe hepatic impairment, genital bleeding of unknown cause, breast CA, estrogen-dependent tumors, thromboembolic disorders, thrombosis, thrombophlebitis **Supplied:** Tabs (estrogen/methyltestosterone) 0.625 mg/5 mg, 1.25 mg/10 mg **SE:** Nausea, bloating, breast enlargement/tenderness, edema, HA, hypertriglyceridemia, gallbladder Dz. See Estrogen, Conjugated **Additional Interactions:** ↑ Effects of insulin

Etanercept (Enbrel) Uses: *Reduces Sxs of RA in Pts who have failed other DMARD (Dz-modifying antirheumatic drug),* Crohn's Dz **Action:** Binds TNF **Dose:** *Adults.* 25 mg SQ 2×/wk (separated by at least 72–96 h). *Peds 4–17 y.* 0.4 mg/kg SQ 2×/wk (max 25 mg) **Caution:** [B, ?] **Contra:** Active infection; caution in conditions that predispose to infection (ie, DM) **Supplied:** Inj 25 mg/vial **SE:** HA, rhinitis, inj site Rxn, URI, rhinitis **Interactions:** ↓ Response to live virus vaccine **NIPE:** Rotate inj sites, ◎ live vaccines

Ethambutol (Myambutol) Uses: *Pulmonary TB* & other mycobacterial infections, MAC **Action:** Inhibits RNA synthesis **Dose:** *Adults & Peds.* >12 y: 15–25 mg/kg/d PO as a single dose; ↓ dose in renal impairment, take w/ food, ◎ antacids **Caution:** [B, +] **Contra:** Optic neuritis **Supplied:** Tabs 100, 400 mg **SE:** HA, hyperuricemia, acute gout, abdominal pain, ↑ LFTs, optic neuritis, GI upset **Interactions:** ↑ Neurotoxicity w/ neurotoxic drugs; ↓ effects w/ Al salts **NIPE:** Monitor visual acuity

Ethinyl Estradiol (Estinyl, Feminone) Uses: *Menopausal vasomotor Sxs; female hypogonadism* **Action:** Estrogen suppl **Dose:** 0.02–1.5 mg/d ÷ daily–tid **Caution:** [X, –] **Contra:** Severe hepatic impairment; genital bleeding of unknown cause, breast CA, estrogen-dependent tumors, thromboembolic disorders, thrombosis, thrombophlebitis **Supplied:** Tabs 0.02, 0.05, 0.5 mg **SE:** Nausea, bloating, breast enlargement/tenderness, edema, HA, hypertriglyceridemia, gallbladder Dz **Interactions:** ↑ Effects of corticosteroids; ↓ effects w/ barbiturates, carbamazepine, hypoglycemics, insulin, phenytoin, primidone, rifampin, ↓ effects of anticoagulants, tamoxifen; **Labs:** ↑ Prothrombin & factors VII, VIII, IX, X, plt aggregbility, thyroid-binding globulin, T_4, triglycerides; ↓ antithrombin III, folate **NIPE:** ◎ PRG, breast-feeding

Ethinyl Estradiol & Levonorgestrel (Preven) Uses: *Emergency contraceptive* ("morning-after pill"); prevent PRG after contraceptive failure or unprotected intercourse **Actions:** Estrogen & progestin; interferes w/ implantation **Dose:** 4 tabs, take 2 tabs q12h × 2 (w/in 72 h of intercourse) **Caution:** [X, M] **Contra:** Known/suspected PRG, abnormal uterine bleeding **Supplied:** Kit ethinyl estradiol (0.05), levonorgestrel (0.25) blister pack w/ 4 pills & urine PRG test **SE:** Peripheral edema, N/V/D, bloating, abdominal pain, fatigue, HA, & menstrual changes **Notes:** Will not induce abortion; may ↑ risk of ectopic PRG. See Ethinyl Estradiol, page 113. **Additional Interactions:** ↑ Effects of ASA, benzodiazepines, metoprolol, TCAs **NIPE:** Monitor for vision changes or ↓ tolerance of contact lens

Ethinyl Estradiol & Norelgestromin (Ortho Evra) Uses: *Contraceptive patch* **Action:** Estrogen & progestin **Dose:** Apply patch to abdomen, buttocks, upper torso (not breasts), or upper outer arm at the beginning of the menstrual cycle; new patch is applied weekly for 3 wk; week 4 is patch-free **Caution:** [X, M] **Contra:** Thrombophlebitis, undiagnosed vaginal bleeding, PRG, carcinoma of breast, estrogen-dependent tumor **Supplied:** 20 cm² patch (6 mg norelgestromin (active metabolite norgestimate) & 0.75 mg of ethinyl estradiol) **SE:** Breast discomfort, HA, application site Rxns, nausea, menstrual cramps; thrombosis risks similar to OCP **Notes:** Less effective in women >90 kg. See Ethinyl Estradiol. **Additional Labs:** ↑ Serum amylase, Na, Ca, protein

Ethosuximide (Zarontin)
Uses: *Absence (petit mal) Szs* **Action:** Anticonvulsant; ↑ Sz threshold **Dose:** *Adults.* Initial, 250 mg PO ÷ bid; ↑ by 250 mg q4–7d PRN (max 1500 mg/d). *Peds.* 3–6 y. *Initial:* 15 mg/kg/d PO ÷ bid. *Maint:* 15–40 mg/kg/d ÷ bid, max 1500 mg/d; use w/ caution in renal/hepatic impairment **Caution:** [C, +] **Contra:** Component sensitivity **Supplied:** Caps 250 mg; syrup 250 mg/5 mL **SE:** Blood dyscrasias, GI upset, drowsiness, dizziness, irritability **Interactions:** ↑ Effects w/ INH, phenobarbital, EtOH; ↑ effects of CNS depressants, phenytoin; ↓ effects w/ carbamazepine, valproic acid, ginkgo biloba; ↓ effects of phenobarbital **NIPE:** Take w/ food, ⊘ EtOH

Etidronate Disodium (Didronel)
Uses: *Hypercalcemia of malignancy, Paget's Dz, & heterotopic ossification* **Action:** Inhibits normal & abnormal bone resorption **Dose:** *Paget's:* 5–10 mg/kg/d PO ÷ doses (for 3–6 mo). *Hypercalcemia:* 7.5 mg/kg/d IV inf over 2 h × 3 d, then 20 mg/kg/d PO on last day of inf × 1–3 mo **Caution:** [B PO (C parenteral), ?] **Contra:** SCr >5 mg/dL **Supplied:** Tabs 200, 400 mg; inj 50 mg/mL **SE:** GI intolerance (↓ by dividing daily doses); hypophosphatemia, hypomagnesemia, bone pain, abnormal taste, fever, convulsions, nephrotoxicity **Notes:** Take PO on empty stomach 2 h before any meal **Interactions:** ↓ Effects w/ antacids, foods that contain Ca **NIPE:** ⊘ Take w/ food, improvement may take 3 mo

Etodolac (Lodine)
Uses: *Osteoarthritis & pain.* RA **Action:** NSAID **Dose:** 200–400 mg PO bid–qid (max 1200 mg/d) **Caution:** [C (D 3rd tri), ?] ↑ bleeding risk w/ ASA, warfarin; ↑ nephrotoxicity w/ cyclosporine; Hx CHF, HTN, renal/hepatic impairment, PUD **Contra:** Active GI ulcer **Supplied:** Tabs 400, 500 mg; ER tabs 400, 500, 600 mg; caps 200, 300 mg **SE:** N/V/D, gastritis, abdominal cramps, dizziness, HA, depression, edema, renal impairment **Notes:** ⊘ Crush tabs **Interactions:** ↑ Risk of bleeding w/ anticoagulants, antiplts; ↑ effects of Li, MRX, digoxin, cyclosporine; ↓ effects w/ ASA; ↓ effects of antihypertensives **Labs:** False + of urine ketones & bilirubin **NIPE:** Take w/ food

Etonogestrel/Ethinyl Estradiol (NuvaRing)
Uses: *Contraceptive* **Action:** Estrogen & progestin combination **Dose:** Rule out PRG first; insert ring vaginally for 3 wk, remove for 1 wk; insert new ring 7 d after last removed (even if still bleeding) at same time of day ring removed. First day of menses is day 1, insert prior to day 5 even if still bleeding. Use other contraception for first 7 d of starting therapy. See insert if converting from other contraceptive; after delivery or 2nd-tri abortion, insert 4 wk postpartum (if not breast-feeding) **Caution:** [X, ?/–]

HTN, gallbladder Dz, ↑ lipids, migraines, sudden HA **Contra**: PRG, heavy smokers >35 y, DVT, PE, cerebro-/CV Dz, estrogen-dependent neoplasm, undiagnosed abnormal genital bleeding, hepatic tumors, cholestatic jaundice **Supplied**: Intravaginal ring: ethinyl estradiol 0.015 mg/d & etonogestrel 0.12 mg/d **Notes**: If ring accidentally removed, rinse w/ cool/lukewarm water (not hot) & reinsert ASAP; if not reinserted w/in 3h, effectiveness decreased; ⊘ use w/ diaphragm. See Ethinyl Estradiol

Etoposide [VP-16] (VePesid, Toposar)
Uses: *Testicular CA, non-small-cell lung CA, Hodgkin's & NHLs, pediatric ALL, & allogeneic/autologous BMT in high doses* **Action**: Topoisomerase II inhibitor **Dose**: 50 mg/m²/d IV for 3–5 d; 50 mg/m²/d PO for 21 d (PO bioavailability = 50% of the IV form); 2–6 g/m² or 25–70 mg/kg used in BMT (refer to specific protocols); ↓ in renal/hepatic impairment **Caution**: [D, –] **Contra**: IT administration **Supplied**: Caps 50 mg; inj 20 mg/mL **SE**: Myelosuppression, N/V, alopecia, hypotension if infused too rapidly, anorexia, anemia, leukopenia, potential for secondary leukemias **Notes**: Emetic potential low (10–30%) **Interactions**: ↑ Bleeding w/ ASA, NSAIDs, warfarin; ↑ bone marrow suppression w/ antineoplastics & radiation; ↑ effects of cisplatin; ↓ effects of live vaccines **Labs**: ↑ Uric acid **NIPE**: ⊘ EtOH, immunizations, PRG, breast-feeding; use contraception, 2–3 L/d fluids

Exemestane (Aromasin)
Uses: *Rx of advanced breast CA in postmenopausal women whose Dz has progressed following tamoxifen therapy* **Action**: An irreversible, steroidal aromatase inhibitor; ↓ circulating estrogens **Dose**: 25 mg PO qd after a meal **Caution**: [D, ?/–] **Contra**: Component sensitivity **Supplied**: Tabs 25 mg **SE**: Hot flashes, nausea, fatigue **Interactions**: ↓ Effects with erythromycin, ketoconazole, phenobarbital, rifampin, other drugs that inhibit P4503A4, St John's wort, black cohosh, dong quai **Labs**: ↑ Alkaline phosphatase, AST, ALT **NIPE**: ⊘ PRG, breast-feeding; take pc and same time each day; monitor BP

Ezetimibe (Zetia)
Uses: *Primary hypercholesterolemia alone or in combination w/ an HMG-CoA reductase inhibitor* **Action**: Inhibits intestinal absorption of cholesterol & phytosterols **Dose**: *Adults & Peds.* >10 y, 10 mg/d PO **Caution**: [C, +/–] Bile acid sequestrants ↓ bioavailability **Contra**: Hepatic impairment **Supplied**: Tabs 10 mg **SE**: HA, diarrhea, abdominal pain, ↑ transaminases in combination w/ an HMG-CoA reductase inhibitor **Interactions**: ↑ Effects w/ cyclosporine; ↓ effects w/ cholestyramine, fenofibrate, gemfibrozil **NIPE**: If used w/ fibrates ↑ risk of cholethiasis

Famciclovir (Famvir)
Uses: *Acute herpes zoster (shingles) & genital herpes* **Action**: Inhibits viral DNA synthesis **Dose**: *Zoster*: 500 mg PO q8h ×7 d. *Simplex*: 125–250 mg PO bid; ↓ in renal impairment **Caution**: [B, –] **Contra**: Component sensitivity **Supplied**: Tabs 125, 250, 500 mg **SE**: Fatigue, dizziness, HA, pruritus, nausea, diarrhea **Interactions**: ↑ Effects w/ cimetidine, probenecid, theophylline; ↑ effects of digoxin **NIPE**: Not affected by food, therapy most effective if taken w/in 72 h of rash

Famotidine (Pepcid) Uses: *Short-term Rx of active duodenal ulcer & benign gastric ulcer; maint for duodenal ulcer, hypersecretory conditions, GERD, & heartburn* **Action:** H$_2$-antagonist; inhibits gastric acid secretion **Dose:** *Adults. Ulcer:* 20 mg IV q12h or 20–40 mg PO qhs × 4–8 wk. *Hypersecretion:* 20–160 mg PO q6h. *GERD:* 20 mg PO bid ×6 wk; maint: 20 mg PO hs. *Heartburn:* 10 mg PO PRN q12h. *Peds.* 0.5–1 mg/kg/d; ↓ dose in severe renal insufficiency **Caution:** [B, M] **Contra:** Component sensitivity **Supplied:** Tabs 10, 20, 40 mg; chew tabs 10 mg; susp 40 mg/5 mL; inj 10 mg/2 mL **SE:** Dizziness, HA, constipation, diarrhea, thrombocytopenia **Notes:** Chewable tablets contain phenylalanine **Interactions:** ↑ Effects of glipizide, glyburide, nifedipine, nitrendipine, nisoldipine, tolbutamide; ↓ effects w/ antacids; ↓ effects of azole antifungals, cefuroxime, enoxacin, diazepam **NIPE:** ⊘ ASA, EtOH, tobacco, caffeine; take hs

Felodipine (Plendil) Uses: *HTN & CHF* **Action:** CCB **Dose:** 2.5–10 mg PO qd; ↓ in hepatic impairment **Caution:** [C, ?] ↑ effect w/ azole antifungals, erythromycin, bioavailability ↑ w/ grapefruit juice **Contra:** Component sensitivity **Supplied:** ER tabs 2.5, 5, 10 mg **SE:** Peripheral edema, flushing, tachycardia, HA, gingival hyperplasia **Notes:** Follow BP in elderly & in ↓ hepatic Fxn; swallow whole **Interactions:** ↑ Effects w/ azole antifungals, cimetidine, cyclosporine, ranitidine, propranolol, EtOH, grapefruit juice; ↑ effects of digoxin, erythromycin; ↓ effects w/ barbiturates, carbamazepine, nafcillin, oxcarbazepine, phenytoin; rifampin; ↓ effects of theophylline **NIPE:** ⊘ DC abruptly

Fenofibrate (Tricor) Uses: *Hypertriglyceridemia* **Action:** Inhibits triglyceride synthesis **Dose:** 54–160 mg qd; ↓ in renal impairment, take w/ meals **Caution:** [C, ?] **Contra:** Hepatic/severe renal insufficiency, 1st-deg biliary cirrhosis, unexplained persistent ↑ LFTs, gallbladder Dz **Supplied:** Tabs 54, 160 mg **SE:** GI disturbances, cholecystitis, arthralgia, myalgia, dizziness **Notes:** Monitor LFTs **Interactions:** ↑ Effects of anticoagulants; ↓ effects w/ BBs, cholestyramine, colestipol, estrogens, resins, rifampin, thiazide diuretics **Labs:** ↑ LFTs, BUN, creatinine; ↓ Hgb, Hct, WBCs, uric acid

Fenoldopam (Corlopam) Uses: *Hypertensive emergency* **Action:** Rapid vasodilator **Dose:** Initial 0.03–0.1 μg/kg/min IV inf, titrate q15min in 0.05–0.1 μg/kg/min increments **Caution:** [B, ?] Hypotension w/ BBs **Contra:** Hypersensitivity to sulfites **Supplied:** Inj 10 mg/mL **SE:** Hypotension, edema, facial flushing, N/V/D, atrial flutter/fibrillation, ↑ intraocular pressure **Notes:** ⊘ Concurrent BBs **Interactions:** ↑ Effects w/ acetaminophen ↓ hypotension w/ BBs **Labs:** ↑ Serum urea nitrogen, creatinine, LFTs, LDH; ↑ K$^+$

Fenoprofen (Nalfon) Uses: *Arthritis & pain* **Action:** NSAID **Dose:** 200–600 mg q4–8h, to 3200 mg/d max; take w/ food **Caution:** [B (D 3rd tri), +/–] CHF, HTN, renal/hepatic impairment, Hx PUD **Contra:** NSAID sensitivity **Supplied:** Caps 200, 300 mg; tabs 600 mg **SE:** GI disturbance, dizziness, HA, rash, edema, renal impairment, hepatitis **Notes:** Take w/ food, swallow whole **Interactions:** ↑ Effects w/ ASA, anticoagulants; ↑ hyperkalemia w/ K-sparing diuretics; ↑

effects of aminoglycoside, anticoagulants, Li, MRX, phenytoin, sulfonamides, sulfonylureas; ↓ effects w/ phenobarbital; ↓ effects of antihypertensives **Labs:** False ↑ free and total T_3 levels, false + urine barbiturates & benzodiazepines; ↑ serum Na & Cl **NIPE:** ⊘ ASA, EtOH, OTC drugs

Fentanyl (Sublimaze) [C-II]

Uses: *Short-acting analgesic* in anesthesia & PCA **Action:** Narcotic analgesic **Dose:** *Adults.* 25–100 μg/kg/dose IV/IM titrated to effect. *Peds.* 1–2 μg/kg IV/IM q1–4h titrated to effect; ↓ in renal impairment **Caution:** [B, +] **Contra:** ↑d ICP, resp depression, severe renal/hepatic impairment **Supplied:** Inj 0.05 mg/mL **SE:** Sedation, hypotension, bradycardia, constipation, nausea, resp depression, miosis **Notes:** 0.1 mg of fentanyl = 10 mg of morphine IM **Interactions:** ↑ Effects w/ CNS depressants, cimetidine, phenothiazines, ritonavir, TCAs, EtOH, grapefruit juice; ↑ risks of HTN crisis w/ MAOIs; ↓ effects w/ buprenorphine, dezocine, nalbuphine, pentazocine **Labs:** False ↑ serum amylase, lipase

Fentanyl, Transdermal (Duragesic) [C-II]

Uses: *Chronic pain* **Action:** Narcotic **Dose:** Apply patch to torso q72h; dose calculated from narcotic requirements in previous 24 h; ↓ in renal impairment **Caution:** [B, +] **Contra:** ↑ ICP, resp depression, severe renal/hepatic impairment **Supplied:** TD patches 25, 50, 75, 100 μg/h **SE:** Sedation, ↓ BP, bradycardia, constipation, nausea, resp depression, miosis **Notes:** 0.1 mg of fentanyl = 10 mg of morphine IM. See Fentanyl. **NIPE:** ↑ Risk of ↑ absorption w/ elevated temperature; cleanse skin only w/ water, ⊘ soap, lotions, or EtOH because they may ↑ absorption; ⊘ use in children <110 lb

Fentanyl, Transmucosal System (Actiq) [C-II]

Uses: *Induction of anesthesia; breakthrough CA pain* **Action:** Narcotic analgesic **Dose:** *Adults.* Anesthesia: 5–15 μg/kg. *Pain:* 200 μg over 15 min, titrate to effect; ↓ in renal impairment **Caution:** [B, +] **Contra:** ↑ ICP, resp depression, severe renal/hepatic impairment **Supplied:** Lozenges on stick 200, 400, 600, 800, 1200, 1600 μg **SE:** Sedation, ↓ BP, bradycardia, constipation, nausea, resp depression, miosis **Notes:** 0.1 mg of fentanyl = 10 mg of morphine IM See Fentanyl. **Additional NIPE:** ⊘ Use for children <33 lb and <2 y old

Ferrous Gluconate (Fergon)

Uses: *Fe deficiency anemia* & Fe suppl **Action:** Dietary suppl **Dose:** *Adults.* 100–200 mg of elemental Fe/d ÷ doses. *Peds.* 4–6 mg/kg/d ÷ doses; take on empty stomach (OK w/ meals if GI upset occurs); ⊘ antacids **Caution:** [A, ?] **Contra:** Hemochromatosis, hemolytic anemia **Supplied:** Tabs 300 (34 mg Fe), 325 mg (36 mg Fe) **SE:** GI upset, constipation, dark stools, discoloration of urine, may stain teeth **Notes:** 12% elemental Fe **Interactions:** ↑ Effects w/ chloramphenicol, citrus fruits or juices; ↓ effects w/ antacids, cimetidine, black cohosh, chamomile, feverfew, gossypol, hawthorn, nettle, plantain, St. John's wort, whole-grain breads, cheese, eggs, milk, coffee, tea, yogurt; ↓ effects of fluoroquinolones, levodopa **Labs:** False + guaiac test **NIPE:** ⊘ Antacids, tetracyclines, take liq form in liquids and through a straw to prevent teeth staining

Ferrous Gluconate Complex (Ferrlecit)   Uses: *Fe deficiency anemia or suppl to erythropoietin therapy* **Action:** Suppl Fe **Dose:** Test dose: 2 mL (25 mg Fe) infused over 1 h. If no Rxn, 125 mg (10 mL) IV over 1 h. Usual cumulative dose 1 g Fe over 8 sessions (until favorable Hct achieved) **Caution:** [B, ?] **Contra:** Anemia not caused by Fe deficiency; CHF; Fe overload **Supplied:** Inj 12.5 mg/mL **SE:** Hypotension, serious hypersensitivity Rxns, GI disturbance, inj site Rxn **Notes:** Dose expressed as mg Fe; may be infused during dialysis. See Ferrous Gluconate

Ferrous Sulfate   Uses: *Fe deficiency anemia & Fe suppl* **Action:** Dietary suppl **Dose:** *Adults.* 100–200 mg of elemental Fe/d in ÷ doses. *Peds.* 1–6 mg/kg/d ÷ daily–tid; take on empty stomach (OK w/ meals if GI upset occurs); ⊘ antacids **Caution:** [A, ?] ↑ absorption w/ vitamin C; ↓ absorption w/ tetracycline, fluoroquinolones, antacids, H_2 blockers, proton pump inhibitors **Contra:** Hemochromatosis, hemolytic anemia **Supplied:** Tabs 187 (60 mg Fe), 200 (65 mg Fe), 324 (65 mg Fe), 325 mg (65 mg Fe); SR caplets & tabs 160 mg (50 mg Fe), 200 mg (65 mg Fe); gtt 75 mg/0.6 mL (15 mg Fe/0.6 mL); elixir 220 mg/5 mL (44 mg Fe/5 mL); syrup 90 mg/5 mL (18 mg Fe/5 mL) **SE:** GI upset, constipation, dark stools, discolored urine. See Ferrous Gluconate

Fexofenadine (Allegra, Allegra-D)   Uses: *Allergic rhinitis* **Action:** Antihistamine **Dose:** *Adults & Peds.* >12 y. 60 mg PO bid or 180 mg/d; ↓ in renal impairment **Caution:** [C, ?] **Contra:** Component sensitivity **Supplied:** Caps 60 mg; tabs 30, 60, 180 mg; Allegra-D (60 mg fexofenadine/120 mg pseudoephedrine) **SE:** Drowsiness (uncommon) **Interactions:** ↑ Effects w/ erythromycin, ketoconazole; ↓ effects w/ antacids **NIPE:** ⊘ EtOH or CNS depressants

Filgrastim [G-CSF] (Neupogen)   Uses: *↓ Incidence of infection in febrile neutropenic Pts; Rx chronic neutropenia* **Action:** Recombinant G-CSF **Dose:** *Adults & Peds.* 5 µg/kg/d SQ or IV single daily dose; DC therapy when ANC >10,000 **Caution:** [C, ?] Drug interactions w/ drugs that potentiate release of neutrophils (eg, Li) **Contra:** Hypersensitivity to *E. coli*-derived proteins or G-CSF **Supplied:** Inj 300 µg/mL **SE:** Fever, alopecia, N/V/D, splenomegaly, bone pain, HA, rash **Notes:** Monitor CBC & plt; monitor for cardiac events; no benefit w/ ANC >10,000/mm^3 **Interactions:** ↑ Interference w/ cytotoxic drugs; ↑ release of neutrophils w/ Li **NIPE:** Monitor CBC & plts

Finasteride (Proscar, Propecia)   Uses: *BPH & androgenetic alopecia* **Action:** Inhibits 5α-reductase **Dose:** *BPH:* 5 mg/d PO. *Alopecia:* 1 mg/d PO; food may reduce absorption **Caution:** [X, –] Caution in hepatic impairment **Contra:** PRG women should ⊘ handling pills **Supplied:** Tabs 1 mg (Propecia), 5 mg (Proscar) **SE:** ↓ PSA levels; ↓ libido, impotence (rare) **Notes:** Reestablish PSA baseline at 6 mo; 3–6 mo for effect on urinary Sxs; continue therapy to maintain new hair **Interactions:** ↑ Effects w/ saw palmetto; ↓ effects w/ anticholinergics, adrenergic bronchodilators, theophylline

Flavoxate (Urispas) Uses: *Symptomatic relief of dysuria, urgency, nocturia, suprapubic pain, urinary frequency, & incontinence* Action: Antispasmodic Dose: 100–200 mg PO tid–qid Caution: [B, ?] Contra: Pyloric or duodenal obstruction, GI hemorrhage, GI obstruction, ileus, achalasia, BPH Supplied: Tabs 100 mg SE: Drowsiness, blurred vision, xerostomia Interactions: ↑ Effects of CNS depressants NIPE: ↑ Risk of heat stroke w/ exercise and in hot weather

Flecainide (Tambocor) Uses: Prevent AF/flutter & PSVT, *prevent/suppress life-threatening ventricular arrhythmias* Action: Class 1C antiarrhythmic Dose: *Adults.* 100 mg PO q12h; ↑ by 50 mg q12h q4d to max 400 mg/d. *Peds.* 3–6 mg/kg/d in 3 ÷ doses; ↓ in renal impairment, monitor in hepatic impairment Caution: [C, +] ↑ conc w/ amiodarone, digoxin, quinidine, ritonavir/amprenavir, BB, verapamil Contra: 2nd-/3rd-degree AV block, RBBB w/ bifascicular or trifascicular block, cardiogenic shock, CAD, ritonavir/amprenavir, alkalinizing agents Supplied: Tabs 50, 100, 150 mg SE: Dizziness, visual disturbances, dyspnea, palpitations, edema, tachycardia, CHF, HA, fatigue, rash, nausea Notes: May cause new/worsened arrhythmias; initiate Rx in hospital; dose q8h if Pt is intolerant/condition is uncontrolled at 12-h intervals Interactions: ↑ Effects w/ alkalinizing drugs, amiodarone, cimetidine, propranolol, quinidine; ↓ effects of digoxin; ↑ risk of arrhythmias w/ CCBs, antiarrhythmics, disopyramide; ↓ effects w/ acidifying drugs, tobacco Labs: ↑ Alkaline phosphatase NIPE: Full effects may take 3–5 d

Floxuridine (FUDR) Uses: *GI adenoma, liver, renal cell carcinoma*; colon & pancreatic CAs Action: Inhibitor of thymidylate synthase; interferes w/ DNA synthesis (S-phase specific) Dose: 0.1–0.6 mg/kg/d for 1–6 wk (refer to specific protocols) Caution: [D, –] Drug intoxication w/ live & rotavirus vaccine Contra: Bone marrow suppression, poor nutritional status, potentially serious infection Supplied: Inj 500 mg SE: Myelosuppression, anorexia, abdominal cramps, N/V/D, mucositis, alopecia, skin rash, & hyperpigmentation; rare neurotoxicity (blurred vision, depression, nystagmus, vertigo, & lethargy); intraarterial catheter-related problems (ischemia, thrombosis, bleeding, & infection) Notes: Need effective birth control; palliative Rx for inoperable/incurable Pts Interactions: ↑ Effects w/ metronidazole Labs: ↑ LFTs, 5-HIAA urine excretion; ↓ plasma albumin NIPE: ↑ Risk of photosensitivity—use sunscreen

Fluconazole (Diflucan) Uses: *Candidiasis (esophageal, oropharyngeal, urinary tract, vaginal, prophylaxis); cryptococcal meningitis* Action: Antifungal; inhibits fungal cytochrome P-450 sterol demethylation. *Spectrum:* All *Candida* sp except *C. krusei* Dose: *Adults.* 100–400 mg/d PO or IV. *Vaginitis:* 150 mg PO daily. *Cryptococcal meningitis:* 400 mg day 1, then 200 mg × 10–12 wk after CSF (–). *Peds.* 3–6 mg/kg/d PO or IV; ↓ in renal impairment Caution: [C, –] Contra: Use w/ terfenadine Supplied: Tabs 50, 100, 150, 200 mg; susp 10, 40 mg/mL; inj 2 mg/mL SE: HA, rash, GI upset, hypokalemia, ↑ LFTs Notes: PO use produces the same blood levels as IV; PO preferred when possible Interactions: ↑ Effects w/ HCTZ, benzodiazepines, anticoagulants; ↑ effects of amitriptyline, carbamazepine, cyclosporine, hypoglycemics, losartan, methadone, phenytoin, quinidine, tacrolimus, TCAs, theophylline, caffeine, zidovudine; ↓ effects w/ cimetidine, rifampin **Labs:** ↓ LFTs

Fludarabine Phosphate (Flamp, Fludara) **Uses:** *Autoimmune hemolytic anemia, CLL, cold agglutinin hemolysis,* low-grade lymphoma, mycosis fungoides **Action:** Inhibits ribonucleotide reductase; blocks DNA polymerase-induced DNA repair **Dose:** 18–30 mg/m^2/d for 5 d, as a 30-min inf (refer to specific protocols) **Caution:** [D, –] Give cytarabine before fludarabine (↓ its metabolism) **Contra:** Severe infections **Supplied:** Inj 50 mg **SE:** Myelosuppression, N/V/D, ↑ LFT, edema, CHF, fever, chills, fatigue, dyspnea, nonproductive cough, pneumonitis, severe CNS toxicity rare in leukemia **Notes:** ⊘ in CrCl <30 mL/min **Interactions:** ↑ Effects w/ other myelosuppressive drugs; ↑ risk of pulmonary effects w/ pentostatin **NIPE:** May take several weeks for full effect, use barrier contraception

Fludrocortisone Acetate (Florinef) **Uses:** *Adrenocortical insufficiency, Addison's Dz, salt-wasting syndrome* **Action:** Mineralocorticoid replacement **Dose:** *Adults.* 0.1–0.2 mg/d PO. *Peds.* 0.05–0.1 mg/d PO **Caution:** [C, ?] **Contra:** Systemic fungal infections; known hypersensitivity **Supplied:** Tabs 0.1 mg **SE:** HTN, edema, CHF, HA, dizziness, convulsions, acne, rash, bruising, hyperglycemia, HPA suppression, cataracts **Notes:** For adrenal insufficiency, must use w/ glucocorticoid suppl; dosage changes based on plasma renin activity **Interactions:** ↑ Risk of hypokalemia w/ amphotericin B, thiazide diuretics, loop diuretics; ↓ effects w/ rifampin, barbiturates, hydantoins; ↓ effects of ASA, INH **Labs:** ↓ Serum K$^+$ **NIPE:** Eval for fluid retention

Flumazenil (Romazicon) **Uses:** *Reverse sedative effects of benzodiazepines & general anesthesia* **Action:** Benzodiazepine receptor antagonist **Dose:** *Adults.* 0.2 mg IV over 15 s; repeat PRN, to 1 mg max (3 mg max in benzodiazepine OD). *Peds.* 0.01 mg/kg (0.2 mg/dose max) IV over 15 s; repeat 0.005 mg/kg at 1-min intervals to max 1 mg total; ↓ in hepatic impairment **Caution:** [C, ?] **Contra:** In TCA OD; if Pts given benzodiazepines to control life-threatening conditions (ICP/status epilepticus) **Supplied:** Inj 0.1 mg/mL **SE:** N/V, palpitations, HA, anxiety, nervousness, hot flashes, tremor, blurred vision, dyspnea, hyperventilation, withdrawal syndrome **Notes:** Does not reverse narcotic Sx or amnesia **Interactions:** ↑ Risk of Szs and arrhythmias when benzodiazepine action is reduced **NIPE:** Food given during IV administration will reduce drug serum level

Flunisolide (AeroBid, Nasalide) **Uses:** *Bronchial asthma in Pts requiring chronic steroid therapy; relief of seasonal/perennial allergic rhinitis* **Action:** Topical steroid **Dose:** *Adults.* Met-dose inhal: 2 inhal bid (max 8/d). *Nasal:* 2 sprays/nostril bid (max 8/d). *Peds.* >6 y. *Met-dose inhal:* 2 inhal bid (max 4/d). *Nasal:* 1–2 sprays/nostril bid (max 4/d) **Caution:** [C, ?] **Contra:** Status asthmaticus **Supplied:** Aerosol 250 mg/actuation; nasal spray 0.025% **SE:** tachycardia, bitter taste, local effects, oral candidiasis **Notes:** Not for acute asthma **NIPE:** Shake well before use

Fluorouracil [5-FU] (Adrucil) Uses: *Colorectal, gastric, pancreatic, breast, basal cell,* head, neck, bladder, CAs* **Action:** Inhibitor of thymidylate synthetase (interferes w/ DNA synthesis, S-phase specific) **Dose:** 370–1000 mg/m²/d for 1–5 d IV push to 24-h cont inf; protracted venous inf of 200–300 mg/m²/d (refer to specific protocol) **Caution:** [D, ?] ↑ toxicity w/ allopurinol; ⊘ give MRX before 5-FU **Contra:** Poor nutritional status, depressed bone marrow Fxn, thrombocytopenia, major surgery w/in past mo, DPD enzyme deficiency, PRG, serious infection, bilirubin >5 mg/dL **Supplied:** Inj 50 mg/mL **SE:** Stomatitis, esophagopharyngitis, N/V/D, anorexia, myelosuppression (leukocytopenia, thrombocytopenia, & anemia); rash/dry skin/photosensitivity, tingling in hands/feet w/pain (palmar–plantar erythrodysesthesia), phlebitis/discoloration at inj sites **Notes:** ↑ thiamine intake; sun sensitivity; daily doses > 800 mg ⊘ **Interactions:** ↑ Effects w/ leucovorin, Ca **Labs:** ↑ LFTs **NIPE:** ⊘ EtOH, ↑ risk of photosensitivity—use sunscreen; ⊘ fluids 2–3 L/d, use barrier contraception

Fluorouracil, Topical [5-FU] (Efudex) Uses: *Basal cell carcinoma; actinic/solar keratosis* **Action:** Inhibitor of thymidylate synthetase (inhibits DNA synthesis, S-phase specific) **Dose:** Apply 5% cream bid × 3–6 wk **Caution:** [D, ?] Irritant chemotherapy **Contra:** Component sensitivity **Supplied:** Cream 1, 5%; soln 1, 2, 5% **SE:** Rash, dry skin, photosensitivity **Notes:** Complete healing may not be evident for 1–2 mo; ⊘ overuse. See Fluorouracil. **Additional NIPE:** ⊘ Use occlusive dressing; wash hands immediately after application

Fluoxetine (Prozac, Sarafem) WARNING: Closely monitor for worsening depression or emergence of suicidality, particularly in pediatric Pts Uses: *Depression, OCD, panic disorder, bulimia, PMDD* (Sarafem) **Action:** SSRI **Dose:** 20 mg/d PO (max 80 mg/d ÷); weekly regimen 90 mg/wk after 1–2 wk of standard dose. *Bulimia:* 60 mg q AM. *Panic disorder:* 20 mg/d. *OCD:* 20–80 mg/d. *PMDD:* 20 mg/d or 20 mg intermittently starting 14 d prior to menses, repeat w/ each cycle; ↓ dose in hepatic failure **Caution:** [B, ?/–] Risk of serotonin syndrome w/ MAOI, SSRI, serotonin agonists, linezolid; risk of QT prolongation w/ phenothiazines **Contra:** MAOI/thioridazine (wait 5 wk after DC before starting MAOI) **Supplied:** *Prozac:* Caps 10, 20, 40 mg; scored tabs 10 mg; SR cap 90 mg; soln 20 mg/5 mL. *Sarafem:* Caps 10, 20 mg **SE:** Nausea, nervousness, weight loss, HA, insomnia **Interactions:** ↑ Effects w/ CNS depressants, MAOIs, EtOH, St. John's wort; ↑ effects of alprazolam, BBs, carbamazepine, clozapine, cardiac glycosides, diazepam, dextromethorphan, loop diuretics, haloperiodol, phenytoin, Li, ritonavir, thioridazine, tryptophan, warfarin, sympathomimetic drugs; ↓ effects w/ cyproheptadine; ↓ effects of buspirone, statins **Labs:** ↑ LFTs, BUN, creatinine, urine albumin **NIPE:** Stop MAOIs 14 d before start of this drug

Fluoxymesterone (Halotestin) Uses: Androgen-responsive metastatic *breast CA, hypogonadism* **Action:** Inhibits secretion of LH & FSH by feedback inhibition **Dose:** *Breast CA:* 10–40 mg/d × × 1–3 mo *Hypogonadism:* 5–20 mg/d **Caution:** [X, ?/–] ↑ effect w/ anticoagulants, cyclosporine, insulin, Li, narcotics

Contra: Serious cardiac, liver, or kidney Dz; PRG **Supplied:** Tabs 2, 5, 10 mg **SE:** Virilization, amenorrhea & menstrual irregularities, hirsutism, alopecia, acne, nausea, & cholestasis. *Hematologic toxicity:* Suppression of clotting factors II, V, VII, & X & polycythemia; ↑ libido, HA, & anxiety **Notes:** ↓ total T_4 levels **Interactions:** ↑ Effects w/ narcotics, EtOH, echinacea; ↑ effects of anticoagulants, cyclosporine, insulin, hypoglycemics, tacrolimus; ↓ effects w/ anticholinergics, barbiturates **Labs:** ↑ Creatinine, creatinine clearance; ↓ thyroxine-binding globulin, serum total T_4 **NIPE:** Radiographic studies of skeletal maturation (hand/wrist) q6mo in prepubertal children; monitor fluid retention

Fluphenazine (Prolixin, Permitil) Uses: *Schizophrenia* **Action:** Phenothiazine antipsychotic; blocks postsynaptic mesolimbic dopaminergic brain receptors **Dose:** 0.5–10 mg/d in ÷ doses PO q6–8h, average maint 5 mg/d; or 1.25 mg IM, then 2.5–10 mg/d in ÷ doses q6–8h PRN; ↓ dose in elderly **Caution:** [C, ?/–] **Contra:** Severe CNS depression, coma, subcortical brain damage, blood dyscrasias, hepatic Dz **Supplied:** Tabs 1, 2.5, 5, 10 mg; conc 5 mg/mL; elixir 2.5 mg/5 mL; inj 2.5 mg/mL; depot inj 25 mg/mL **SE:** Drowsiness, extrapyramidal effects **Notes:** Monitor LFTs; less sedative/hypotensive than chlorpromazine; ◌ administer conc w/ caffeine, tannic acid, or pectin-containing products **Interactions:** ↑ Effects w/ antimalarials, BBs, CNS depressants, EtOH, kava kava; ↑ effects of anticholinergics, BBs, nitrates; ↓ effects w/ antacids, caffeine, tobacco; ↓ effects of anticonvulsants, guanethidine, levodopa, sympathomimetics **Labs:** False + urine PRG test; ↑ serum cholesterol, glucose, LFTs, ↓ uric acid **NIPE:** Photosensitivity—use sunscreen, urine may turn pink or red in color, ↑ risk of heatstroke in hot weather

Flurazepam (Dalmane) [C-IV] Uses: *Insomnia* **Action:** Benzodiazepine **Dose:** *Adults & Peds.* >15 y. 15–30 mg PO qhs PRN; ↓ in elderly **Caution:** [X, ?/–] Caution in elderly, low albumin, hepatic impairment **Contra:** Narrow-angle glaucoma; PRG **Supplied:** Caps 15, 30 mg **SE:** "Hangover" due to accumulation of metabolites, apnea **Notes:** May cause dependency

Flurbiprofen (Ansaid) Uses: *Arthritis* **Action:** NSAID **Dose:** 50–300 mg/d ÷ bid–qid, max 300 mg/d **Caution:** [B (D in 3rd tri), +] **Contra:** PRG (3rd tri); ASA allergy **Supplied:** Tabs 50, 100 mg **SE:** Dizziness, GI upset, peptic ulcer Dz **Notes:** Take w/ food to ↓ GI upset **Interactions:** ↑ Effects w/ amprenavir, anticonvulsants, azole antifungals, BBs, CNS depressants, cimetidine, ciprofloxin, clozapine, digoxin, disulfiram, diltiazem, INH, levodopa, macrolides, oral contraceptives, rifampin, ritonavir, SSRIs, valproic acid, verapamil, EtOH, grapefruit juice, kava kava, valerian; ↓ effects w/ aminophylline, carbamazepine, rifampin, rifabutin, theophylline; ? ↓ effects of levodopa **Labs:** ↑ LFTs, false – urine glucose **NIPE:** ◌ PRG, breast-feeding

Flutamide (Eulexin) **WARNING:** Liver failure & death reported. Measure LFT before, monthly, & periodically after; DC immediately if ALT 2× upper limits of normal or jaundice develops Uses: Advanced *CAP* (in combination w/ LHRH agonists, (eg, leuprolide or goserelin); w/ radiation & GnRH for localized CAP **Action:** Nonsteroidal antiandrogen **Dose:** 250 mg PO tid (750 mg total) **Caution:** [D, ?] **Contra:** Severe hepatic impairment **Supplied:** Caps 125 mg **SE:** Hot flashes, loss of libido, impotence, diarrhea, N/V, gynecomastia **Interactions:** ↑ Effects w/ anticoagulants **Labs:** ↑ LFTs, BUN **NIPE:** Urine amber/yellow-green in color

Fluticasone, Nasal (Flonase) **Uses:** *Seasonal allergic rhinitis* **Action:** Topical steroid **Dose:** *Adults & Adolescents.* Nasal: 2 sprays/nostril/d. *Peds.* 4–11 y. Nasal: 1–2 sprays/nostril/d **Caution:** [C, M] **Contra:** Primary Rx of status asthmaticus **Supplied:** Nasal spray 50 μg/activation **SE:** HA, dysphonia, oral candidiasis **Interactions:** ↑ Effects w/ ketoconazole **Labs:** ↑ Cholesterol **NIPE:** Clear nares of exudate before use

Fluticasone, Oral (Flovent, Flovent Rotadisk) **Uses:** Chronic *asthma* **Action:** Topical steroid **Dose:** *Adults & Adolescents.* 2–4 puffs bid. *Peds.* 4–11 y. 50 μg bid **Caution:** [C, M] **Contra:** Primary Rx of status asthmaticus **Supplied:** Met-dose inhal 44, 110, 220 μg/activation; Rotadisk dry powder: 50, 100, 250 μg/activation **SE:** HA, dysphonia, oral candidiasis **Notes:** Risk of thrush; counsel Pts on use of device **Interactions:** ↑ Effects w/ ketoconazole **Labs:** ↑ Cholesterol **NIPE:** Rinse mouth after use, ⊘ & report exposure to measles & chickenpox

Fluticasone Propionate & Salmeterol Xinafoate (Advair Diskus) **Uses:** *Maint therapy for asthma* **Action:** Corticosteroid w/ long-acting bronchodilator **Dose:** *Adults & Peds.* >12 y. 1 inhal bid q 12 h **Caution:** [C, M] **Contra:** Not for acute attack or in conversion from PO steroids; status asthmaticus **Supplied:** Met-dose inhal powder(fluticasone/salmeterol in μg) 100/50, 250/50, 500/50 **SE:** Upper resp infection, pharyngitis, HA **Notes:** Combination of Flovent & Serevent; ⊘ use w/ spacer, ⊘ wash mouthpiece, ⊘ exhale into device **Interactions:** ↑ Bronchospasm w/ BBs; ↑ hypokalemia w/ loop and thiazide diuretics; ↑ effects w/ ketoconazole, MAOIs, TCAs **Labs:** ↑ Cholesterol **NIPE:** ⊘ & report exposure to measles & chickenpox, rinse mouth after use

Fluvastatin (Lescol) **Uses:** *Atherosclerosis, primary hypercholesterolemia, hypertriglyceridemia* **Action:** HMG-CoA reductase inhibitor **Dose:** 20–80 mg PO qhs; ↓ dose w/ hepatic impairment **Caution:** [X, –] **Contra:** Active liver Dz, ↑ LFTs, PRG, breast-feeding **Supplied:** Caps 20, 40 mg; XL 80 mg **SE:** HA, dyspepsia, nausea, diarrhea, abdominal pain **Interactions:** ↑ Effects w/ azole antifungals, cimetidine, danazol, glyburide, macrolides, phenytoin, ritonavir, EtOH, grapefruit juice; ↑ effects of diclofenac, glyburide, phenytoin, warfarin; ↓ effects w/ cholestyramine, colestipol, isradipine, rifampin **Labs:** ↑ LFTs, CPK, thyroid Fxn **NIPE:** Take hs, ↑ photosensitivity—use sunscreen

Fluvoxamine (Luvox) **WARNING:** Closely monitor for worsening depression or emergence of suicidality, particularly in pediatric Pts **Uses:** *OCD* **Action:** SSRI **Dose:** Initial 50 mg as single qhs dose, ↑ to 300 mg/d in ÷ doses; ↓ dose in elderly/hepatic impairment, titrate slowly **Caution:** [C, ?/–] Numerous interactions (MAOIs, phenothiazines, SSRIs, serotonin agonists) **Supplied:** Tabs 25, 50, 100 mg **SE:** HA, nausea, diarrhea, somnolence, insomnia **Notes:** ÷ doses >100 mg **Interactions:** ↑ Effects w/ melatonin, MAOIs; ↑ effects of BBs, benzodiazepines, methadone, carbamazepine, haloperidol, Li, phenytoin, TCAs, theophylline, warfarin, St. John's wort; ↑ risks of serotonin syndrome w/ buspirone, dexfenfluramine, fenfluramine, tramadol, nefazodone, sibutramine, tryptophan; ↓ effects w/ buspirone, cyproheptadine, tobacco; ↓ effects of buspirone, HMG-CoA reductase inhibitors **NIPE:** ⊘ MAOIs for 14 d before start of drug; ⊘ EtOH

Folic Acid **Uses:** *Megaloblastic anemia; folate deficiency* **Action:** Dietary suppl **Dose:** *Adults.* Suppl: 0.4 mg/d PO. *PRG:* 0.8 mg/d PO. *Folate deficiency:* 1 mg PO daily–tid. *Peds.* Suppl: 0.04–0.4 mg/24 h PO, IM, IV, or SQ. *Folate deficiency:* 0.5–1 mg/24 h PO, IM, IV, or SQ **Caution:** [A, +] **Contra:** Pernicious, aplastic, normocytic anemias **Supplied:** Tabs 0.4, 0.8, 1 mg; inj 5 mg/mL **SE:** Well tolerated **Notes:** Recommended for all women of childbearing age; ↓ fetal neural tube defects by 50%; no effect on normocytic anemias **Interactions:** ↓ Effects w/ anticonvulsants, sulfasalazine, aminosalicylic acid, chloramphenicol, MRX, oral contraceptives, pyrimethamine, triamterene, trimethoprim; ↓ effects of phenobarbital, phenytoin

Fondaparinux (Arixtra) **WARNING:** When epidural/spinal anesthesia or spinal puncture is used, Pts anticoagulated or scheduled to be anticoagulated w/ LMW heparins, heparinoids, or fondaparinux for prevention of thromboembolic complications are at risk for epidural or spinal hematoma, which can result in long-term or permanent paralysis **Uses:** *DVT prophylaxis* in hip fracture or replacement or knee replacement **Action:** Synthetic, specific inhibitor of activated factor X; an LMW heparin **Dose:** 2.5 mg SQ daily, up to 5–9 d; start at least 6 h postop **Caution:** [B, ?] ↑ bleeding risk w/ anticoagulants, antiplts, drotrecogin alfa, NSAIDs **Contra:** Wt <50 kg, CrCl <30 mL/min, active bleeding, bacterial endocarditis, thrombocytopenia associated w/ antiplt antibody **Supplied:** Prefilled syringes 2.5 mg/0.5mL **SE:** Thrombocytopenia, anemia, fever, nausea **Notes:** DC if plts <100,000 mm^3; only give SQ; may monitor anti-factor Xa levels **Interactions:** ↑ Effects w/ anticoagulants, cephalosporins, NSAIDs, penicillins, salicylates **Labs:** ↑ LFTs

Formoterol (Foradil Aerolizer) **Uses:** Maint Rx of *asthma & prevention of bronchospasm* w/ reversible obstructive airway Dz; exercise-induced bronchospasm **Action:** Long-acting β$_2$-adrenergic agonist, bronchodilator **Dose:** *Adults & Peds.* >5 y. Asthma: Inhale one 12-µg cap q12h w/ aerolizer, 24 µg/d max. *Adults & Peds.* > 12 y. Exercise-induced bronchospasm: 1 inhal 12-µg cap 15 min before exercise **Caution:** [C, ?] **Contra:** Need for acute bronchodilation; use w/in 2 wk of MAOI **Supplied:** 12-µg blister pack for use in aerolizer **SE:** Paradoxical bronchospasm; URI, pharyngitis, back pain **Notes:** ⊘ swallow caps—for use only w/ inhaler; ⊘ start w/ significantly worsening or acutely deteriorating asthma, which may be life-threatening **Interactions:** ↑ Effects w/ adrenergics; ↑ effects of

BBs; ↑ risk of hypokalemia w/ corticosteroids, diuretics, xanthines; ↑ risk of arrhythmias w/ MAOIs, TCAs

Fosamprenavir (Lexiva) WARNING: ⊘ Use w/ severe liver dysfunction, reduce dose w/ mild–moderate liver impairment (fosamprenavir 700 mg bid **w/o** ritonavir) Uses: HIV infection Action: Protease inhibitor Dose: 1400 mg bid w/o ritonavir; if given w/ ritonavir, fosamprenavir 1400 mg + ritonavir 200 mg qd or fosamprenavir 700 mg + ritonavir 100 mg bid. If given w/ efavirenz & ritonavir, then fosamprenavir 1400 mg + ritonavir 300 mg qd Caution: [C, ?/–]; Contra: Cannot be given w/ ergot alkaloids, midazolam, triazolam, or pimozide; ⊘ if sulfa allergy Supplied: Tabs 700 mg SE: N/V/D, HA, fatigue, rash Notes: Numerous drug interactions because of hepatic metabolism Interactions: ↑ Effects with indinavir, nelfinavir; ↑ effects of antiarrhythmics, amitriptyline, atorvastatin, benzodiazepine, bepridil, CCBs, cyclosporine, ergotamine, ethinyl estradiol, imipramine, itraconazole, ketoconazole, midazolam, norethindrone, rapamycin, rifabutin, sildenafil, tacrolimus, TCA, vardenafil, warfarin; ↓ effects with antacids, carbamazepine, dexamethasone, didanosine, efavirenz, H₂-receptor antagonists, nevirapine, phenobarbital, phenytoin, proton pump inhibitors, rifampin St. John's wort; ↓ effects of methadone; Labs: ↑ ALT, AST, triglycerides, glucose, lipase NIPE: Take w/o regard to food, use barrier contraception, monitor for opportunistic infection, inform about fat redistribution/accumulation

Foscarnet (Foscavir) Uses: *CMV retinitis*; acyclovir-resistant *herpes infections* Action: Inhibits viral DNA polymerase & RT Dose: *CMV retinitis: Induction:* 60 mg/kg IV q8h or 100 mg/kg q12h × 14–21 d. *Maint:* 90–120 mg/kg/d IV (Monday–Friday). *Acyclovir-resistant HSV induction:* 40 mg/kg IV q8–12h × 14–21 d; ↓ w/ renal impairment Caution: [C, –] ↑ Sz potential w/ flouroquinolones; ⊘ nephrotoxic Rx (cyclosporine, aminoglycosides, ampho B, protease inhibitors) Contra: Significant renal impairment (CrCl <0.4 mL/min/kg) Supplied: Inj 24 mg/mL SE: Nephrotoxicity, causes electrolyte abnormalities Notes: Na loading (500 mL 0.9% NaCl) before & after helps minimize nephrotoxicity; monitor ionized Ca; administer through central line Interactions: ↑ Risks of Sz w/ quinolines; ↑ risks of nephrotoxicity w/ aminoglycosides, amphotericin B, didanosine, pentamidine, vancomycin Labs: ↑ LFTs, CPK, BUN, SCr; ↓ Hmg, Hct, Ca²⁺, Mg²⁺, K⁺, P NIPE: ↑ Fluids; perioral tingling, extremity numbness & paresthesia indicates electrolyte imbalance

Fosfomycin (Monurol) Uses: *Uncomplicated UTI* Action: Inhibits bacterial cell wall synthesis. *Spectrum:* Gram(+) (staph, pneumococci); gram(–) (*E. coli, Enterococcus, Salmonella, Shigella, H. influenzae, Neisseria,* indole-negative *Proteus, Providencia*); *B. fragilis* & anaerobic gram(–) cocci are resistant Dose: 3 g PO dissolved in 90–120 mL of water single dose; ↓ in renal impairment Caution: [B, ?] ↓ absorption w/ antacids/Ca salts Contra: Component sensitivity Supplied: Granule packets 3 g SE: HA, GI upset Notes: May take 2–3 d for Sxs to improve Interactions: ↓ Effects w/ antacids, metoclopramide Labs: ↑ LFTs; ↓ Hmg, Hct NIPE: May take w/o regard to food

Fosinopril (Monopril) Uses: *HTN, CHF.* DN Action: ACEI Dose: 10 mg/d PO initial; max 40 mg/d PO; ↓ dose in elderly; ↓ in renal impairment Caution: [D, +] ↑ K+ w/ K suppls, ARBs, K-sparing diuretics; ↑ renal AE w/ NSAIDs, diuretics, hypovolemia Contra: Hereditary/idiopathic angioedema or angioedema w/ ACEI, bilateral renal artery stenosis Supplied: Tabs 10, 20, 40 mg SE: Nonproductive cough, dizziness, angioedema, hyperkalemia Interactions: ↑ Effects w/ antihypertensives, diuretics; ↑ effects of Li; ↑ risk of hyperkalemia w/ K sparing diuretics, salt substitutes; ↑ cough w/ capsaicin; ↓ effects w/ antacids, ASA, NSAIDs Labs: ↓ Hmg, Hct NIPE: ⊘ PRG, breast-feeding

Fosphenytoin (Cerebyx) Uses: *Status epilepticus* Action: Inhibits Sz spread in motor cortex Dose: Dosed as phenytoin equivalents (PE). Load: 15–20 mg PE/kg. Maint: 4–6 mg PE/kg/d; ↓ dosage monitor levels in hepatic impairment Caution: [D, +] May ↑ phenobarbital Contra: Sinus bradycardia, SA block, 2nd-/3rd-degree AV block, Adams–Stokes syndrome, rash during Rx Supplied: Inj 75 mg/mL SE: ↓ BP, dizziness, ataxia, pruritus, nystagmus Notes: 15 min to convert fosphenytoin to phenytoin; admin <150 mg PE/min to prevent hypotension; administer w/ BP monitoring Interactions: ↑ Effects w/ amiodarone, chloramphenicol, cimetidine, diazepam, disulfiram, estrogens, INH, omeprazole, phenothiazines, salicylates, sulfonamides, tolbutamide; ↓ effects w/ TCAs, antituberculosis drugs, carbamazepine, EtOH, nutritional suppls, ginkgo biloba; ↓ effects of anticoagulants, corticosteroids, digitoxin, doxycycline, oral contraceptives, folic acid, Ca, vitamin D, rifampin, quinidine, theophylline Labs: ↑ Serum glucose, alkaline phosphatase; ↓ serum thyroxine, Ca NIPE: Breast-feeding, for short-term use

Frovatriptan (Frova) See Table 11, page 283

Fulvestrant (Faslodex) Uses: Hormone receptor-+ metastatic *breast CA* in postmenopausal women w/ Dz progression following antiestrogen therapy Action: Estrogen receptor antagonist Dose: 250 mg IM monthly, either a single 5-mL inj or two concurrent 2.5-mL IM inj into buttocks Caution: [X, ?/–] ↑ effects w/ CYP3A4 inhibitors (amiodarone, clarithromycin, fluoxetine, grapefruit juice, ketoconazole, ritonavir, etc), w/ hepatic impairment Contra: PRG Supplied: Prefilled syringes 50 mg/mL (single 5 mL, dual 2.5 mL) SE: N/V/D, constipation, abdominal pain, HA, back pain, hot flushes, pharyngitis, inj site Rxns Notes: Only use IM; caution in hepatic impairment Interactions: ↑ Risk of bleeding w/ anticoagulants NIPE: ⊘ PRG, breast-feeding; use barrier contraception

Furosemide (Lasix) Uses: *CHF, HTN, edema,* ascites Action: Loop diuretic; inhibits Na & Cl reabsorption in ascending loop of Henle & distal tubule Dose: Adults. 20–80 mg PO or IV daily bid. Peds. 1 mg/kg/dose IV q6–12h; 2 mg/kg/dose PO q12–24h (max 6 mg/kg/dose) Caution: [C, +] Hypokalemia may ↑ risk of digoxin toxicity; ↑ risk of ototoxicity w/ aminoglycosides, cisplatinum (esp in renal dysfunction) Contra: Hypersensitivity to sulfonylureas; anuria; hepatic coma/severe electrolyte depletion Supplied: Tabs 20, 40, 80 mg; soln 10 mg/mL, 40 mg/5 mL; inj 10 mg/mL SE: Hypotension, hyperglycemia, hypokalemia **Notes:** Monitor electrolytes, renal Fxn; high doses IV may cause ototoxicity **Interactions:** ↑ Nephrotoxic effects w/ cephalosporins; ↑ ototoxicity w/ aminoglycosides, cisplatin; ↑ risk of hypokalemia w/ antihypertensives, carbenoxolone, corticosteroids, digitalis glycosides, terbutaline; ↓ effects w/ barbiturates, cholestyramine, colestipol, NSAIDs, phenytoin, dandelion, ginseng; ↓ effects of hypoglycemics **Labs:** ↑ BUN, serum amylase, cholesterol, glucose, triglycerides, uric acid, ↓ serum K^+, Na^+, Ca^{2+}, Mg^{2+} **NIPE:** Risk of photosensitivity—use sunscreen

Gabapentin (Neurontin) **Uses:** Adjunct therapy in the Rx of *partial Szs; postherpetic neuralgia (PHN)*; chronic pain syndromes **Action:** Anticonvulsant **Dose:** *Anticonvulsant:* 300–1200 mg PO tid (max 3600 mg/d). *PHN:* 300 mg day 1, 300 mg bid day 2, 300 mg tid day 3, titrate (1800–3600 mg/d); ↓ in renal impairment **Caution:** [C, ?] **Contra:** Component sensitivity **Supplied:** Caps 100, 300, 400 mg; soln 250 mg/5mL; tab 600, 800 mg **SE:** Somnolence, dizziness, ataxia, fatigue **Notes:** Not necessary to monitor levels **Interactions:** ↑ Effects w/ cimetidine, CNS depressants; ↑ effects of phenytoin; ↓ effects w/ antacids, ginkgo biloba **Labs:** False + urinary protein **NIPE:** Take w/o regard to food

Galantamine (Reminyl) **Uses:** *Alzheimer's Dz* **Action:** Acetylcholinesterase inhibitor **Dose:** 4 mg PO bid, ↑ to 8 mg bid after 4 wk; may ↑ to 12 mg bid in 4 wk **Caution:** [B, ?] ↑ effect w/ succinylcholine, amiodarone, diltiazem, verapamil, NSAIDs, digoxin; ↓ effect w/ anticholinergics **Contra:** Severe renal/hepatic impairment **Supplied:** Tabs 4, 8, 12 mg; soln 4 mg/mL **SE:** GI disturbances, weight loss, sleep disturbances, dizziness, HA **Notes:** Caution w/ urinary outflow obstruction, Parkinson's, severe asthma/COPD, severe heart Dz or hypotension **Interactions:** ↑ Effects w/ amitriptyline, cimetidine, erythromycin, fluoxetine, fluvoxamine, ketoconazole, paroxetine, quinidine **Labs:** ↑ Alkaline phosphatase **NIPE:** ↑ Dosage q4wk, if DC several days then restart at lowest dose; take w/ food and maintain adequate fluid intake

Gallium Nitrate (Ganite) **Uses:** *Hypercalcemia of malignancy*; bladder CA **Action:** Inhibits bone resorption of Ca^{2+} **Dose:** *Hypercalcemia:* 200 mg/m²/day × 5 d. *CA:* 350 mg/m² cont inf × 5 d to 700 mg/m² rapid IV inf q2wk in antineoplastic settings (refer to specific protocols) **Caution:** [C, ?] ⊘ give w/ live vaccines or rotavirus vaccine **Supplied:** SCr >2.5 mg/dL **Supplied:** Inj 25 mg/mL **SE:** Renal insufficiency, ↓ Ca^{2+}, hypophosphatemia, ↓ bicarbonate, <1% acute optic neuritis **Notes:** Bladder CA: use in combination w/ vinblastine & ifosfamide **Interactions:** ↑ Risks of nephrotoxicity w/ amphotericin B, aminoglycosides, vancomycin **NIPE:** Monitor SCr, adequate fluids

Ganciclovir (Cytovene, Vitrasert) **Uses:** *Rx & prevent CMV retinitis, prevent CMV Dz* in transplant recipients **Action:** Inhibits viral DNA synthesis **Dose:** *Adults & Peds.* IV: 5 mg/kg IV q12h for 14–21 d, then maint 5 mg/kg/d IV × 7 d/wk or 6 mg/kg/d IV × 5 d/wk. *Ocular implant:* One implant q5–8mo. *Adults.* PO: Following induction, 1000 mg PO tid. *Prevention:* 1000 mg PO tid; take w/

food; ↓ in renal impairment **Caution:** [C, –] ↑ effect w/ immunosuppressives, imipenem/cilastatin, zidovudine, didanosine, other nephrotoxic Rx **Contra:** Neutropenia (ANC <500), thrombocytopenia (plt <25,000), intravitreal implant **Supplied:** Caps 250, 500 mg; inj 500 mg; ocular implant 4.5 mg **SE:** Granulocytopenia & thrombocytopenia, fever, rash, GI upset **Notes:** Not a cure for CMV; inj should be handled w/ cytotoxic cautions; implant confers no systemic benefit **Interactions:** ↑ Effects w/ cytotoxic drugs, immunosuppressive drugs, probenecid; ↑ risks of nephrotoxicity w/ amphotericin B, cyclosporine ; ↑ effects w/ didanosine **Labs:** ↑ LFTs; ↓ blood glucose **NIPE:** Take w/ food, ⊘ PRG, breast-feeding, EtOH, NSAIDs; photosensitivity—use sunscreen

Gatifloxacin (Tequin) Uses: *Bronchitis, sinusitis, community-acquired pneumonia, UTI, uncomplicated skin/soft tissue infection* **Action:** Quinolone antibiotic, inhibits DNA-gyrase. **Spectrum:** Gram(+) (except MRSA, *Listeria*), gram(–) (not *Pseudomonas*), atypicals, some anaerobes (*Clostridium*, not *C. difficile*) **Dose:** 400 mg/d PO or IV; ↓ in renal impairment **Caution:** [C, M] **Contra:** Prolongation of QT interval, uncorrected hypokalemia, use w/ other Rx that prolong QT interval (Class Ia & III antiarrhythmics, erythromycin, antipsychotics, TCA); children <18 y or in PRG/lactating women **Supplied:** Tabs 200, 400 mg; inj 10 mg/mL; premixed infuse D₅W 200 mg, 400 mg **SE:** Prolonged QT interval, HA, nausea & diarrhea, tendon rupture, photosensitivity **Notes:** Reliable activity against *S. pneumoniae*; take 4 h after antacids containing Mg, Al, Fe, or Zn and drink plenty of fluids; ⊘ direct sunlight **Interactions:** ↑ Effects w/ antiarrhythmics, antipsychotics, cimetidine, erythromycin, loop diuretics, probenecid, TCAs; ↑ CNS effects and Szs w/ NSAIDs; ↑ effects of digoxin, warfarin; ↓ effects w/ antacids, didanosine, H₂ antagonists, proton pump inhibitors, Fe

Gefitinib (Iressa) Uses: *Rx locally advanced or metastatic non-small-cell lung CA after failure of both platinum-based & docetaxel chemotherapies* **Action:** Inhibits intracellular phosphorylation of tyrosine kinases **Dose:** 250 mg/d PO **Caution:** [D, –] **Supplied:** Tabs 250 mg **SE:** Diarrhea, rash, acne, dry skin, N/V, interstitial lung Dz, ↑↓ liver transaminases **Notes:** Follow LFTs **Interactions:** ↑ Effects w/ ketoconazole, itraconazole, and other CYP3A4 inhibitors; ↑ risk of bleeding w/ warfarin; ↓ effects w/ cimetidine, ranitidine and other H₂ receptor antagonists; ↓ effects w/ phenytoin, rifampin, and other CYP3A4 inducers **Labs:** ↑ ALT, AST, PT **NIPE:** ⊘ PRG or breast-feeding; take w/o regard to food; ↑ risk of corneal erosion/ulcer

Gemcitabine (Gemzar) Uses: *Pancreatic CA, brain mets, NSCLC,* gastric CA **Action:** Antimetabolite; inhibits ribonucleotide reductase; produces false nucleotide base-inhibiting DNA synthesis **Dose:** 1000 mg/m² over 30 min–1 h IV inf/wk × 3–4 wk or 6–8 wk; dose modifications based on hematologic Fxn (refer to specific protocol) **Caution:** [D, ?/–] **Contra:** PRG **Supplied:** Inj 200 mg, 1 g **SE:** Myelosuppression, N/V/D, drug fever, skin rash **Notes:** Reconsituted soln has concn of 38 mg/mL (not 40 mg/mL as earlier labeling); monitor hepatic & renal Fxn prior & during Rx **Interactions:** ↑ Bone marrow depression w/ radiation therapy, antineoplastic drugs; ↓ live virus vaccines **Labs:** ↑ LFTs, BUN, SCr **NIPE:** ⊘ EtOH, NSAIDs, immunizations, PRG?

Gemfibrozil (Lopid)
Uses: *Hypertriglyceridemia, coronary heart Dz* **Action:** Fibric acid **Dose:** 1200 mg/d PO ÷ bid 30 min ac AM & PM **Caution:** [C, ?] Enhances the effect of warfarin, sulfonylureas; ↑ risk of rhabdomyopathy w/ HMG-CoA reductase inhibitors; ↓ effects w/ cyclosporine **Contra:** Renal/hepatic impairment (SCr >2.0 mg/dL), gallbladder Dz, primary biliary cirrhosis **Supplied:** Tabs 600 mg **SE:** Cholelithiasis, GI upset **Notes:** ⊘ Concurrent use w/ the HMG-CoA reductase inhibitors; monitor LFTs & serum lipids **Interactions:** ↑ Effects of anticoagulants, sulfonylureas; ↓ effects w/ rifampin; ↓ effects of cyclosporine **Labs:** ↑ LFTs, + ANA, ↓ Hmg, Hct, WBCs

Gemtuzumab Ozogamicin (Mylotarg)
WARNING: Can cause severe hypersensitivity Rxns & other inf-related Rxns including severe pulmonary events; hepatotoxicity, including severe hepatic venoocclusive Dz (VOD) reported **Uses:** *Relapsed CD33+ AML in Pts > 60 who are poor candidates for chemotherapy* **Action:** Monoclonal antibody linked to calicheamicin; selective for myeloid cells **Dose:** Refer to specific protocol **Contra:** Component sensitivity **Supplied:** 5 mg/20 mL vial **SE:** Myelosuppression, hypersensitivity (including anaphylaxis), inf Rxns (chills, fever, N/V, HA), pulmonary events, hepatotoxicity **Notes:** Only use as single-agent chemo & not in combination w/ other agents; premedicate w/ diphenhydramine & acetaminophen **Interactions:** ↑ Risk for allergic or hypersensitive reaction and thrombocytopenia w/ abciximab; ↓ effects with abciximab **Labs:** Monitor before & after therapy CBC, ALT, AST, electrolytes **NIPE:** Mmonitor for bleeding, myelosuppression, BP; ⊘ ASA, PRG, breast-feeding

Gentamicin (Garamycin, G-Mycitin, others)
Uses: *Serious infections* caused by *Pseudomonas, Proteus, E. coli, Klebsiella, Enterobacter,* & *Serratia* & initial Rx of gram(–) sepsis **Action:** Bactericidal; inhibits protein synthesis. *Spectrum:* Synergy w/ penicillins; gram(–) (not *Neisseria, Legionella, Acinetobacter*) **Dose:** *Adults.* 3–7 mg/kg/24h IV ÷ q8–24h. *Synergy:* 1 mg/kg q8h. *Peds.* Infants <7 d <1200 g: 2.5 mg/kg/dose q18–24h. *Infants >1200 g:* 2.5 mg/kg/dose q12–18h. *Infants >7 d:* 2.5 mg/kg/dose IV q8–12h. *Children:* 2.5 mg/kg/d IV q8h; ↓ w/ renal insufficiency **Caution:** [C, +/–] ⊘ other nephrotoxic Rxns **Contra:** Aminoglycoside sensitivity **Supplied:** Premixed infus 40, 60, 70, 80, 90, 100, 120 mg; ADD-Vantage inj vials 10 mg/mL; inj 40 mg/mL; IT preservative-free 2 mg/mL **SE:** Nephrotoxic/ototoxic/neurotoxic **Notes:** Follow CrCl & serum conc for dosage adjustments (see Table 2, page 265); once daily dosing becoming popular; follow SCr; use IBW to dose (use adjusted if obese >30% IBW) **Interactions:** ↑ Ototoxicity, neurotoxicity, nephrotoxicity w/ aminoglycosides, amphotericin B, cephalosporins, loop diuretics, penicillins; ↑ effects w/ NSAIDs; ↓ effects w/ carbenicillin; **Labs:** False ↑ AST, urine protein; ↑ urine amino acids **NIPE:** Photosensitivity—use sunscreen

Gentamicin & Prednisolone, Ophthalmic (Pred-G Ophthalmic)

Uses: *Steroid-responsive ocular & conjunctival infections* sensitive to gentamicin (eg, *Staphylococcus, E. coli, H. influenzae, Klebsiella, Neisseria, Pseudomonas, Proteus,* & *Serratia* sp) Action: Bactericidal; inhibits protein synthesis plus antiinflammatory Dose: *Oint:* ½ in. in conjunctival sac qd–tid. *Susp:* 1 gt bid–qid, up to 1 gt/h for severe infections Contra: Aminoglycoside sensitivity Caution: [C, ?] Supplied: *Oint, ophth:* Prednisolone acetate 0.6% & gentamicin sulfate 0.3% (3.5 g). *Susp, ophth:* Prednisolone acetate 1% & gentamicin sulfate 0.3% (2, 5, 10 mL) SE: Local irritation. See Gentamicin. Additional NIPE: Systemic effects w/ long-term use

Gentamicin, Ophthalmic (Garamycin, Genoptic, Gentacidin, Gentak, others)

Uses: *Conjunctival infections* Action: Bactericidal; inhibits protein synthesis Dose: *Oint:* Apply ½ in. bid–tid. *Soln:* 1–2 gtt q2–4h, up to 2 gtt/h for severe infection Caution: [C, ?] Contra: Aminoglycoside sensitivity Supplied: Soln & oint 0.3% SE: Local irritation Notes: ⊘ Use of other eye drops w/in 5–10 mins; ⊘ touch dropper to eye. See Gentamicin. NIPE: ⊘ Other eye drops for 10 min after administering this drug

Gentamicin, Topical (Garamycin, G-Mycitin)

Uses: *Skin infections* caused by susceptible organisms Action: Bactericidal; inhibits protein synthesis Dose: *Adults & Peds.* >1 y: Apply tid–qid Caution: [C, ?] Contra: Aminoglycoside sensitivity Supplied: Cream & oint 0.1% SE: Irritation. See Gentamicin. NIPE: ⊘ Apply to large denuded areas

Glimepiride (Amaryl)

Uses: *Type 2 DM* Action: Sulfonylurea; stimulates pancreatic insulin release; ↑ peripheral insulin sensitivity; ↓ hepatic glucose output & production Dose: 1–4 mg/d, max 8 mg Caution: [C, –] Contra: DKA Supplied: Tabs 1, 2, 4 mg SE: HA, nausea, hypoglycemia Notes: Give w/ 1st meal of day Interactions: ↑ Effects w/ ACEIs, adrenergic antagonists, BBs, chloramphenicol, MAOIs, NSAIDs, probenecid, salicylates, sulfonamides, warfarin, ginseng, garlic; ↓ effects w/ corticosteroids, estrogens, INH, oral contraceptives, nicotinic acid, phenytoin, sympathomimetics, thiazide diuretics, thyroid hormones NIPE: Antabuse-like effect w/ EtOH

Glipizide (Glucotrol, Glucotrol XL)

Uses: *Type 2 DM* Action: Sulfonylurea; stimulates pancreatic insulin release; ↑ peripheral insulin sensitivity Dose: ↓ hepatic glucose output & production; ↓ intestinal absorption of glucose Dose: 5 mg initial, ↑ by 2.5–5 mg/d, max 40 mg/d; XL max 20 mg Caution: [C, ?/–] Severe liver Dz Contra: DKA, Type 1 DM, sensitivity to sulfonamides Supplied: Tabs 5, 10 mg; XL tabs 2.5, 5, 10 mg SE: HA, anorexia, N/V/D, constipation, fullness, rash, urticaria, photosensitivity Notes: Counsel Pt about diabetes management; wait several days before adjusting dose; monitor glucose; give 30 min before meal; hold dose if Pt NPO Interactions: ↑ Effects w/ azole antifungals, anabolic steroids, chloramphenicol, cimetidine, clofibrate, MAOIs, NSAIDs, probenecid, salicylates, sulfonamides, TCAs, warfarin, celery, coriander, dandelion root, fenugreek, ginseng, garlic, juniper berries; ↓ effects w/ amphetamines, corticosteroids, epinephrine, estrogens, glucocorticoids, oral contraceptives, phenytoin, rifampin, sympathomimetics, thiazide diuretics, thyroid hormones, tobacco **NIPE:** Antabuse-like effect w/ EtOH

Glucagon Uses: Severe *hypoglycemic* Rxns in DM w/ sufficient liver glycogen stores or BB OD **Action:** Accelerates liver gluconeogenesis **Dose:** *Adults.* 0.5–1 mg SQ, IM, or IV; repeat in 20 min PRN. *BB OD:* 3–10 mg IV; repeat in 10 min PRN; may give as cont infus 1–5 mg/h. *Peds.* Neonates: 0.3 mg/kg/dose SQ, IM, or IV q4h PRN. *Children:* 0.025–0.1 mg/kg/dose SQ, IM, or IV; repeat in 20 min PRN **Caution:** [B, M] **Contra:** Known pheochromocytoma **Supplied:** Inj 1 mg **SE:** N/V, hypotension **Notes:** Administration of glucose IV necessary; ineffective in states of starvation, adrenal insufficiency, or chronic hypoglycemia **Interactions:** ↑ Effect w/ epinephrine, phenytoin; ↑ effects of anticoagulants; **Labs:** ↓ Serum K⁺; **NIPE:** Response w/in 20 min after inj

Glyburide (DiaBeta, Micronase, Glynase) Uses: *Type 2 DM* **Action:** Sulfonylurea: stimulates pancreatic insulin release; ↑ peripheral insulin sensitivity; ↓ hepatic glucose output & production; ↑ intestinal absorption of glucose **Dose:** 1.25–10 mg qd–bid, max 20 mg/d. *Micronized:* 0.75–6 mg qd–bid, max 12 mg/d **Caution:** [C, ?] Renal impairment **Contra:** DKA, Type I DM **Supplied:** Tabs 1.25, 2.5, 5 mg; micronized tabs 1.5, 3, 6 mg **SE:** HA, hypoglycemia **Notes:** ⊘ for CrCl <50 mL/min; hold dose if Pt NPO **Interactions:** ↑ Effects w/ anticoagulants, anabolic steroids, BBs, chloramphenicol, cimetidine, clofibrate, MAOIs, NSAIDs, probenecid, salicylates, sulfonamides, TCAs, EtOH, celery, coriander, dandelion root, fenugreek, ginseng, garlic, juniper berries; ↓ effects w/ amphetamines, corticosteroids, baclofen, epinephrine, glucocorticoids, oral contraceptives, phenytoin, rifampin, sympathomimetics, thiazide diuretics, thyroid hormones, tobacco **Labs:** False ↑ urine protein **NIPE:** Antabuse-like effect w/ EtOH

Glyburide/Metformin (Glucovance) Uses: *Type 2 DM* **Action:** *Sulfonylurea:* Stimulates pancreatic insulin release *Metformin:* ↑ Peripheral insulin sensitivity; ↓ hepatic glucose output & production; ↓ intestinal absorption of glucose **Dose:** 1st line (naive Pts), 1.25/250 mg PO qd–bid; 2nd line, 2.5/500 mg or 5/500 mg bid (max 20/2000 mg); take w/ meals, ↑ dose gradually **Caution:** [C, –] **Contra:** SCr >1.4 in females or >1.5 in males; hypoxemic conditions (CHF, sepsis, recent MI); alcoholism; metabolic acidosis; liver Dz; hold dose prior to & 48 h after ionic contrast media **Supplied:** Tabs 1.25/250 mg, 2.5/500 mg, 5/500 mg **SE:** HA, hypoglycemia, lactic acidosis, anorexia, N/V, rash **Notes:** ⊘ EtOH; hold dose if NPO; monitor folate levels for megaloblastic anemia. See Glyburide. **Additional Interactions:** ↑ Effects w/ amiloride, ciprofloxacin cimetidine, digoxin, miconazole, morphine, nifedipine, procainamide, quinidine, quinine, ranitidine, triamterene, trimethoprim, vancomycin; ↓ effects w/ CCBs, INH, phenothiazines

Glycerin Suppository Uses: *Constipation* **Action:** Hyperosmolar laxative **Dose:** *Adults.* 1 adult supp PR PRN. *Peds.* 1 infant supp PR qd–bid PRN **Cau-**

tion: [C, ?] **Supplied:** Supp (adult, infant); liq 4 mL/applicatorful **SE:** Can cause diarrhea **Interactions:** ↑ Effects w/ diuretics **Labs:** ↑ Serum triglycerides, phosphatidylglycerol in amniotic fluid; ↓ serum Ca **NIPE:** Insert and retain for 15 min

Gonadorelin (Lutrepulse) Uses: *Primary hypothalamic amenorrhea* **Action:** Stimulates the pituitary to release the gonadotropins LH & FSH **Dose:** 5 µg IV q 90 min × 21 d using Lutrepulse pump kit **Caution:** [B, M] ↑ levels w/ androgens, estrogens, progestins, glucocorticoids, spironolactone, levodopa; ↓ levels w/ OCP, digoxin, dopamine antagonists **Contra:** Any condition exacerbated by PRG, ovarian cysts, causes of anovulation other than hypothalamic, conditions worsened by reproductive hormones, hormone-dependent tumor **Supplied:** Inj 100 µg **SE:** Risk of multiple pregnancies; inj site pain **Notes:** Monitor LH, FSH **Interactions:** ↑ Effects w/ androgens, estrogens, glucocorticoids, levodopa, progestins, spironolactone; ↓ effects w/ digoxin, dopamine antagonists, oral contraceptives, phenothiazines

Goserelin (Zoladex) Uses: Advanced *CAP* & w/ radiation for localized CAP, *endometriosis, breast CA* **Action:** LHRH agonist, inhibits LH, resulting in ↓ testosterone **Dose:** 3.6 mg SQ (implant) q 28d or 10.8 mg SQ q3mo; usually into lower abdominal wall **Caution:** [X, −] **Contra:** PRG, breast-feeding, 10.8-mg implant not for women **Supplied:** Subcutaneous implant 3.6 (1 mo), 10.8 mg (3 mo) **SE:** Hot flashes, ↓ libido, gynecomastia, & transient exacerbation of CA-related bone pain ("flare Rxn" 7–10 d after 1st dose) **Notes:** Inject SQ into fat in abdominal wall; ⊘ aspirate; females must use contraception **Interactions:** None noted **Labs:** ↑ Alkaline phosphatase, estradiol, HDL, LDL, triglycerides; initial ↑ then ↓ after 1–2 wk FSH, LH, testosterone

Granisetron (Kytril) Uses: *Prevention of N/V* **Action:** Serotonin receptor antagonist **Dose:** *Adults & Peds.* 10 µg/kg/dose IV 30 min prior to initiation of chemotherapy *Adults.* 2 mg PO 1 h prior to chemotherapy, then 12 h later. *Postop N/V:* 1 mg IV before end of operative case **Caution:** [B, +/−] St. John's wort may ↓ levels **Contra:** Liver Dz, children <2 y **Supplied:** Tabs 1 mg; inj 1 mg/mL; soln 2 mg/10 mL **SE:** HA, constipation **Interactions:** ↑ Serotonergic effects w/ horehound; ↑ extrapyramidal Rxns w/ drugs causing these effects **Labs:** ↑ ALT, AST **NIPE:** May cause anaphylactic Rxn

Guaifenesin (Robitussin, others) Uses: *Symptomatic relief of dry, nonproductive cough* **Action:** Expectorant **Dose:** *Adults.* 200–400 mg (10–20 mL),PO q4h (max 2.4 g/d). *Peds.* <2 y: 12 mg/kg/d in 6 ÷ doses. 2–5 y: 50–100 mg (2.5–5 mL) PO q4h (max 600 mg/d). 6–11 y: 100–200 mg (5–10 mL) PO q4h (max 1.2 g/d) **Caution:** [C, ?] **Supplied:** Tabs 100, 200; SR tabs 600, 1200 mg; caps 200 mg; SR caps 300 mg; liq 100 mg/5 mL **SE:** GI upset **Notes:** Give w/ large amount of water; some dosage forms contain EtOH **Interactions:** ↑ Bleeding w/ heparin **Labs:** False results of urine 5-HIAA, VMA **NIPE:** ↑ Fluid intake

Guaifenesin & Codeine (Robitussin AC, Brontex, others) [C-V] Uses: *Symptomatic relief of dry, nonproductive cough* **Action:** Antitussive w/ expectorant **Dose:** *Adults.* 5–10 mL or 1 tab PO q6–8h (max 60 mL/24 h). *Peds.* 2–6 y: 1–1.5 mg/kg codeine/d ÷ dose q4–6h (max 30 mg/24 h). *6–12 y:* 5 mL q4h (max 30 mL/24 h) **Caution:** [C, +] **Supplied:** Brontex tab 10 mg codeine/300 mg guaifenesin; liq 2.5 mg codeine/75 mg guaifenesin/5 mL; others 10 mg codeine/100 mg guaifenesin/5 mL **SE:** Somnolence **Interactions:** ↑ CNS depression w/ barbiturates, antihistamines, glutethimide, methocarbamol, cimetidine, EtOH; ↓ effects w/ quinidine **Labs:** ↑ Urine morphine; false ↑ amylase, lipase **NIPE:** Take w/ food

Guaifenesin & Dextromethorphan (many OTC brands)
Uses: *Cough* due to upper resp tract irritation **Action:** Antitussive w/ expectorant **Dose:** *Adults & Peds.* >12 y: 10 mL PO q6–8h (max 40 mL/24 h). *Peds.* 2–6 y: Dextromethorphan 1–2 mg/kg/24 h ÷ 3–4 × d (max 10 mL/d). *6–12 y:* 5 mL q6–8h (max 20 mL/d) **Caution:** [C, +] **Contra:** Administration w/ MAOI **Supplied:** Many OTC formulations **SE:** Somnolence **Notes:** Give w/ plenty of fluids **Interactions:** ↑ Effects w/ quinidine, terbinafine; ↑ effects of isocarboxazid, MAOIs, phenelzine; ↑ risk of serotonin syndrome w/ sibutramine

Haemophilus B Conjugate Vaccine (ActHIB, HibTITER, PedvaxHIB, Prohibit, others)
Uses: Routine *immunization* of children against *H. influenzae* type B Dzs **Action:** Active immunization against *Haemophilus* B **Dose:** *Peds.* 0.5 mL (25 mg) IM in deltoid or vastus lateralis **Caution:** [C, +] **Contra:** Febrile illness, immunosuppression, hypersensitivity to thimerosal **Supplied:** Inj 7.5, 10, 15, 25 µg/0.5 mL **SE:** Observe for anaphylaxis; edema, ↑ risk of *Haemophilus* B infection in the week after vaccination **Notes:** Booster not required; report all serious adverse Rxn to VAERS: 1-800-822-7967 **Interactions:** ↓ Effects w/ immunosuppressives, steroids

Haloperidol (Haldol)
Uses: *Psychotic disorders, agitation, Tourette's disorders, & hyperactivity in children* **Action:** Antipsychotic, neuroleptic **Dose:** *Adults.* Moderate Sxs: 0.5–2.0 mg PO bid–tid. *Severe Sxs/agitation:* 3–5 mg PO bid–tid or 1–5 mg IM q4h PRN (max 100 mg/d). *Peds.* 3–6 y: 0.01–0.03 mg/kg/24 h PO qd. *6–12 y:* Initially, 0.5–1.5 mg/24 h PO; ↑ by 0.5 mg/24 h to maintenance of 2–4 mg/24 h (0.05–0.1 mg/kg/24 h) or 1–3 mg/dose IM q4–8h to a max of 0.1 mg/kg/24 h; Tourette's may require up to 15 mg/24 h PO; ↓ dose in elderly **Caution:** [C, ?] ↑ effects w/ SSRIs, CNS depressants, TCA, indomethacin, metoclopramide; ⊘ levodopa (inhibits antiparkinsonian effects of levodopa) **Contra:** Narrow-angle glaucoma, severe CNS depression, Parkinson's, bone marrow suppression, severe cardiac/hepatic Dz, coma **Supplied:** Tabs 0.5, 1, 2, 5, 10, 20 mg; conc liq 2 mg/mL; inj 5 mg/mL; decanoate inj 50, 100 mg/mL **SE:** Extrapyramidal Sxs (EPS), hypotension, anxiety, dystonias **Notes:** ⊘ administer decanoate IV; dilute PO conc liq w/ water/juice; monitor for EPS **Interactions:** ↑ Effects w/ CNS depressants, quinidine, EtOH; ↑ hypotension w/ antihypertensives, nitrates; ↑ anticholinergic effects w/ antihistamines, antidepressants, atropine, phenothiazines, quinidine, disopyramide; ↓ effects w/ antacids, carbamazepine, Li, nutmeg, to-

bacco; ↓ effects of anticoagulants, levodopa, guanethidine **Labs:** False + PRG test, ↓ serum cholesterol **NIPE:** ↑ Risk of photosensitivity—use sunscreen

Haloprogin (Halotex) **Uses:** *Topical Rx of tinea pedis, tinea cruris, tinea corporis, tinea manus* **Action:** Topical antifungal **Dose:** *Adults.* Apply bid for up to 2 wk; intertriginous Sxs may require up to 4 wk **Caution:** [B, ?] **Contra:** Component sensitivity **Supplied:** 1% cream; soln **SE:** Local irritation **Notes:** ⊘ Contact w/ eyes; improvement should occur w/in 4 wk

Heparin **Uses:** *Rx & prevention of DVT & PE,* unstable angina, AF w/ emboli formation, & acute arterial occlusion **Action:** Acts w/ antithrombin III to inactivate thrombin & inhibit thromboplastin formation **Dose:** *Adults.* Prophylaxis: 3000–5000 units SQ q8–12h. *Thrombosis Rx:* Loading dose 50–80 units/kg IV, then 10–20 units/kg IV qh (adjusted based on PTT). *Peds.* Infants: Loading dose 50 units/kg IV bolus, then 20 units/kg/h IV by cont inf. *Children:* Loading dose 50 units/kg IV, then 15–25 units/kg cont inf or 100 units/kg/dose q4h IV intermittent bolus (adjust based on PTT) **Caution:** [B, +] ↑ risk of hemorrhage w/ anticoagulants, ASA, antiplts, cephalosporins that contain MTT side chain **Contra:** Uncontrolled bleeding, severe thrombocytopenia, suspected ICH **Supplied:** Inj 10, 100, 1000, 2000, 2500, 5000, 7500, 10,000, 20,000, 40,000 units/mL **SE:** Bruising, bleeding, thrombocytopenia **Notes:** Follow PTT, thrombin time, or activated clotting time to assess effectiveness; little effect on the PT; therapeutic PTT is 1.5–2 × control for most conditions; monitor for thrombocytopenia (HIT); follow plt counts **Interactions:** ↑ Effects w/ anticoagulants, antihistamines, ASA, clopidogrel, cardiac glycosides, cephalosporins, pyridamole, NSAIDs, quinine, tetracycline, ticlopidine, ferverfew, ginkgo biloba, ginger, valerian; ↓ effects w/ nitroglycerine, ginseng, goldenseal, ↓ effects of insulin **Labs:** ↑ LFTs, TFTs

Hepatitis A Vaccine (Havrix, Vaqta) **Uses:** *Prevent hepatitis A* in high-risk individuals (eg, travelers, certain professions, or high-risk behaviors) **Action:** Provides active immunity **Dose:** (Expressed as ELISA units [EL. U.]) *Havrix: Adults.* 1440 EL. U. single IM dose. *Peds.* >2 y: 720 EL. U. single IM dose. *Vaqta: Adults.* 50 units single IM dose. *Peds.* 25 units single IM dose **Caution:** [C, +] **Contra:** Hypersensitivity to any component of formulation **Supplied:** Inj 720 EL.U./0.5 mL, 1440 EL.U./1 mL.; 50 units/mL **SE:** Fever, fatigue, pain at inj site, HA **Notes:** Booster recommended 6–12 mo after primary vaccination; report all serious adverse Rxns to VAERS: 1-800-822-7967 **Interactions:** None noted **NIPE:** ⊘ if Pt febrile

Hepatitis A (Inactivated) & Hepatitis B (Recombinant) Vaccine (Twinrix) **Uses:** *Active immunization against hepatitis A/B* **Action:** Active immunity **Dose:** 1 mL IM at 0, 1, & 6 mo **Caution:** [C, +] **Contra:** Component sensitivity **Supplied:** Single-dose vials, syringes **SE:** Fever, fatigue, pain at inj site, HA **Notes:** Booster recommended 6–12 mo after primary vaccination; report all serious adverse Rxns to VAERS: 1-800-822-7967 **Interactions:** ↓ Immune response w/ corticosteroids, immunosuppressants **NIPE:** ↑ Response if inj in deltoid vs gluteus

Hepatitis B Immune Globulin (HyperHep, H-BIG)   Uses: *Exposure to HBsAg+ materials,* eg, blood, plasma, or serum (accidental needlestick, mucous membrane contact, or PO ingestion) **Action:** Passive immunization **Dose: Adults & Peds.** 0.06 mL/kg IM to a max of 5 mL; w/in 24 h of needle-stick or percutaneous exposure; w/in 14 d of sexual contact; repeat 1 & 6 mo after exposure **Caution:** [C, ?] **Contra:** Allergies to γ-globulin or antiimmunoglobulin antibodies; allergies to thimerosal, IgA deficiency **Supplied:** Inj **SE:** Pain at site, dizziness **Notes:** Administered IM in gluteal or deltoid; if exposure continues, Pt should also receive the hepatitis B vaccine **Interactions:** ↓ Immune response if given w/ live virus vaccines

Hepatitis B Vaccine (Engerix-B, Recombivax HB)   Uses: *Prevention of hepatitis B* **Action:** Active immunization **Dose: Adults.** 3 IM doses of 1 mL each, the 1st 2 doses given 1 mo apart, the 3rd 6 mo after the 1st. **Peds.** 0.5 mL IM given on the same schedule as for adults **Caution:** [C, +] ↓ effect w/ immunosuppressives **Contra:** Yeast hypersensitivity **Supplied:** *Engerix-B:* Inj 20 μg/mL; peds inj 10 μg/0.5 mL. *Recombivax HB:* Inj 10 & 40 μg/mL; peds inj 5 μg/0.5 mL **SE:** Fever, inj site soreness **Notes:** IM inj for adults & older peds in the deltoid; in other peds, administer in the anterolateral thigh; derived from recombinant DNA technology **Interactions:** ↓ Immune response w/ corticosteroids, immunosuppressants **NIPE:** ↑ Response inj in deltoid vs gluteus

Hetastarch (Hespan)   Uses: *Plasma volume expansion* as adjunct in the Rx of shock & leukapheresis **Action:** Synthetic colloid w/ actions similar to albumin **Dose:** *Volume expansion:* 500–1000 mL (1500 mL/d max) IV at a rate not to exceed 20 mL/kg/h. *Leukapheresis:* 250–700 mL; ↓ in renal failure **Caution:** [C, +] **Contra:** Severe bleeding disorders, CHF, or renal failure w/ oliguria or anuria **Supplied:** Inj 6 g/100 mL **SE:** Bleeding side effect (prolongs PT, PTT, bleed time, etc) **Notes:** Not a substitute for blood or plasma **NIPE:** Monitor CBC, PT, PTT; observe for anaphylactic Rxns

Hydralazine (Apresoline, others)   Uses: *Moderate to severe HTN; CHF* (w/ Isordil) **Action:** Peripheral vasodilator **Dose: Adults.** Begin at 10 mg PO qid, then ↑ to 25 mg qid to max of 300 mg/d. **Peds.** 0.75–3 mg/kg/24 h PO ÷ q6–12h; ↓ in renal impairment; check CBC & ANA before starting **Caution:** [C, +] ↓ hepatic Fxn & CAD; ↑ toxicity w/ MAOI, indomethacin, BBs **Contra:** Dissecting aortic aneurysm, mitral heart rheumatic heart Dz **Supplied:** Tabs 10, 25, 50, 100 mg; inj 20 mg/mL **SE:** Chronically high doses cause SLE-like syndrome; SVT following IM administration, peripheral neuropathy **Notes:** Compensatory sinus tachycardia eliminated w/ use of a BB **Interactions:** ↑ Effects w/ antihypertensives, diazoxide, diuretics, MAOIs, nitrates, EtOH; ↓ pressor response w/ epinephrine; ↓ effects w/ NSAIDs **NIPE:** Take w/ food

Hydrochlorothiazide (HydroDIURIL, Esidrix, others) Uses: *Edema, HTN* **Action:** Thiazide diuretic; inhibits Na reabsorption in the distal tubule **Dose:** *Adults.* 25–100 mg/d PO in single or ÷ doses. *Peds.* <6 mo: 2–3 mg/kg/d in 2 ÷ doses. >6 mo: 2 mg/kg/d in 2 ÷ doses **Caution:** [D, +] **Contra:** Anuria, sulfonamide allergy, renal decompensation **Supplied:** Tabs 25, 50, 100 mg; caps 12.5 mg; PO soln 50 mg/5 mL **SE:** ↓ K+, hyperglycemia, hyperuricemia, hyponatremia **Interactions:** ↑ Hypotension w/ ACEIs, antihypertensives, carbenoxolone, ↑ hypokalemia w/ carbenoxolone, corticosteroids; ↑ hyperglycemia w/ BBs, diazoxide, hypoglycemic drugs; ↑ effects of Li, MRX; ↓ effects w/ amphetamines, cholestyramine, colestipol, NSAIDs, quinidine, dandelion **Labs:** False ↓ urine estriol **NIPE:** Monitor uric acid, take w/ food, ↑ risk of photosensitivity—use sunscreen

Hydrochlorothiazide & Amiloride (Moduretic) Uses: *HTN* **Action:** Combined effects of a thiazide diuretic & a K-sparing diuretic **Dose:** 1–2 tabs/d PO **Caution:** [D, ?] **Contra:** ⊘ Give to Pts w/ renal failure, sulfonamide allergy **Supplied:** Tabs (amiloride/HCTZ) 5 mg/50 mg **SE:** Hypotension, photosensitivity, hyper-/hypokalemia, hyperglycemia, hyponatremia, hyperlipidemia, hyperuricemia

Hydrochlorothiazide & Spironolactone (Aldactazide) Uses: *Edema, HTN* **Action:** Combined thiazide diuretic & a K-sparing diuretic **Dose:** 25–200 mg each component/d in ÷ doses **Caution:** [D, +] **Contra:** Sulfonamide allergy **Supplied:** Tabs (HCTZ/spironolactone) 25 mg/25 mg, 50 mg/50 mg **SE:** Photosensitivity, hypotension, hyper-/hypokalemia, hyperglycemia, hyponatremia, hyperlipidemia, hyperuricemia. See Hydrochlorothiazide **Additional Interactions:** ↑ Risk of hyperkalemia w/ ACEIs, K-sparing diuretics, K suppls, salt substitutes; ↓ effects of digoxin **NIPE:** DC drug 3 d before glucose tolerance test

Hydrochlorothiazide & Triamterene (Dyazide, Maxzide) Uses: *Edema & HTN* **Action:** Combined thiazide diuretic & a K-sparing diuretic **Dose:** *Dyazide:* 1–2 caps PO qd–bid. *Maxzide:* 1 tab/d PO **Caution:** [D, +/–] **Contra:** Sulfonamide allergy **Supplied:** (Triamterene/HCTZ) 37.5 mg/25 mg, 50 mg/25 mg, 75 mg/50 mg **SE:** Photosensitivity, hypotension, hyper-/hypokalemia, hyperglycemia, hyponatremia, hyperlipidemia, hyperuricemia **Notes:** HCTZ component in Maxzide more bioavailable than in Dyazide. See Hydrochlorothiazide. **Additional Interactions:** ↑ Risk of hyperkalemia w/ ACEIs, K-sparing diuretics, K suppls, salt substitutes; ↑ effects w/ cimetidine, licorice root, ↓ effects of digoxin **Labs:** ↑ Serum glucose, BUN, creatinine K+, Mg^{2+}, uric acid, urinary Ca^{2+}; interference w/ assay of quinidine & lactic dehydrogenase **NIPE:** Urine may turn blue

Hydrocodone & Acetaminophen (Lorcet, Vicodin, others) [C-III] Uses: *Moderate to severe pain*; hydrocodone has antitussive properties **Action:** Narcotic analgesic w/ nonnarcotic analgesic **Dose:** 1–2 caps or tabs PO q4–6h PRN **Caution:** [C, M] **Contra:** CNS depression, severe resp depression **Supplied:** Many different combinations; specify hydrocodone/APAP dose; caps 5/500; tabs 2.5/500, 5/400, 5/500, 7.5/400, 10/400, 7.5/500, 7.5/650, 7.5/750,

10/325, 10/400, 10/500, 10/650; elixir & soln (fruit punch flavor) 2.5 mg hydrocodone/167 mg APAP/5 mL **SE:** GI upset, sedation, fatigue **Notes:** ⊘ Exceed >4 g acetaminophen/d **Interactions:** ↑ Effects w/ antihistamines, cimetidine, CNS depressants, dextroamphetamines, glutethimide, MAOIs, protease inhibitors, TCAs, EtOH, St. John's wort; ↑ effects of warfarin; ↓ effects w/ phenothiazines **Labs:** False ↑ amylase, lipase **NIPE:** Take w/ food, ↑ fluid intake

Hydrocodone & Aspirin (Lortab ASA, others) [C-III] Uses: *Moderate to severe pain* **Action:** Narcotic analgesic w/ NSAID **Dose:** 1–2 PO q4–6h PRN **Caution:** [C, M] ↓ renal Fxn, gastritis/PUD, ⊘ use in children for chickenpox (Reye's syndrome) **Contra:** Component sensitivity **Supplied:** 5 mg hydrocodone/500 mg ASA/tab **SE:** GI upset, sedation, fatigue **Notes:** Give w/ food/milk; monitor for GI bleed. See Hydrocodone and Acetaminophen

Hydrocodone & Guaifenesin (Hycotuss Expectorant, others) [C-III] Uses: *Nonproductive cough* associated w/ resp infection **Action:** Expectorant plus cough suppressant **Dose:** *Adults & Peds.* >12 y: 5 mL q4h pc & hs. *Peds.* < 2 y: 0.3 mg/kg/d ÷ qid. *2–12 y:* 2.5 mL q4h pc & hs **Caution:** [C, M] **Contra:** Component sensitivity **Supplied:** Hydrocodone 5 mg/guaifenesin 100 mg/5 mL **SE:** GI upset, sedation, fatigue. See Hydrocodone and Acetaminophen. **Additional Interactions:** ↑ Bleeding w/ heparin **Labs:** False results of urine 5-HIAA, VMA

Hydrocodone & Homatropine (Hycodan, Hydromet, others) [C-III] Uses: *Relief of cough* **Action:** Combination antitussive **Dose:** (Dose based on hydrocodone) *Adults.* 5–10 mg q4–6h. *Peds.* 0.6 mg/kg/d ÷ tid–qid **Caution:** [C, M] **Contra:** Narrow-angle glaucoma, ↑ ICP, depressed ventilation **Supplied:** Syrup 5 mg hydrocodone/5 mL; tabs 5 mg hydrocodone **SE:** Sedation, fatigue, GI upset **Notes:** ⊘ Give >q4h; see individual Rx monographs. See Hydrocodone and Acetaminophen. **Additional Labs:** ↑ ALT, AST

Hydrocodone & Ibuprofen (Vicoprofen) [C-III] Uses: *Moderate to severe pain (<10 d)* **Action:** Narcotic w/ NSAID **Dose:** 1–2 tabs q4–6h PRN **Caution:** [C, M] Renal insufficiency; ↓ effect w/ ACEIs & diuretics; ↑ effect w/ CNS depressants, EtOH, MAOI, ASA, TCA, anticoagulants **Contra:** Component sensitivity **Supplied:** Tabs 7.5 mg hydrocodone/200 mg ibuprofen **SE:** Sedation, fatigue, GI upset. See Hydrocodone and Acetaminophen **Additional Interactions:** ↓ Effects of ACEIs, diuretics

Hydrocodone & Pseudoephedrine (Detussin, Histussin-D, others) [C-III] Uses: *Cough & nasal congestion* **Action:** Narcotic cough suppressant w/ decongestant **Dose:** 5 mL qid, PRN **Caution:** [C, M] **Contra:** MAOIs **Supplied:** 5 mg hydrocodone/60 mg pseudoephedrine/5 mL **SE:** ↑ BP, GI upset, sedation, fatigue. See Hydrocodone and Acetaminophen **Additional Interactions:** ↑ Effects w/ sympathomimetics

Hydrocodone, Chlorpheniramine, Phenylephrine, Acetaminophen, & Caffeine (Hycomine Compound)[C-III] Uses:

Cough & Sxs of URI **Action:** Narcotic cough suppressant w/ decongestants & analgesic **Dose:** 1 tab PO q4h PRN **Caution:** [C, M] **Contra:** Narrow-angle glaucoma **Supplied:** Hydrocodone 5 mg/chlorpheniramine 2 mg/phenylephrine 10 mg/APAP 250 mg/caffeine 30 mg/tab **SE:** ↑ BP, GI upset, sedation, fatigue. See Hydrocodone and Acetaminophen

Hydrocortisone, Rectal (Anusol-HC Suppository, Cortifoam Rectal, Proctocort, others)
Uses: *Painful anorectal conditions,* radiation proctitis, management of ulcerative colitis **Action:** Antiinflammatory steroid **Dose:** *Adults.* *Ulcerative colitis:* 10–100 mg PR 1–2×/d for 2–3 wk **Caution:** [B, ?/–] **Contra:** Component sensitivity **Supplied:** *Hydrocortisone acetate:* Rectal aerosol 90 mg/applicator; supp 25 mg. *Hydrocortisone base:* Rectal 1%; rectal susp 100 mg/60 mL **SE:** Minimal systemic effect **NIPE:** Administer after BM, insert supp blunt end first, admin enema w/ Pt lying on side and retain for 1 h

Hydrocortisone, Topical & Systemic (Cortef, Solu-Cortef)
Caution: [B, –] **Contra:** Viral, fungal, or tubercular skin lesions; serious infections (except septic shock or tuberculous meningitis) **SE:** Systemic forms: ↑d appetite, insomnia, hyperglycemia, bruising **Notes:** May cause HPA axis suppression **Interactions:** ↑ Effects w/ cyclosporine, estrogens; ↑ effects of cardiac glycosides, cyclosporine; ↑ risk of GI bleed w/ NSAIDs; ↓ effects w/ aminoglutethimide, antacids, barbiturates, cholestyramine, colestipol, ephedrine, phenobarbital, phenytoin, rifampin; ↓ effects of anticoagulants, hypoglycemics, insulin, INH, salicylates **Labs:** False – in skin allergy tests **NIPE:** ⊘ EtOH, live virus vaccines, abrupt DC of drug; take w/ food; may mask S/Sxs infection

Hydromorphone (Dilaudid) [C–II]
Uses: *Moderate/severe pain* **Action:** Narcotic analgesic **Dose:** 1–4 mg PO, IM, IV, or PR q4–6h PRN; 3 mg PR q6–8h PRN; ↓ w/ hepatic failure **Caution:** [B (D if prolonged use or high doses near term), ?] ↑ effects w/ CNS depressants, phenothiazines, TCA **Contra:** Component sensitivity **Supplied:** Tabs 1, 2, 3, 4, 8 mg; liq 5 mg/mL; inj 1, 2, 4, 10 mg/mL; supp 3 mg **SE:** Sedation, dizziness, GI upset **Notes:** Morphine 10 mg IM = hydromorphone 1.5 mg IM **Interactions:** ↑ Effects w/ CNS depressants, phenothiazines, TCAs, EtOH, St. John's wort; ↓ effects w/ nalbuphine, pentazocine **Labs:** ↑ Serum amylase, lipase **NIPE:** Take w/ food, ↑ fluids & fiber to prevent constipation

Hydroxyurea (Hydrea, Droxia)
Uses: *CML, head & neck, ovarian & colon CA, melanoma, acute leukemia, sickle cell anemia, polycythemia vera, HIV* **Action:** Inhibitor of the ribonucleotide reductase system **Dose:** (Refer to individual protocols) 50–75 mg/kg for WBC counts of >100,000 cells/mL; 20–30 mg/kg in refractory CML. *HIV:* 1000–1500 mg/d in single or ÷ doses; ↓ in renal insufficiency **Caution:** [D, –] ↑ effects w/ zidovudine, zalcitabine, didanosine, stavudine, fluorouracil **Contra:** Severe anemia, severe bone marrow suppression, WBC <2500 or plt <100,000, PRG **Supplied:** Caps 200, 300, 400, 500 mg; tabs

1000 mg **SE:** Myelosuppression (primarily leukopenia), N/V, rashes, facial erythema, radiation recall Rxns, & renal dysfunction **Notes:** Capsules can be opened & emptied into water **Interactions:** ↑ Risk of pancreatitis w/ didanosine, indinavir, stavudine; ↑ bone marrow depression w/ antineoplastic drugs or radiation therapy **Labs:** ↑ Serum uric acid, BUN, creatinine **NIPE:** ↑ Fluids 10–12 glasses/d, use barrier contraception, ↑ risk of infertility

Hydroxyzine (Atarax, Vistaril)
Uses: *Anxiety, sedation, itching* **Action:** Antihistamine, antianxiety **Dose:** *Adults.* Anxiety or sedation: 50–100 mg PO or IM qid or PRN (max 600 mg/d). *Itching:* 25–50 mg PO or IM tid–qid. *Peds.* 0.5–1.0 mg/kg/24 h PO or IM q6h; ↓ in hepatic failure **Caution:** [C, +/–] ↑ effects w/ CNS depressants, anticholinergics, EtOH **Contra:** Component sensitivity **Supplied:** Tabs 10, 25, 50, 100 mg; caps 25, 50, 100 mg; syrup 10 mg/5 mL; susp 25 mg/5 mL; inj 25, 50 mg/mL **SE:** Drowsiness & anticholinergic effects **Notes:** Useful in potentiating effects of narcotics; not for IV/SQ use due to thrombosis & digital gangrene **Interactions:** ↑ Effects w/ antihistamines, anticholinergics, CNS depressants, EtOH **Labs:** False – skin allergy tests; false ↑ in urinary 17-hydroxycorticosteroid levels

Hyoscyamine (Anaspaz, Cystospaz, Levsin, others)
Uses: *Spasm associated w/ GI & bladder disorders* **Action:** Anticholinergic **Dose:** *Adults.* 0.125–0.25 mg (1–2 tabs) SL/PO tid–qid, ac & hs; 1 SR cap q12h **Caution:** [C, +] ↑ effects w/ amantadine, antihistamines, antimuscarinics, haloperidol, phenothiazines, TCA, MAOI **Contra:** Obstructive uropathy, GI obstruction, glaucoma, MyG, paralytic ileus, severe ulcerative colitis, MI **Supplied:** (Cystospaz-M, Levsinex): cap timed release 0.375 mg; elixir (EtOH); soln 0.125 mg/5 mL; inj 0.5 mg/mL; tab 0.125 mg; tab (Cystospaz) 0.15 mg; XR tab (Levbid): 0.375 mg; SL (Levsin SL) 0.125 mg **SE:** Dry skin, xerostomia, constipation, anticholinergic SE **Notes:** Administer tabs ac/food; heat prostration may occur in hot weather **Interactions:** ↑ Effects w/ amantadine, antimuscarinics, haloperidol, phenothiazines, quinidine, TCAs, MAOIs; ↓ effects w/ antacids, antidiarrheals; ↓ effects of levodopa **NIPE:** ↑ Risk of heat intolerance, photophobia

Hyoscyamine, Atropine, Scopolamine, & Phenobarbital (Donnatal, others)
Uses: *Irritable bowel, spastic colitis, peptic ulcer, spastic bladder* **Action:** Anticholinergic, antispasmodic **Dose:** 0.125–0.25 mg (1–2 tabs) tid–qid, 1 cap q12h (SR), 5–10 mL elixir tid–qid or q8h **Caution:** [D, M] **Contra:** Narrow-angle glaucoma **Supplied:** Many combinations/manufacturers available; *Cap* (Donnatal, others): Hyoscyamine 0.1037 mg/atropine 0.0194 mg/scopolamine 0.0065 mg/phenobarbital 16.2 mg. *Tabs* (Donnatal, others): Hyoscyamine 0.1037 mg/atropine 0.0194 mg/scopolamine 0.0065 mg/phenobarbital 16.2 mg. *Long-acting* (Donnatal): Hyoscyamine 0.311 mg/atropine 0.0582 mg/scopolamine 0.0195 mg/phenobarbital 48.6 mg. *Elixirs* (Donnatal, others): Hyoscyamine 0.1037 mg/atropine 0.0194 mg/scopolamine 0.0065 mg/phenobarbital 16.2 mg/5 mL **SE:** Sedation, xerostomia, constipation **Interactions:** ↑ Effects

w/ anticoagulants, amantadine, antihistamines, antidiarrheals, anticonvulsants, CNS depressants, corticosteroids, digitalis, griseofulvin, MAOIs, phenothiazides, tetracyclines, TCAs **NIPE:** ↑ Risk of photophobia, constipation, urinary hesitancy

Ibuprofen (Motrin, Rufen, Advil, others) [OTC]
Uses: *Arthritis & pain* **Action:** NSAID **Dose:** *Adults.* 200–800 mg PO bid–qid (max 2.4 g/d). *Peds.* 30–40 mg/kg/d in 3–4 ÷ doses (max 40 mg/kg/d); best taken w/ food, caution when combined w/ other NSAIDs **Caution:** [B, +] **Contra:** Severe hepatic impairment, hypersensitivity to NSAIDs, UGI bleed, or ulcers, 3rd tri PRG **Supplied:** Tabs 100, 200, 400, 600, 800 mg; chew tabs 50, 100 mg; caps 200 mg; susp 100 mg/2.5 mL, 100 mg/5 mL, 40 mg/mL (200 mg is OTC prep) **SE:** Dizziness, peptic ulcer, plt inhibition, worsening of renal insufficiency **Interactions:** ↑ Effects w/ ASA, corticosteroids, probenecid, EtOH; ↑ effects of aminoglycosides, anticoagulants, digoxin, hypoglycemics, Li, MRX; ↑ risks of bleeding w/ abciximab, cefotetan, valproic acid, thrombolytic drugs, warfarin, ticlopidine, garlic, ginger, ginkgo biloba; ↓ effects w/ feverfew; ↓ effects of antihypertensives **Labs:** ↑ BUN, creatinine; ↓ Hmg, Hct, BS, plts **NIPE:** Take w/ food

Ibutilide (Corvert)
Uses: *Rapid conversion of AF or flutter* **Action:** Class III antiarrhythmic agent **Dose:** 0.01 mg/kg (max 1 mg) IV inf over 10 min; may be repeated once **Caution:** [C, –] ⊘ administer class I or III antiarrhythmics concurrently or w/in 4 h of ibutilide inf **Contra:** QTc > 440 ms **Supplied:** Inj 0.1 mg/mL **SE:** Arrhythmias, HA **Notes:** Observe Pt w/ continuous ECG monitoring **Interactions:** ↑ Refractory effects w/ amiodarone, disopyramide, procainamide, quinidine, sotalol; ↑ QT interval w/ antihistamines, antidepressants, erythromycin, phenothiazines, TCAs

Idarubicin (Idamycin)
Uses: *Acute leukemias* (AML, ALL, ANLL), *CML* in blast crisis, breast CA* **Action:** DNA intercalating agent; inhibits DNA topoisomerases I & II **Dose:** (Refer to individual protocols) 10–12 mg/m²/d for 3–4 d; ↓ in renal/hepatic dysfunction **Caution:** [D, –] **Contra:** Bilirubin >5 mg/dL, PRG **Supplied:** Inj 1 mg/mL (5-, 10-, 20-mg vials) **SE:** Myelosuppression, cardiotoxicity, N/V, mucositis, alopecia, & irritation at sites of IV administration, rare changes in renal/hepatic Fxn **Notes:** ⊘ Extravasation—potent vesicant; only given IV **Interactions:** ↑ Myelosuppression w/ antineoplastic drugs and radiation therapy; ↓ effects of live virus vaccines **NIPE:** ⊘ Fluids to 2–3 L/d

Ifosfamide (Ifex, Holoxan)
Uses: Lung, breast, pancreatic & gastric CA, HL/NHL, soft tissue sarcoma **Action:** Alkylating agent **Dose:** (Refer to individual protocols) 1.2 g/m²/d for 5 d by bolus or cont inf; 2.4 g/m²/d for 3 d; w/ mesna uroprotection; ↓ in renal/hepatic impairment **Caution:** [D, M] ↑ Clear w/ phenobarbital, carbamazepine, phenytoin; St. John's wort may ↓ levels **Contra:** Severely depressed bone marrow Fxn, PRG **Supplied:** Inj 1, 3 g **SE:** Hemorrhagic cystitis, nephrotoxicity, N/V, mild to moderate leukopenia, lethargy & confusion, alopecia, & ↑ hepatic enzyme **Notes:** Administer w/ mesna to prevent hemorrhagic cystitis **Interactions:** ↑ Effects w/ allopurinol, chloral hydrate, phenobarbital,

phenytoin, grapefruit juice; ↑ myelosuppression w/ antineoplastic drugs and radiation therapy; ↓ effects of live virus vaccines **NIPE:** ↑ Fluids to 2–3 L/d

Imatinib (Gleevec) *Uses:* *Rx of CML, blast crisis, gastrointestinal stromal tumors (GIST)* *Action:* Inhibits BCL-ABL tyrosine kinase (signal transduction) *Dose:* *Chronic phase CML:* 400–600 mg PO qd. *Accelerated/blast crisis*: 600–800 mg PO qd. *GIST:* 400–600 mg qd *Caution:* [D, ?/–] Metabolized by CYP3A4 (caution w/ warfarin, cyclosporine, azole antifungals, erythromycin, phenytoin, rifampin, carbamazepine) *Contra:* Component sensitivity *Supplied:* Caps 100 mg *SE:* GI upset, fluid retention, muscle cramps, musculoskeletal pain, arthralgia, rash, HA, neutropenia, thrombocytopenia *Notes:* Follow CBCs & LFTs baseline & monthly *Additional Interactions:* ↓ Effects w/ St. John's wort *NIPE:* Take w/ food, ↑ fluids, use barrier contraception

Imipenem–Cilastatin (Primaxin) *Uses:* *Serious infections* caused by a wide variety of susceptible bacteria *Action:* Bactericidal; interferes w/ cell wall synthesis. *Spectrum*: Gram(+) (inactive against *S. aureus*, group A & B streptococci), gram(–) (not *Legionella*), anaerobes *Dose:* *Adults.* 250–1000 mg (imipenem) IV q6–8h. *Peds.* 60–100 mg/kg/24 h IV ÷ q6h; ↓ in renal Dz if calculated CrCl is <70 mL/min *Caution:* [C, +/–] Probenecid may ↑ risk for toxicity *Contra:* Pediatric Pts w/ CNS infection (↑ Sz risk) & <30 kg w/ renal impairment *Supplied:* Inj (imipenem/cilastatin) 250/250 mg, 500/500 mg *SE:* Szs may occur if drug accumulates, GI upset, thrombocytopenia *Interactions:* ↑ Risks of Szs w/ ganciclovir, theophylline; ↓ effects w/ aztreonam, cephalosporins, chloramphenicol, penicillins, probenicid *Labs:* ↑ LFTs, BUN, creatinine; ↓ Hmg, Hct *NIPE:* Eval for superinfection

Imipramine (Tofranil) *Uses:* *Depression, enuresis,* panic attack, chronic pain *Action:* TCA; ↑ synaptic conc of serotonin or norepinephrine in the CNS *Dose:* *Adults.* Hospitalized: Initial 100 mg/24 h PO in ÷ doses; can ↑ over several wks to max 300 mg/d. *Outpatient:* Maint 50–150 mg PO hs, 300 mg/24 h max. *Peds.* Antidepressant: 1.5–5 mg/kg/24 h ÷ qd–qid. *Enuresis:*>6 y: 10–25 mg PO qhs; ↑ by 10–25 mg at 1–2-wk intervals (max 50 mg for 6–12 y, 75 mg for >12 y); treat for 2–3 mo, then taper *Caution:* [D, ?/–] *Contra:* Use w/ MAOIs, narrow-angle glaucoma, acute recovery phase of MI, PRG, CHF, angina, CVD, arrhythmias *Supplied:* Tabs 10, 25, 50 mg; caps 75, 100, 125, 150 mg *SE:* CV Sxs, dizziness, xerostomia, discolored urine *Notes:* Less sedation than w/ amitriptyline *Interactions:* ↑ Effects w/ amiodarone, anticholinergics, BBs, cimetidine, diltiazem, Li, oral contraceptives, quinidine, phenothiazines, ritonavir, verapamil, EtOH, evening primrose oil; ↑ effects of CNS depressants, hypoglycemics, warfarin; ↑ risk of serotonin syndrome w/ MAOIs; ↓ effects w/ carbamazepine, phenobarbital, rifampin, tobacco; ↓ effects of clonidine, guanethidine, methyldopa, reserpine *Labs:* ↑ Serum glucose, bilirubin, alkaline phosphatase *NIPE:* DC 48 h before surgery, DC MAOIs 2 wk before admin this drug, 4–6 wk for full effects, take w/ food

Imiquimod Cream, 5% (Aldara) **Uses:** *Anogenital warts, HPV, condylomata acuminata* **Action:** Unknown; may induce cytokines **Dose:** Applied 3×/wk, leave on skin for 6–10 h & wash off w/ soap & water, continue therapy for a max of 16 wk **Caution:** [B, ?] **Contra:** Component sensitivity **Supplied:** Single-dose packets 5% (250 mg of the cream) **SE:** Local skin Rxns common **Notes:** Not a cure; wash hands before & after application of cream **NIPE:** Condoms & diaphragms may be weakened—○ contact

Immune Globulin, IV (Gamimune N, Sandoglobulin, Gammar IV) **Uses:** *IgG antibody deficiency Dz states, (eg, congenital agammaglobulinemia, CVH, & BMT), HIV, hepatitis A prophylaxis, ITP* **Action:** IgG supplation **Dose:** *Adults & Peds.* Immunodeficiency: 100–200 mg/kg/mo IV at a rate of 0.01–0.04 mL/kg/min to a max of 400 mg/kg/dose. *ITP:* 400 mg/kg/dose IV qd × 5 d. *BMT:* 500 mg/kg/wk; ↓ in renal insufficiency **Caution:** [C, ?] Separate administration of live vaccines by 3 mo **Contra:** Isolated immunoglobulin A deficiency w/ antibodies to IgA, severe thrombocytopenia or coagulation disorders **Supplied:** Inj **SE:** Adverse effects associated mostly w/ rate of inf, GI upset **Interactions:** ↓ Effects of live virus vaccines **NIPE:** Give live virus vaccines 3 mo after this drug; rapid inf can cause anaphylactoid Rxn

Inamrinone [Amrinone] (Inocor) **Uses:** *Acute CHF, ischemic cardiomyopathy* **Action:** + inotrope w/ vasodilator activity **Dose:** Initial IV bolus 0.75 mg/kg over 2–3 min, then maint dose 5–10 μg/kg/min; 10 mg/kg/d max; ↓ if ClCr <10 mL/min **Caution:** [C, ?] **Contra:** Hypersensitivity to bisulfites **Supplied:** Inj 5 mg/mL **SE:** Monitor for fluid, electrolyte, & renal changes **Notes:** Incompatible w/ dextrose-containing solns **Interactions:** Precipitates form if contact made w/ furosemide; diuretics cause significant hypovolemia; ↑ effects of digitalis **Labs:** Monitor ALT, AST, BUN, creatinine, electrolytes, plts **NIPE:** Monitor I&O, daily weights, BP, pulse

Indapamide (Lozol) **Uses:** *HTN, edema, CHF* **Action:** Thiazide diuretic; enhances Na, Cl, & water excretion in the proximal segment of the distal tubule **Dose:** 1.25–5 mg/d PO **Caution:** [D, ?] ↑ effect w/ loop diuretics, ACEIs, cyclosporine, digoxin, Li **Contra:** Anuria, thiazide/sulfonamide allergy, renal decompensation, PRG **Supplied:** Tabs 1.25, 2.5 mg **SE:** Hypotension, dizziness, photosensitivity **Notes:** Doses >5 mg do not have additional effects on ↓ BP; take early in day to avoid nocturia; use sunscreen; may take w/ food/milk **Interactions:** ↑ Effects w/ antihypertensives, diazoxide, nitrates, EtOH; ↑ effects of ACEIs, Li; ↑ risk of gout w/ cyclosporine, thiazides; ↑ risk of hypokalemia w/ amphotericin B, corticosteroids, mezlocillin, piperacillin, ticarcillin; ↓ effects w/ cholestyramine, colestipol, NSAIDs; ↓ effects of hypoglycemics **Labs:** ↑ Serum glucose, uric acid, ↓ K⁺, Na, Cl **NIPE:** ↑ Risk photosensitivity—use sunscreen, take w/ food

Indinavir (Crixivan) **Uses:** *HIV infection* **Action:** Protease inhibitor; inhibits maturation of immature noninfectious virions to mature infectious virus **Dose:** 800 mg PO q8h; use in combination w/ other antiretroviral agents; take on an empty stomach; ↓ in hepatic impairment **Caution:** [C, ?] Numerous drug interactions **Contra:** Concomitant use w/ triazolam, midazolam, pimozide, ergot alkaloids; ⊘ use simvastatin, lovastatin, sildenafil, St. John's wort **Supplied:** Caps 100, 200, 333, 400 mg **SE:** Nephrolithiasis, dyslipidemia, lipodystrophy, GI effects **Interactions:** ↑ Effects w/ aldesleukin, azole antifungals, clarithromycin, delavirdine, interleukins, quinidine, zidovudine; ↑ effects of amiodarone, cisapride, clarithromycin, ergot alkaloids, fentanyl, HMG-CoA reductase inhibitors, INH, oral contraceptives, phenytoin, rifabutin, ritonavir, sildenafil, stavudine, zidovudine; ↓ effects w/ efavirenz, fluconazole, phenytoin, rifampin, St. John's wort, high-fat/protein foods, grapefruit juice; ↓ effects of midazolam, triazolam **Labs:** ↑ Serum glucose, LFTs, ↓ Hmg, plts, neutrophils **NIPE:** ↑ Fluids 1–2 L/d, capsules moisture sensitive—keep dessicant in container

Indomethacin (Indocin) **Uses:** *Arthritis; closure of the ductus arteriosus; ankylosing spondylitis* **Action:** Inhibits prostaglandins **Dose:** *Adults.* 25–50 mg PO bid–tid, max 200 mg/d. *Infants.* 0.2–0.25 mg/kg/dose IV; may repeat in 12–24 h up to 3 doses; take w/ food **Caution:** [B, +] **Contra:** ASA/NSAID sensitivity, peptic ulcer Dz/active GI bleed, precipitation of asthma/urticaria/rhinitis by NSAIDs/ASA, premature neonates w/ necrotizing enterocolitis, ↓ renal Fxn, active bleeding, thrombocytopenia, 3rd tri PRG **Supplied:** Inj 1 mg/vial; caps 25, 50 mg; SR caps 75 mg; susp 25 mg/5 mL **SE:** GI bleeding or upset, dizziness, edema **Notes:** Monitor renal Fxn; must swallow SR caps whole **Interactions:** ↑ Effects w/ acetaminophen, antiinflammatories, gold compounds, diflunisal, probenicid; ↑ effects of aminoglycosides, anticoagulants, digoxin, hypoglycemics, Li, MRX, nifedipine, phenytoin, penicillamine, verapamil; ↓ effects w/ ASA; ↓ effects of antihypertensives **Labs:** ↑ Serum K⁺, BUN, creatinine, AST, ALT, urine glucose, protein, PT; ↓ Hmg, Hct, leukocytes, plts **NIPE:** Take w/ food

Infliximab (Remicade) **WARNING:** TB, invasive fungal infections, and other opportunistic infections reported, some fatal; TB skin testing must be performed prior to therapy **Uses:** *Moderate/severe Crohn's Dz; fistulizing Crohn's Dz; RA (combination w/ MTX)* **Action:** IgG1K neutralizes TNFα (human and murine regions) **Dose:** *Crohn's: Induction:* 5 mg/kg IV inf, follow w/doses at 2 and 6 wk after. *Maint:* 5 mg/kg IV inf q8wk. *RA:* 3 mg/kg IV inf at 0, 2, 6 wk, then q8wk **Caution:** [B, ?/–] Active infection **Contra:** Murine hypersensitivity, moderate–severe CHF **Supplied:** Inj **SE:** hypersensitivity Rxns,; Pts are predisposed to infection (especially TB); HA, fatigue, GI upset, inf Rxns **Interactions:** May ↓ effects of live virus vaccines; **Labs:** May ↑ + ANA **NIPE:** ↑ Susceptibility to infection

Influenza Vaccine (Fluzone, FluShield, Fluvirin) **Uses:** *Prevent influenza*; all adults >50 y, children 6–23 mo, PRG women (2nd/3rd tri during flu season), nursing home residents, chronic Dzs, health care workers and household contacts of high-risk Pts, children < 9 y receiving vaccine for the first time **Action:** Active immunization **Dose:** *Adults.* 0.5 mL/dose IM. *Peds.* ≥ 3 y: 0.5-mL IM;

6–35 mo: 0.25 mL IM; *6 mo–< 9 y* (first-time vaccination): 2 doses > 4 wk apart, 2nd dose before Dec if possible **Caution:** [C, +] **Contra:** Egg, gentamicin, or thimerosal allergy, infection at site; high risk of influenza complications, Hx of Guillain–Barré, asthma, children 5–17 y on ASA **Supplied:** Based on specific manufacturer, 0.25- and 0.5- mL prefilled syringes **SE:** Soreness at inj site, fever, myalgia, malaise, Guillain–Barré syndrome (controversial) **Notes:** Optimal in U.S.: Oct–Nov, protection begins 1-2 wk after, lasts up to 6 mo; each year, vaccines manufactured based on predictions of flu active in flu season (December–Spring in U.S.); whole or split virus given to adults; Peds <13 y split virus or purified surface antigen to ↓ febrile Rxns **Interactions:** ↑ Effects of theophylline, warfarin; ↓ effects w/ corticosteroids, immunosuppressants; ↓ effects of aminopyrine, phenytoin

Influenza Virus Vaccine Live, Intranasal (FluMist) Uses:
Prevention of influenza **Action:** Live-attenuated vaccine **Dose:** *Adults 9–49 y.* 1 dose (0.5 mL) per season **Caution:** [C,?/–] **Contra:** Egg allergy, PRG, Hx Guillain–Barré syndrome, known/suspected immune deficiency, asthma or reactive airway Dz **Supplied:** Prefilled, single-use, intranasal sprayer **SE:** Runny nose, nasal congestion, HA, cough **Notes:** 0.25 mL into each nostril; ⊘ administer concurrently w/ other vaccines; ⊘ contact w/ immunocompromised individuals for 21 days **NIPE:** ⊘ Take w/ antivirals, ASA, NSAIDs, immunosuppressants, corticosteroids, radiation therapy

Insulin Uses:
Type 1 or type 2 DM refractory to diet change or PO hypoglycemic agents; management of acute life-threatening hyperkalemia **Action:** Insulin suppl **Dose:** Based on serum glucose levels; usually SQ but can be given IV (only regular)/IM; typical starting dose for type 1 0.5–1 U/kg/d; type 2 0.3–0.4 Units/kg/d; renal failure may ↓ insulin needs **Caution:** [B, +] **Contra:** Hypoglycemia **Supplied:** See Table 6, page 275 **SE:** Highly purified insulins ↑ free insulin; monitor Pts closely for several wks when changing doses/agents **Interactions:** ↑ Hypoglycemic effects w/ α-blockers, anabolic steroids, BBs, clofibrate, fenfluramine, guanethidine, MAOIs, NSAIDs, pentamidine, phenylbutazone, salicylates, sulfinpyrazone, tetracyclines, EtOH, celery, coriander, dandelion root, fenugreek, ginseng, garlic, juniper berries; ↓ hypoglycemic effects w/ corticosteroids, dextrothyroxine, diltiazem, dobutamine, epinephrine, niacin, oral contraceptives, protease inhibitor antiretrovirals, rifampin, thiazide diuretics, thyroid preps, marijuana, tobacco **NIPE:** If mixing insulins, draw up short-acting preps first in syringe

Interferon Alfa (Roferon-A, Intron A) Uses:
Hairy cell leukemia, Kaposi's sarcoma, melanoma, CML, chronic hepatitis C, follicular NHL, condylomata acuminata, multiple myeloma, renal cell carcinoma, and bladder CA **Action:** Antiproliferative against tumor cells; modulation of the host immune response **Dose:** See specific protocols. *Adults.* Hairy cell leukemia: Alfa-2a (Roferon-A): 3 MUNITS/d for 16–24 wk SQ or IM. Alfa-2b (Intron A): 2

MUNITS/m² IM or SQ 3×/wk for 2–6 mo **Peds. CML:** Alfa-2a (Roferon-A): 2.5–5 MUNITS/m² IM or SQ 3×/wk. **Chronic hepatitis B:** Alfa-2b (Intron A): 3–10 MUNITS/m² SQ 3×/wk **Contra:** Benzyl EtOH sensitivity, decompensated liver Dz, autoimmune Dz, rapidly progressing AIDS-related Kaposi's sarcoma **Supplied:** Injectable forms **SE:** Flu-like Sxs; fatigue common; anorexia in 20–30%; neurotoxicity at high doses; neutralizing antibodies in up to 40% of Pts receiving prolonged systemic therapy **Interactions:** ↑ Effects of antineoplastics, CNS depressants, doxorubicin, theophylline; ↓ effects of live virus vaccine **Labs:** ↑ LFTs, BUN, SCr, glucose, phosphorus, ↓ Hmg, Hct, Ca **NIPE:** ASA & EtOH use may cause GI bleed, ↑ fluids to 2–3 L/d

Interferon Alfa-2b and Ribavirin Combination (Rebetron)
WARNING: Contraindicated in PRG females and their male partners **Uses:** *Chronic hepatitis C in Pts w/ compensated liver Dz who have relapsed following α-interferon therapy* **Action:** Combination antiviral agents **Dose:** 3 MUNITS Intron A SQ 3×/wk w/ 1000–1200 mg of Rebetron PO ÷ bid dose for 24 wk. **Pts <75 kg:** 1000 mg of Rebetron/d **Caution:** [X, ?] **Contra:** PRG, males w/ PRG female partner, autoimmune hepatitis, creatinine clearance < 50 mL/min **Supplied:** **Pts <75 kg:** Combination packs: 6 vials Intron A (3 MUNITS/0.5 mL) w/ 6 syringes and EtOH swabs, 70 Rebetron caps; one 18 MUNITS multidose vial of Intron A inj (22.8 MUNITS/3.8 mL; 3 MUNITS/0.5 mL) and 6 syringes and swabs, 70 Rebetron caps; one 18 MUNITS Intron A inj multidose pen (22.5 MUNITS/1.5 mL; 3 MUNITS/0.2 mL) and 6 disposable needles and swabs, 70 Rebetron caps. **Pts <75 kg:** Identical except 84 Rebetron caps/pack **SE:** Flu-like syndrome, HA, anemia **Notes:** Negative PRG test required monthly; instruct Pts in self-administration of SQ Intron A. See Interferon Alfa **Additional Labs:** ↑ Uric acid

Interferon Alfacon-1 (Infergen)
Uses: *Management of chronic hepatitis C* **Action:** Biologic response modifier **Dose:** 9 μg SQ 3×/wk × 24 wk **Caution:** [C, M] **Contra:** Hypersensitivity to E. coli-derived products **Supplied:** Inj 9, 15 μg **SE:** Flu-like syndrome, depression, blood dyscrasias **Notes:** Allow at least 48 h between inj **Interactions:** ↑ Effects of theophylline **Labs:** ↑ Triglycerides, TSH; ↓ Hmg, Hct **NIPE:** Refrigerate, ⊘ shake, use barrier contraception

Interferon β-1b (Betaseron)
Uses: *MS, relapsing-remitting and secondary progressive* **Action:** Biologic response modifier **Dose:** 0.25 mg SQ qod **Caution:** [C, ?] **Contra:** Hypersensitivity to human albumin products **Supplied:** Powder for inj 0.3 mg **SE:** Flu-like syndrome, depression, blood dyscrasias **Interactions:** ↑ Effects of theophylline, zidovudine **Labs:** ↑ LFTs, BUN, urine protein **NIPE:** ↑ Risk of photosensitivity—use sunscreen, abortion; ↑ fluid intake, use barrier contraception

Interferon γ-1b (Actimmune)
Uses: *↓ incidence of serious infections in chronic granulomatous Dz (CGD), osteopetrosis* **Action:** Biologic response modifier **Dose:** **Adults.** CGD: 50 μg/m² SQ (1.5 MU/m²) BSA >0.5 m²; if BSA <0.5 m², give 1.5 μg/kg/dose; given 3×/wk. **Peds.** BSA ≤ 0.5 m²: 1.5 μg/kg/ SQ tid;

BSA > 0.5 m²: 50 μg/m² SQ tid **Caution:** [C, ?] **Contra:** Hypersensitivity to *E. coli*-derived products **Supplied:** Inj 100 μg (2 MU) **SE:** Flu-like syndrome, depression, blood dyscrasias

Ipecac Syrup **Uses:** *Drug OD and certain cases of poisoning* **Action:** Irritation of the GI mucosa; stimulation of the chemoreceptor trigger zone **Dose:** **Adults.** 15–30 mL PO, followed by 200–300 mL of water; if no emesis in 20 min, repeat once. **Peds.** *6–12 y:* 5–10 mL PO, followed by 10–20 mL/kg of water; if no emesis in 20 min, repeat once. *1–12 y:* 15 mL PO followed by 10–20 mL/kg of water; if no emesis in 20 min, repeat once **Caution:** [C, ?] **Contra:** Ingestion of petroleum distillates, strong acid, base, or other caustic agents; in comatose or unconscious Pts **Supplied:** Syrup 15, 30 mL (OTC) **SE:** Lethargy, diarrhea, cardiotoxicity, protracted vomiting **Notes:** Caution in CNS depressant OD; usage is falling out of favor and is no longer recommended by some sources (www.clintox.org/Pos_Statements/Ipecac.html) **Interactions:** ↑ Effects of myelosuppressives, theophylline, zidovudine **NIPE:** ↑ Fluids to 2–3 L/d, ⊘ EtOH, CNS depressants

Ipratropium (Atrovent) **Uses:** *Bronchospasm w/ COPD, rhinitis, and rhinorrhea* **Action:** Synthetic anticholinergic agent similar to atropine **Dose:** **Adults & Peds.** >12 y. 2–4 puffs qid. Nasal: 2 sprays/nostril bid–tid **Caution:** [B, +/–] **Contra:** Hypersensitivity to soya lecithin or related foods **Supplied:** Metdose inhaler 18 μg/dose; soln for inhal 0.02%; nasal spray 0.03%, 0.06%; nasal inhaler 20 μg/dose **SE:** Nervousness, dizziness, HA, cough, bitter taste, nasal dryness **Notes:** Not for acute bronchospasm **Interactions:** ↑ Effects w/ albuterol; ↑ effects of anticholinergics, antimuscarinics; ↓ effects w/ jaborandi tree, pill-bearing spurge **NIPE:** Adequate fluids, separate inhalation of other drugs by 5 min

Irbesartan (Avapro) **Uses:** *HTN*, DN, CHF* **Action:** Angiotensin II receptor antagonist **Dose:** 150 mg/d PO, may ↑ to 300 mg/d **Caution:** [C (1st tri; D 2nd/3rd), ?/–] **Supplied:** Tabs 75, 150, 300 mg **SE:** Fatigue, hypotension **Interactions:** ↑ Risk of hyperkalemia w/ K-sparing diuretics, trimethoprim, K suppls; ↑ effects of Hmg **Labs:** ↑ BUN, SCr; ↓ Hmg **NIPE:** ⊘ PRG, breast-feeding

Irinotecan (Camptosar) **Uses:** *Colorectal* and lung CA* **Action:** Topoisomerase I inhibitor; interferes w/ DNA synthesis **Dose:** Per protocol; 125–350 mg/m² weekly to every 3 wk (↓ hepatic dysfunction, as tolerated per toxicities) **Caution:** [D, –] **Contra:** Hypersensitivity to component **Supplied:** Inj 20 mg/mL **SE:** Myelosuppression, N/V/D, abdominal cramping, alopecia; diarrhea is dose-limiting; Rx acute diarrhea w/ atropine; Rx subacute diarrhea w/ loperamide **Notes:** Diarrhea correlated to levels of metabolite SN-38 **Interactions:** ↑ Effects of antineoplastics; ↑ risk of akathisia w/ prochlorperazine **Labs:** ↑ LFTs **NIPE:** Use barrier contraception, ⊘ exposure to infection

Iron Dextran (Dexferrum, INFeD) **Uses:** *Fe deficiency when PO suppl not possible** **Action:** Parenteral Fe suppl **Dose:** Estimate Fe deficiency, given IM/IV. A 0.5-mL test dose. Total replacement dose (mL) = 0.0476 × weight (kg) ×

[desired hemoglobin (g/dL) – measured hemoglobin (g/dL)] + 1 mL/5 kg weight (max 14 mL). *Adults.* Max daily dose: 100 mg Fe. *Peds.* Max daily dose: <5 kg: 25 mg Fe. *5–10 kg:* 50 mg Fe. *10–50 kg:* 100 mg Fe **Caution:** [C, M] **Contra:** Anemia w/o Fe deficiency. **Supplied:** Inj 50 mg (Fe)/mL **SE:** Anaphylaxis, flushing, dizziness, inj site and inf Rxns, metallic taste **Notes:** Give deep IM using "Z-track" technique; IV route preferred **Interactions:** ↓ Effects w/ chloramphenicol, ↓ absorption of oral Fe **Labs:** False ↓ serum Ca; false + guaiac test **NIPE:** ⊘ Take oral Fe

Iron Sucrose (Venofer) Uses: *Fe deficiency anemia in chronic hemodialysis in those receiving erythropoietin* **Actions:** Fe replacement. **Dose:** 5 mL (100 mg) IV during dialysis, no faster than 1 mL (20 mg)/min. **Caution:** [C, M] **Contra:** Anemia w/o Fe deficiency **Supplied:** 20 mg elemental Fe per mL, 5-mL vials. **SE:** Anaphylaxis, hypotension, cramps, N/V/D, HA **Notes:** Most Pts require cumulative doses of 1000 mg; ensure drug administered at slow rate

Isoniazid (INH) Uses: *Rx and prophylaxis of TB* **Action:** Bactericidal; interferes w/ mycolic acid synthesis (disrupts cell wall) **Dose:** *Adults.* Active TB: 5 mg/kg/24 h PO or IM (usually 300 mg/d). *Prophylaxis:* 300 mg/d PO for 6–12 mo. *Peds.* Active TB: 10–20 mg/kg/24 h PO or IM to a max of 300 mg/d. *Prophylaxis:* 10 mg/kg/24 h PO; ↓ in hepatic/renal dysfunction **Caution:** [C, +] Liver Dz, dialysis; ⊘ EtOH **Contra:** Acute liver Dz, Hx INH hepatitis **Supplied:** Tabs 100, 300 mg; syrup 50 mg/5 mL; inj 100 mg/mL **SE:** Hepatitis, peripheral neuropathy, GI upset, anorexia, dizziness, skin Rxn **Notes:** Give w/ 2–3 other drugs for active TB, based on INH resistance patterns when TB acquired and sensitivity results; prophylaxis generally is INH alone. IM route rarely used. To prevent peripheral neuropathy, give pyridoxine 50–100 mg/d. Check CDC guidelines (in MMWR) for specific Rx recommendations **Interactions:** ↑ Effects of acetaminophen, anticoagulants, carbamazepine, cycloserine, diazepam, meperidine, hydantoins, theophylline, valproic acid, EtOH; ↑ effects w/ rifampin; ↓ effects w/ Al salts; ↓ effects of anticoagulants, ketoconazole **Labs:** False + urine glucose, false ↑ AST, uric acid, false ↓ serum glucose **NIPE:** Only take w/ food if GI upset

Isoproterenol (Isuprel) Uses: *Shock, bronchospasm, cardiac arrest, and AV nodal block* **Action:** β_1- and β_2-receptor stimulant **Dose:** *Adults.* 2–10 µg/min IV inf; titrate to effect. *Inhal:* 1–2 inhal 4–6×/d. *Peds.* 0.2–2 µg/kg/min IV inf; titrate to effect. *Inhal:* 1–2 inhal 4–6×/d **Caution:** [C, ?] **Contra:** Angina, tachyarrhythmias (digitalis-induced or others) **Supplied:** Met-inhaler; soln for neb 0.5%, 1%; inj 0.02 mg/mL, 0.2 mg/mL **SE:** Insomnia, arrhythmias, HA, trembling, dizziness **Notes:** Pulse > 130 bpm may induce ventricular arrhythmias **Interactions:** ↑ Eeffects w/ albuterol, guanethidine, oxytocic drugs, sympathomimetics, TCAs; ↑ risk of arrhythmias w/ amitriptyline, bretylium, cardiac glycosides, K-depleting drugs, theophylline; ↓ effects w/ BBs **Labs:** False ↑ serum AST, bilirubin, glucose **NIPE:** Saliva may turn pink in color, ↑ fluids to 2–3 L/d

Isosorbide Dinitrate (Isordil, Sorbitrate, Dilatrate-SR) Uses: *Rx and prevention of angina,* CHF (w/ hydralazine) **Action:** Relaxes vascular smooth muscle **Dose:** *Acute angina:* 5–10 mg PO (chew tabs) q2–3h or 2.5–10 mg SL PRN q5–10min; >3 doses should not be given in a 15630- min period. *Angina prophylaxis:* 5–40 mg PO q6h; ⊘ give nitrates on a chronic q6h or qid basis >7–10 d because tolerance may develop; provide 10–12-h drug-free intervals **Caution:** [C, ?] Sildenafil, tadalafil, vardenafil **Contra:** Severe anemia, closed-angle glaucoma, postural hypotension, cerebral hemorrhage, head trauma (can ↑ ICP); w/ sildenafil, tadalafil, vardenafil **Supplied:** Tabs 5, 10, 20, 30, 40 mg; SR tabs 40 mg; SL tabs 2.5, 5, 10 mg; chew tabs 5, 10 mg; SR caps 40 mg **SE:** HA, ↓ BP, flushing, tachycardia, dizziness **Notes:** Higher PO dose usually needed to achieve same results as SL forms **Interactions:** ↑ Hypotension w/ antihypertensives, ASA, CCBs, phenothiazines, sildenafil, EtOH **Labs:** False ↓ serum cholesterol **NIPE:** ⊘ Nitrates for a 8–12-h period/d to avoid tolerance

Isosorbide Mononitrate (Ismo, Imdur) Uses: *Prevention/Rx of angina pectoris* **Action:** Relaxes vascular smooth muscle **Dose:** 20 mg PO bid, w/ the 2 doses 7 h apart or XR (Imdur) 30–120 mg/d PO **Caution:** [C, ?] ⊘ coadminister w/ sildenafil **Contra:** Head trauma or cerebral hemorrhage (can ↑ ICP), w/ sildenafil, tadalafil, vardenafil **Supplied:** Tabs 10, 20 mg; XR 30, 60, 120 mg **SE:** HA, dizziness, ↓ BP **Interactions:** ↑ Hypotension w/ ASA, CCB, nitrates, sildenafil, EtOH **Labs:** False ↓ serum cholesterol

Isotretinoin [13-*cis* Retinoic Acid] (Accutane, Amnesteem, Claravis, Sotret) WARNING: Must not be used by PRG females; Pt must be capable of complying w/ mandatory contraceptive measures; prescribed according to product-specific risk management system **Uses:** *Refractory severe acne* **Action:** Retinoic acid derivative **Dose:** 0.5–? mg/kg/d PO ÷ bid (↓ in hepatic Dz, take w/ food) **Caution:** [X, –] ⊘ tetracyclines **Contra:** Retinoid sensitivity, PRG **Supplied:** Caps 10, 20, 40 mg **SE:** Isolated reports of depression, psychosis, suicidal thoughts; dermatologic sensitivity, xerostomia, photosensitivity, ↑ LFTs, ↑ triglycerides **Notes:** Risk management program requires 2 – PRG tests before therapy and use of 2 forms of contraception 1 mo before, during, and 1 mo after therapy; informed consent recommended; monitor LFTs and lipids **Interactions:** ↑ Effects w/ corticosteroids, phenytoin, vitamin A ; ↑ risk of pseudotumor cerebri w/ tetracyclines; ↑ triglyceride levels w/ EtOH; ↓ effects of carbamazepine **NIPE:** ↑ Risk of photosensitivity—use sunscreen, take w/ food, ⊘ PRG

Isradipine (DynaCirc) Uses: *HTN* **Action:** CCB **Dose:** *Adults.* 2.5–10 mg PO bid. *Peds.* 0.05–0.15 mg/kg PO tid–qid, up to 20 mg/d (⊘ crush or chew) **Caution:** [C, ?] **Contra:** Severe heart block sinus bradycardia, CHF, dosing w/in several hours of IV BBs **Supplied:** Caps 2.5, 5 mg; tabs CR 5, 10 mg **SE:** HA, edema, flushing, fatigue, dizziness, palpitations **Interactions:** ↑Effects w/ azole antifungals, BBs, cimetidine; ↑ effects of carbamazepine, cyclosporine, digitalis glycosides, prazosin, quinidine; ↓ effects w/ Ca, rifampin; ↓ effects of lovastatin **Labs:** ↑ LFTs **NIPE:** ⊘ DC abruptly

Itraconazole (Sporanox) **WARNING:** Potential for negative inotropic effects on the heart; if signs or Sxs of CHF occur during administration, continued use should be assessed **Uses:** *Fungal infections (aspergillosis, blastomycosis, histoplasmosis, candidiasis)* **Action:** Inhibits synthesis of ergosterol **Dose:** 200 mg PO or IV qd–bid (capsule w/ meals or cola/grapefruit juice); PO soln on empty stomach; ⊘ antacids **Caution:** [C, ?] Numerous drug interactions **Contra:** CrCl <30 mL/min, Hx of CHF or ventricular dysfunction, or w/ H₂-antagonist, omeprazole **Supplied:** Caps 100 mg; soln 10 mg/mL; inj 10 mg/mL **SE:** nausea, rash, hepatitis, hypokalemia, CHF **Notes:** PO soln and caps not interchangeable; useful in Pts who cannot take amphotericin B, watch for signs/Sxs of CHF w/ IV use **Interactions:** ↑ Effects w/ clarithromycin, erythromycin; ↑ effects of alprazolam, anticoagulants, atevirdine, atorvastatin, buspirone, cerivastatin, chlordiazepoxide, cyclosporine, diazepam, digoxin, felodipine, fluvastatin, indinavir, lovastatin, methadone, methylprednisolone, midazolam, nelfinavir, pravastatin, ritonavir, saquinavir, simvastatin, tacrolimus, tolbutamide, triazolam, warfarin; ↑ QT prolongation w/ astemizole, cisapride, pimozide, quinidine, terfenadine; ↓ effects w/ antacids, Ca, cimetidine, didanosine, famotidine, lansoprazole, Mg, nizatidine, omeprazole, phenytoin, rifampin, sucralfate, grapefruit juice **Labs:** ↑ LFTs, BUN, SCr **NIPE:** Take capsule w/ food & soln w/o food, ⊘ PRG or breast-feeding, ↑ risk of disulfiram-like response w/ EtOH

Kaolin-Pectin (Kaodene, Kao-Spen, Kapectolin, Parepectolin) **Uses:** *Diarrhea* **Action:** Absorbent demulcent **Dose:** *Adults.* 60–120 mL PO after each loose stool or q3–4h PRN. *Peds.* 3–6 y: 15–30 mL/dose PO PRN. *6–12 y:* 30–60 mL/dose PO PRN **Caution:** [C, +] **Contra:** Diarrhea secondary to pseudomembranous colitis **Supplied:** Multiple OTC forms; also available w/ opium (Parepectolin) **SE:** Constipation, dehydration **Interaction:** ↓ Effects of ciprofloxacin, clindamycin, digoxin, lincomycin, lovastatin, penicillamine, quinidine, tetracycline **NIPE:** Take other meds 2–3 h before or after this drug

Ketoconazole (Nizoral, Nizoral AD Shampoo) [OTC] **Uses:** *Systemic fungal infections; topical for local fungal infections due to dermatophytes and yeast; shampoo for dandruff,* short term in CAP when rapid reduction of testosterone needed (ie, cord compression) **Action:** Inhibits fungal cell wall synthesis **Dose:** *Adults.* PO: 200 mg PO qd; ↑ to 400 mg PO qd for serious infection; CAP 400 mg PO tid (short term). *Topical:* Apply to area qd (cream or shampoo). *Peds.* >2 y: 5–10 mg/kg/24 h PO ÷ q12–24h (↓ in hepatic Dz) **Caution:** [C, +/–] Any agent ↑ gastric pH prevents absorption; may enhance PO anticoagulants; w/ EtOH (disulfiram-like Rxn; numerous drug interactions) **Contra:** CNS fungal infections (poor CNS penetration), concurrent astemizole, cisapride, PO triazolam **Supplied:** Tabs 200 mg; topical cream 2%; shampoo 2% **SE:** Monitor LFTs w/ systemic use; can cause nausea **Notes:** PO form multiple drug interactions **Interactions:** ↑ Effects of alprazolam, anticoagulants, atevirdine, atorvastatin, buspirone, chlordiazepoxide, cyclosporine, diazepam, felodipine, fluvastatin, indinavir, lovastatin, methadone, methylprednisolone, midazolam, nelfinavir, pravastatin, ritonavir, saquinavir, simvastatin, tacrolimus, tolbutamide, triazolam, warfarin; ↑ QT prolongation w/ astemizole, cisapride, quinidine, terfenadine; ↓ effects w/ antacids, Ca, cimetidine, didanosine, famotidine, lansoprazole, Mg, nizatidine, omeprazole, phenytoin, rifampin, sucralfate **Labs:** ↑ LFTs **NIPE:** Take tabs w/ citrus juice, take w/ food; shampoo wet hair 1 min, rinse, repeat for 3 min; ⊘ PRG or breast-feeding

Ketoprofen (Orudis, Oruvail) **Uses:** * Arthritis, pain* **Action:** NSAID; inhibits prostaglandins **Dose:** 25–75 mg PO tid–qid, 300 mg/d/max; take w/ food **Caution** [B (D 3rd tri), ?] **Contra:** NSAID/ASA sensitivity **Supplied:** Tabs 12.5 mg; caps 25, 50, 75 mg; caps, SR 100, 150, 200 mg **SE:** GI upset, peptic ulcers, dizziness, edema, rash **Interactions:** ↑ Effects w/ ASA, corticosteroids, NSAIDs, probenicid, EtOH; ↑ effects of antineoplastics, hypoglycemics, insulin, Li, MRX; ↑ risk of nephrotoxicity w/ aminoglycosides, cyclosporines; ↑ risk of bleeding w/ anticoagulants, defamandole, cefotetan, cefoperazone, clopidogrel, eptifibatide, plicamycin, thrombolytics, tirofiban, valproic acid, dong quai, feverfew, garlic, ginkgo biloba, ginger, horse chestnut, red clover; ↓ effects of antihypertensives, diuretics **Labs:** ↑ LFTs, BUN, serum Na$^+$, creatinine, Cl$^-$, K$^+$, PT; ↑ or ↓ glucose; ↓ Hmg, Hct, plts, leukocytes **NIPE:** ↑ Risk of photosensitivity—use sunscreen, take w/ food

Ketorolac (Toradol) **WARNING:** Indicated for short-term (≥ 5 d) Rx of moderately severe acute pain that requires analgesia at opioid level **Uses:** *Pain* **Action:** NSAID; inhibits prostaglandins **Dose:** 15–30 mg IV/IM q6h or 10 mg PO qid; max IV/IM 120 mg/d, max PO 40 mg/d; ⊘ use for > 5 d; ↓ for age and renal dysfunction **Caution** [B (D 3rd tri), –] **Contra:** Peptic ulcer Dz, NSAID sensitivity, advanced renal Dz, CNS bleeding, anticipated major surgery, labor and delivery, nursing mothers **Supplied:** Tabs 10 mg; inj 15 mg/mL, 30 mg/mL **SE:** Bleeding, peptic ulcer Dz, renal failure, edema, dizziness, hypersensitivity **Notes:** PO only as continuation of IM/IV therapy **Interactions:** ↑ Effects w/ ASA, corticosteroids, NSAIDs, probenicid, EtOH; ↑ effects of antineoplastics, hypoglycemics, insulin, Li, MRX; ↑ risk of nephrotoxicity w/ aminoglycosides, cyclosporines; ↑ risk of bleeding w/ anticoagulants, defamandole, cefotetan, cefoperazone, clopidogrel, eptifibatide, plicamycin, thrombolytics, tirofiban, valproic acid, dong quai, feverfew, garlic, ginkgo biloba, ginger, horse chestnut, red clover; ↓ effects of antihypertensives, diuretics **Labs:** ↑ LFTs, PT, BUN, SCr, Na$^+$, Cl$^-$, K$^+$ **NIPE:** 30-mg dose equals comparative analgesia of meperidine 100 mg or morphine 12 mg

Ketorolac Ophthalmic (Acular) **Uses:** *Ocular itching caused by seasonal allergies* **Action:** NSAID **Dose:** 1 gt qid **Caution:** [C, +] **Supplied:** Soln 0.5% **SE:** Local irritation. See Ketorolac **NIPE:** ⊘ Soft contact lenses

Ketotifen (Zaditor) Uses: *Allergic conjunctivitis* Action: H₁-receptor antagonist and mast cell stabilizer Dose: *Adults & Peds.* 1 gt in eye(s) q8–12h Caution: [C,?/–] Supplied: Soln 0.025%/5 mL SE: Local irritation, HA, rhinitis NIPE: Insert soft contact lenses 10 min after drug use

Labetalol (Trandate, Normodyne) Uses: *HTN* and hypertensive emergencies Action: α- and β-Adrenergic blocking agent Dose: *Adults.* HTN: Initial, 100 mg PO bid, then 200–400 mg PO bid. *Hypertensive emergency:* 20–80 mg IV bolus, then 2 mg/min IV inf, titrate to effect. *Peds.* PO: 3–20 mg/kg/d in ÷ doses. *Hypertensive emergency:* 0.4–1.5 mg/kg/h IV cont inf Caution: [C (D in 2nd or 3rd tri), +] Contra: Asthma/COPD, cardiogenic shock, uncompensated CHF, heart block Supplied: Tabs 100, 200, 300 mg; inj 5 mg/mL SE: Dizziness, nausea, ↓ BP, fatigue, CV effects Interactions: ↑ Effects w/ cimetidine, diltiazem, nitroglycerine, quinidine, paroxetine, verapamil; ↑ tremors w/ TCAs; ↓ effects w/ glutethimide, NSAIDs, salicylates; ↓ effects of antihypertensives, β-adrenergic bronchodilators, sulfonylureas Labs: False + urine catecholamines NIPE: May have transient tingling of scalp

Lactic Acid & Ammonium Hydroxide [Ammonium Lactate] (Lac-Hydrin) Uses: *Severe xerosis and ichthyosis* Action: Emollient moisturizer Dose: Apply bid Caution: [B, ?] Supplied: Lactic acid 12% w/ ammonium hydroxide SE: Local irritation

Lactobacillus (Lactinex Granules) [OTC] Uses: Control of diarrhea, especially after antibiotic therapy Action: Replaces normal intestinal flora Dose: *Adults & Peds.* >3 y: 1 packet, 2 caps, or 4 tabs tid–qid (w/ meals or liq) Caution: [A, +] Contra: Milk/lactose allergy Supplied: Tabs; caps; EC caps; powder in packets (all OTC) SE: Flatulence

Lactulose (Chronulac, Cephulac, Enulose) Uses: *Hepatic encephalopathy; constipation* Action: Acidifies the colon, allowing ammonia to diffuse into the colon Dose: *Acute hepatic encephalopathy:* 30–45 mL PO q1h until soft stools, then tid–qid. *Chronic laxative therapy:* 30–45 mL PO tid–qid; adjust q1–2d to produce 2–3 soft stools/d. *Rectally:* 200 g in 700 mL of water PR. *Peds. Infants:* 2.5–10 mL/24 h ÷ tid–qid. *Peds:* 40–90 mL/24 h ÷ tid–qid Caution: [B, ?] Contra: Galactosemia Supplied: Syrup 10 g/15 mL, soln 10 g/15 mL, 10 g/packet SE: Severe diarrhea, flatulence; may cause severe diarrhea and life-threatening electrolyte disturbances Interactions: ↓ Effects w/ antacids, neomycin Labs: ↓ Serum ammonia NIPE: May take 24–48 h for results

Lamivudine (Epivir, Epivir-HBV) WARNING: Lactic acidosis and severe hepatomegaly w/ steatosis reported w/ nucleoside analogs Uses: *HIV infection, chronic hepatitis B* Action: Inhibits HIV RT and hepatitis B viral polymerase, resulting in viral DNA chain termination Dose: *HIV: Adults & Peds.* >12 y: 150 mg PO bid. *Peds.* <12 y: 4 mg/kg bid. *HBV: Adults.* 100 mg/d. *Peds.* 2–17 y: 3 mg/kg/d PO, 100 mg max; ↓ in renal impairment Caution: [C, ?] Contra: Hypersensitivity to any component **Supplied:** Tabs 100, 150 mg (HBV); soln 5 mg/mL, 10 mg/mL **SE:** HA, pancreatitis, anemia, GI upset, lactic acidosis **Interactions:** ↑ Effects w/ co-trimoxazole, trimethoprim/sulfamethoxazole; ↑ risk of lactic acidosis w/ antiretrovirals, reverse transcriptase inhibitors **Labs:** ↑ LFTs

Lamotrigine (Lamictal)

WARNING: Serious rashes requiring hospitalization and DC of Rx reported; rash less frequent in adults **Uses:** *Partial Szs, bipolar disorder, Lennox–Gastaut syndrome* **Action:** Phenyltriazine antiepileptic **Dose:** *Adults.* Szs: Initial 50 mg/d PO, then 50 mg PO bid for 2 wk, then maint 300–500 mg/d in 2 ÷ doses. *Bipolar:* Initial 25 mg/d PO, then 50 mg PO qd for 2 wk, then 100 mg PO qd for 1 wk; maint 200 mg/d. *Peds.* 0.15 mg/kg in 1–2 ÷ doses for wk 1 and 2, then 0.3 mg/kg for wk 3 and 4, then maint 1 mg/kg/d in 1–2 ÷ doses (↓ in hepatic Dz or if w/ enzyme inducers or valproic acid) **Caution:** [C,] Interactions w/ other antiepileptics **Supplied:** Tabs 25, 100, 150, 200 mg; chew tabs 5, 25 mg **SE:** HA, GI upset, dizziness, ataxia, rash (potentially life-threatening in children > adults) **Notes:** Value of therapeutic monitoring not established **Interactions:** ↑ Effects valproic acid; ↑ effects of carbamazepine; ↓ effects w/ phenobarbital, phenytoin, primidone; **NIPE:** ↑ Risk of photosensitivity—use sunscreen

Lansoprazole (Prevacid)

Uses: *Duodenal ulcers, prevent and Rx NSAID gastric ulcers,* *H. pylori* infection, erosive esophagitis, and hypersecretory conditions **Action:** Proton pump inhibitor **Dose:** 15–30 mg/d PO; NSAID ulcer prevention 15 mg/d PO ≤ 12 wk, NSAID ulcers 30 mg/d PO, ×8 wk; ↓ in severe hepatic impairment **Caution:** [B, ?/–] **Supplied:** Caps 15, 30 mg **SE:** HA, fatigue **Interactions:** ↑ Effects of hypoglycemics, nifedipine; ↓ effects w/ sucralfate; ↓ effects of ampicillin, cefpodoxime, cefuroxime, digoxin, enoxacin, ketoconazole, theophylline **Labs:** ↑ LFTs, SCr, LDH, gastrin, lipids **NIPE:** Take ac

Latanoprost (Xalatan)

Uses: *Refractory glaucoma* **Action:** Prostaglandin **Dose:** 1 gt eye(s) hs **Caution:** [C, ?] **Supplied:** 0.005% soln **SE:** May darken light irises; blurred vision, ocular stinging, and itching **Interactions:** ↑ Risk of precipitation if mixed w/ eye drops w/ thimerosal

Leflunomide (Arava)

WARNING: PRG must be excluded prior to start of Rx **Uses:** *Active RA* **Action:** Inhibits pyrimidine synthesis **Dose:** Initial 100 mg/d PO for 3 d, then 10–20 mg/d **Caution:** [X, –] **Contra:** PRG **Supplied:** Tabs 10, 20, 100 mg **SE:** Monitor LFTs during initial therapy; diarrhea, infection, HTN, alopecia, rash, nausea, joint pain, hepatitis **Interactions:** ↑ Effects w/ rifampin; ↑ risk of hepatotoxicity w/ hepatotoxic drugs, MRX; ↑ effects of NSAIDs; ↓ effects w/ activated charcoal, cholestyramine **Labs:** ↑ LFTs **NIPE:** ⊘ PRG, breast-feeding, live virus vaccines

Lepirudin (Refludan)

Uses: *Heparin-induced thrombocytopenia* **Action:** Direct inhibitor of thrombin **Dose:** Bolus 0.4 mg/kg IV, then 0.15 mg/kg inf (↓ dose and inf rate if CrCl <60 mL/min) **Caution:** [B, ?/–] Hemorrhagic event or severe HTN **Contra:** Active major bleeding **Supplied:** Inj 50 mg **SE:** Bleeding, anemia, hematoma **Notes:** Adjust dose based on aPTT ratio, maintain aPTT ratio of 1.5–2.0 **Interactions:** ↑ Risk of bleeding w/ antiplt drugs, cephalosporins, NSAIDs, thrombolytics, salicylates, feverfew, ginkgo biloba, ginger, valerian

Letrozole (Femara) **Uses:** *Advanced breast CA* **Action:** Nonsteroidal aromatase inhibitor **Dose:** 2.5 mg/d PO **Caution:** [D, ?] **Contra:** PRG **Supplied:** Tabs 2.5 mg **SE:** Requires periodic CBC, thyroid Fxn, electrolyte, LFT, and renal monitoring; anemia, nausea, hot flashes, arthralgia **Interactions:** ↑ Risk of interference w/ action of drug w/ estrogens and oral contraceptives **Labs:** ↑ LFTs, cholesterol, Ca, ↓ lymphocytes

Leucovorin (Wellcovorin) **Uses:** *OD of folic acid antagonist; augmentation of 5-FU, ↓ MTX elimination* **Action:** Reduced folate source; circumvents action of folate reductase inhibitors (eg, MTX) **Dose:** *Adults & Peds.* MTX rescue: 10 mg/m²/dose IV or PO q6h for 72 h until MTX level <10⁻⁸. *5-FU:* 200 mg/m²/d IV 1–5 d during daily 5-FU Rx or 500 mg/m²/wk w/ weekly 5-FU therapy. *Adjunct to antimicrobials:* 5–15 mg/d PO **Caution:** [C, ?/–] **Contra:** Pernicious anemia **Supplied:** Tabs 5, 15, 25 mg; inj **SE:** Allergic Rxn, N/V/D, fatigue **Notes:** Many dosing schedules for leucovorin rescue following MTX therapy; should not be administered intrathecally/intraventrically **Interactions:** ↑ Effects of fluorouracil; ↓ effects of MRX, phenobarbital, phenyotin, primidone, trimethoprim/sulfamethoxazole **NIPE:** ↑ Fluids to 3 L/d

Leuprolide (Lupron, Lupron DEPOT, Lupron DEPOT-Ped, Viadur, Eligard) **Uses:** *Advanced CAP (all products), endometriosis (Lupron), uterine fibroids (Lupron), and CPP (Lupron-Ped)* **Action:** LHRH agonist; paradoxically inhibits release of gonadotropin, resulting in ↓ pituitary gonadotropins (↓ LH); in men ↓ testosterone **Dose:** *Adults.* CAP: 7.5 mg IM q28d or 22.5 mg IM q3mo or 30 mg IM q4mo of depot; Viadur (CAP only): insert in inner upper arm using local anesthesia, replace q12mo. *Endometriosis (Lupron DEPOT):* 3.75 mg IM qmo ×6. *Fibroids:* 3.75 mg IM qmo ×3. *Peds.* CPP (Lupron-Ped): 50 μg/kg/d daily SQ inj; ↑ by 10 μg/kg/d until total down-regulation achieved. *DEPOT:* <25 kg: 7.5 mg IM q4wk. >25–37.5 kg: 11.25 mg IM q4wk. >37.5 kg: 15 mg IM q4wk **Caution:** [X, ?] **Contra:** Undiagnosed vaginal bleeding, implant dosage form in women and peds; PRG **Supplied:** Inj 5 mg/mL; Lupron DEPOT 3.75 (1 mo for fibroids, endometriosis); Lupron DEPOT for CAP: 7.5 mg (1 mo), 22.5 (3 mo), 30 mg (4 mo); Eligard depot for CAP: 7.5 mg (1 mo); Viadur 12-mo SQ implant, Lupron-Ped 7.5, 11.25, 15 mg **SE:** Hot flashes, gynecomastia, N/V, alopecia, anorexia, dizziness, HA, insomnia, paresthesias, depression exacerbation, peripheral edema, and bone pain (transient "flare Rxn" at 7–14 d after the 1st dose due to LH and testosterone surge before suppression) **Notes:** Nonsteroidal antiandrogen can block flare **Interactions:** ↓ Effects w/ androgens, estrogens **Labs:** ↑ LFTs, BUN, serum Ca, uric acid, glucose, lipids, WBC, PT; ↓ serum K⁺, plts

Levalbuterol (Xopenex) **Uses:** *Asthma (Rx and prevention of bronchospasm)* **Action:** Sympathomimetic bronchodilator **Dose:** 0.63 mg neb q6–8h

Caution: [C, ?] **Supplied:** Soln for inhal 0.63, 1.25 mg/3 mL **SE:** Tachycardia, nervousness, trembling, flu syndrome **Notes:** *R*-isomer of albuterol; potential for lower incidence of CV side effects compared with albuterol **Interactions:** ↑ Effects w/ MAOIs, TCAs; ↑ risk of hypokalemia w/ loop & thiazide diuretics; ↓ effects w/ BBs; ↓ effects of digoxin **Labs:** ↑ Serum glucose, ↓ serum K⁺ **NIPE:** Use other inhalants 5 min after this drug

Levamisole (Ergamisol) **Uses:** *Adjuvant therapy of Dukes C colon CA (in combination w/ 5-FU)* **Action:** Poorly understood immunostimulatory effects **Dose:** 50 mg PO q8h for 3 d q14d during 5-FU therapy; ↓ in hepatic dysfunction **Caution:** [C, ?/–] **Supplied:** Tabs 50 mg **SE:** N/V/D, abdominal pain, taste disturbance, anorexia, hyperbilirubinemia, disulfiram-like Rxn on EtOH ingestion, minimal bone marrow depression, fatigue, fever, conjunctivitis **Interactions:** ↑ Effects of phenytoin, warfarin **NIPE:** ⊘ Exposure to infection

Levetiracetam (Keppra) **Uses:** *Partial onset Szs* **Action:** Unknown **Dose:** *Adults.* 500 mg PO bid, may ↑ to max 3000 mg/d; *Peds.* 4–16 y: 10–20 mg/kg/d ÷ in 2 doses, up to 60 mg/kg/d (↓ in renal insufficiency) **Caution:** [C, ?/–] **Contra:** Component hypersensitivity **Supplied:** Tabs 250, 500, 750 mg **SE:** May cause dizziness and somnolence; may impair coordination **Interactions:** ↑ Effects w/ antihistamines, TCAs, benzodiazepines, narcotics, EtOH **NIPE:** May take w/ food

Levobunolol (A-K Beta, Betagan) **Uses:** * Glaucoma* **Action:** β-Adrenergic blocker **Dose:** 1–2 gtt/d 0.5% or 1–2 gtt 0.25% bid **Caution:** [C, ?] **Supplied:** Soln 0.25, 0.5% **SE:** Ocular stinging or burning **Notes:** Possible systemic effects if absorbed **Interactions:** ↑ Effects w/ BBs; ↑ risk of hypotension & bradycardia w/ quinidine, verapamil; ↓ intraocular pressure w/ carbonic anhydrase inhibitors, epinephrine, pilocarpine **NIPE:** Night vision and acuity may be decreased

Levocabastine (Livostin) **Uses:** *Allergic seasonal conjunctivitis* **Action:** Antihistamine **Dose:** 1 gt in eye(s) qid ≤ 4 wk **Caution:** [C, +/–] **Supplied:** 0.05% drops **SE:** Ocular discomfort **NIPE:** ⊘ Insert soft contact lenses

Levofloxacin (Levaquin, Quixin Ophthalmic) **Uses:** *Lower resp tract infections, sinusitis, UTI; topical for bacterial conjunctivitis, skin infections* **Action:** Quinolone antibiotic, inhibits DNA gyrase. *Spectrum:* Excellent gram(+) except MRSA and *E. faecium*; excellent gram(–) except *S. maltophilia* and *Acinetobacter* sp; poor anaerobic **Dose:** 250–500 mg/d PO or IV; community-acquired pneumonia 750 mg/day for 5 days; ophth 1–2 gtt in eye(s) q2h while awake for 2 d, then q4h while awake for 5 d; ↓ in renal insufficiency; ⊘ antacids if PO **Caution:** [C, –] Interactions w/ cation-containing products (eg antacids) **Contra:** Quinolone sensitivity **Supplied:** Tabs 250, 500 mg; premixed IV 250, 500 mg; Leva-Pak 750 mg × 5 days; ophth 0.5% soln **SE:** N/D, dizziness, rash, GI upset, photosensitivity **Interactions:** ↑ Effects of cyclosporine, digoxin, theophylline, warfarin, caffeine; ↑ risk of Szs w/ foscarnet, NSAIDs; ↑ risk of hyper- or hypoglycemia w/ hypoglycemic drugs; ↓ effects w/ antacids, antineoplastics, Ca, cimetidine, didanosine, famotidine, Fe, lansoprazole, Mg, nizatidine, omeprazole, phenytoin, ranititdine, NaHCO₃, sucralfate, Zn **NIPE:** Risk of tendon rupture & tendonitis—DC if pain or inflammation; ↑ fluids, use sunscreen, antacids 2 h before or after this drug

Levonorgestrel (Plan B) Uses: *Emergency contraceptive ("morning-after pill")*; prevents PRG if taken < 72 h after unprotected sex (contraceptive fails or if no contraception used) **Action:** Progestin **Dose:** 1 pill q12h × 2 **Caution:** [X, M] **Contra:** Known/suspected PRG, abnormal uterine bleeding **Supplied:** Tab. 0.75 mg, 2 blister pack **SE:** N/V, abdominal pain, fatigue, HA, menstrual changes **Notes:** Will not induce abortion; may ↑ risk of ectopic PRG **Interactions:** ↓ Effects w/ barbiturates, carbamazepine, modafinil, phenobarbital, phenytoin, pioglitazone, rifabutin, rifampin, ritonavir, topiramate

Levonorgestrel Implant (Norplant) Uses: *Contraceptive* **Action:** Progestin **Dose:** Implant 6 caps in the midforearm **Caution:** [X, +/–] **Contra:** Undiagnosed abnormal uterine bleeding, hepatic Dz, thromboembolism, Hx of intracranial HTN, breast CA, renal impairment **Supplied:** Kits containing 6 implantable caps, each containing 36 mg **SE:** Uterine bleeding, HA, acne, nausea **Notes:** Prevents PRG for up to 5 y; removed if PRG desired **Interactions:** ↓ Effects w/ barbiturates, carbamazepine, modafinil, phenobarbital, phenytoin, pioglitazone, rifabutin, rifampin, ritonavir, topiramate **Labs:** ↑ uptake of T₃, ↓ T₄ sex hormone-binding globulin levels **NIPE:** Menstrual irregularities 1st y after implant, use barrier contraception if taking anticonvulsants, may cause vision changes or contact lens tolerability

Levorphanol (Levo-Dromoran) [C-II] Uses: *Moderate/severe pain; chronic pain* **Action:** Narcotic analgesic **Dose:** 2 mg PO or SQ PRN q6–8h (↓ in hepatic failure) **Caution:** [B/D (prolonged use or high doses at term), ?] **Contra:** Component hypersensitivity **Supplied:** Tabs 2 mg; inj 2 mg/mL **SE:** Tachycardia, hypotension, drowsiness, GI upset, constipation, resp depression, pruritus **Interactions:** ↑ CNS effects w/ antihistamines, cimetidine, CNS depressants, glutethimide, methocarbamol, EtOH, St. John's wort **Labs:** False ↑ amylase, lipase **NIPE:** ↑ Fluids & fiber, take w/ food

Levothyroxine (Synthroid, Levoxyl, others) Uses: *Hypothyroidism, myxedema coma* **Action:** Suppl of L-thyroxine **Dose:** *Adults.* Initial, 25–50 μg/d PO or IV; ↑ by 25–50 μg/d every mo; usual 100–200 μg/d. *Peds.* 0–1 y: 8–10 μg/kg/24 h PO or IV. *1–5 y:* 4–6 μg/kg/24 h PO or IV. *>5 y:* 3–4 μg/kg/24 h PO or IV; titrate based on response and thyroid tests; dosage can ↑ more rapidly in young to middle-aged Pts **Caution:** [A, +] **Contra:** Recent MI, uncorrected adrenal insufficiency **Supplied:** Tabs 25, 50, 75, 88, 100, 112, 125, 137, 150, 175, 200. 300 μg; inj 200, 500 μg **SE:** Insomnia, weight loss, alopecia, arrhythmia **Interactions:** ↑ Effects of anticoagulants, sympathomimetics, TCAs, warfarin; ↓ effects w/ antacids, BBs, carbamazepine, cholestyramine, estrogens, Fe salts, phenytoin, phenobarbital, rifampin, simethicone, sucralfate, ↓ effects of digoxin, hypoglycemics, theophylline **Labs:** False $\uparrow$ serum T_3; drug alters thyroid uptake of radioactive I—DC drug 4 wk before studies **NIPE:** $\oslash$ Switch brands due to different bioavailabilities

Lidocaine (Anestacon Topical, Xylocaine, others) **Uses:** Local

anesthetic; Rx cardiac arrhythmias **Action:** Anesthetic; class IB antiarrhythmic **Dose:** *Adults.* Antiarrhythmic, ET: 5 mg/kg; follow w/ 0.5 mg/kg in 10 min if effective. *IV load:* 1 mg/kg/dose bolus over 2–3 min; repeat in 5–10 min; 200–300 mg/h max; cont inf 20–50 µg/kg/min or 1–4 mg/min. *Peds.* Antiarrhythmic, ET, load: 1 mg/kg; repeat in 10–15 min max total 5 mg/kg, then IV inf 20–50 µg/kg/min. *Topical:* Apply max 4.5 mg/kg/dose. *Local inj anesthetic:* Max 4.5 mg/kg (see Table 2, page 265) **Caution:** [C, +] **Contra:** $\oslash$ Use lidocaine w/ epinephrine on the digits, ears, or nose because vasoconstriction may cause necrosis; heart block **Supplied:** *Inj local.* 0.5, 1, 1.5, 2, 4, 10, 20%. *Inj IV:* 1% (10 mg/mL), 2% (20 mg/mL); admixture 4, 10, 20%. *IV inf:* 0.2%, 0.4%; cream 2%; gel 2, 2.5%; oint 2.5, 5%; liq 2.5%; soln 2, 4%; viscous 2% **SE:** Dizziness, paresthesias, and convulsions associated w/ toxicity **Notes:** 2nd line to amiodarone in ECC; dilute ET dose 1–2 mL w/ NS; epinephrine may be added for local anesthesia to $\uparrow$ effect and $\downarrow$ bleeding; for IV forms, $\downarrow$ w/ liver Dz or CHF; see Table 2, page 265, for drug levels **Interactions:** $\uparrow$ Effects w/ amprenavir, BBs, cimetidine; $\uparrow$ neuromuscular blockade w/ aminoglycosides, tubocuraine, pareira; $\uparrow$ cardiac depression w/ procainamide, tocainide; $\uparrow$ effects of succinylcholine **Labs:** False $\uparrow$ SCr, $\uparrow$ CPK for 48 h after IM inj **NIPE:** Oral spray/soln may impair swallowing

Lidocaine/Prilocaine (EMLA, LMX) **Uses:** *Topical anesthetic*; ad-

junct to phlebotomy or dermal procedures **Action:** Topical anesthetic **Dose:** *Adults.* EMLA cream, anesthetic disc (1 g/10 cm²): Thick layer 2–2.5 g to intact skin and cover w/ occlusive dressing (eg, Tegaderm) for at least 1 h. *Anesthetic disc:* 1 g/10 cm² for at least 1 h. *Peds.* Max dose: <3 mo or <5 kg: 1 g/10 cm² for 1 h. *3–12 mo and >5 kg:* 2 g/20 cm² for 4 h. *1–6 y and >10 kg:* 10 g/100 cm² for 4 h. *7–12 y and >20 kg:* 20 g/200 cm² for 4 h **Caution:** [B, +] Methemoglobinemia **Contra:** Use on mucous membranes, broken skin, eyes; hypersensitivity to amide-type anesthetics **Supplied:** Cream 2.5% lidocaine/2.5% prilocaine; anesthetic disc (1 g) **SE:** Burning, stinging, methemoglobinemia **Notes:** Longer contact time gives greater effect.See Lidocaine **NIPE:** Low risk of systemic adverse effects

Lindane (Kwell) **Uses:** *Head lice, crab lice, scabies* **Action:** Ectoparasiti-

cide and ovicide **Dose:** *Adults & Peds.* Cream or lotion: Thin layer after bathing, leave for 8–12 h, pour on laundry. *Shampoo:* Apply 30 mL, develop a lather w/ warm water for 4 min, comb out nits **Caution:** [C, +/–] **Contra:** Open wounds, Sz disorder **Supplied:** Lotion 1%; shampoo 1% **SE:** Arrhythmias, Szs, local irritation, GI upset **Notes:** Caution w/ overuse; may be absorbed into blood; may repeat Rx in 7 days **Interactions:** Oil-based hair creams $\uparrow$ drug absorption **NIPE:** Apply to dry hair/dry, cool skin

Linezolid (Zyvox) Uses: *Infections caused by gram(+) bacteria (including vancomycin-resistant enterococcus, VRE), pneumonia, skin infections* **Action:** Unique, binds ribosomal bacterial RNA; bactericidal for strep, bacteriostatic for enterococci and staph. *Spectrum:* Excellent gram(+) activity including VRE and MRSA **Dose:** *Adults.* 400–600 mg IV or PO q12h. *Peds.* 10 mg/kg IV or PO q8h (q12h in preterm neonates) **Caution:** [C, ?/–] W/ reversible MAOI, ⊘ foods containing tyramine and cough and cold products containing pseudoephedrine; myelosuppression **Supplied:** Inj 2 mg/mL; tabs 400, 600 mg; susp 100 mg/5 mL **SE:** HTN, N/D, HA, insomnia, GI upset **Notes:** Follow weekly CBC **Interactions:** ↑ Risk of serotonin syndrome w/ SSRIs, sibutramine, trazodone, venlafaxine; ↑ HTN w/ amphetamines, dextromethorphan, dopamine, epinephrine, levodopa, MAOIs, meperidine, metaraminol, phenylephrine, phenylpropanolamine, pseudoephedrine, tyramine, ginseng, ephedra, ma huang, tyramine containing foods; ↑ risk of bleeding w/ antiplts **NIPE:** Take w/o regard to food, ⊘ tyramine-containing foods

Liothyronine (Cytomel) Uses: *Hypothyroidism, goiter, myxedema coma, thyroid suppression therapy* **Action:** T_3 replacement **Dose:** *Adults.* Initial 25 μg/24 h, titrate q1–2wk to response and TFT to maint of 25–100 μg/d PO. *Myxedema coma:* 25–50 μg IV. *Peds.* Initial dose of 5 μg/24 h, then titrate by 5-μg/24 h increments at 1–2-wk intervals; maint 25–75 μg/24 h PO qd; ↓ dose in elderly **Caution:** [A, +] **Contra:** Recent MI, uncorrected adrenal insufficiency, uncontrolled HTN **Supplied:** Tabs 5, 12.5, 25, 50 μg; inj 10 μg/mL **SE:** Alopecia, arrhythmias, CP, HA, sweating **Notes:** Monitor TFT pain **Interactions:** ↑ Effects of anticoagulants; ↓ effects w/ bile acid sequestrants, carbamazepine, estrogens, phenytoin, rifampin; ↓ effects of hypoglycemics, theophylline **NIPE:** Monitor cardiac status, take in AM

Lisinopril (Prinivil, Zestril) Uses: *HTN, CHF, prevent DN and AMI* **Action:** ACEI **Dose:** 5–40 mg/24 h PO qd–bid. *AMI:* 5 mg w/in 24 h of MI, followed by 5 mg after 24 h, 10 mg after 48 h, then 10 mg/d; ↓ in renal insufficiency **Caution:** [D, –] **Contra:** ACEI sensitivity **Supplied:** Tabs 2.5, 5, 10, 20, 30, 40 mg **SE:** Dizziness, HA, cough, hypotension, angioedema, hyperkalemia **Notes:** To prevent DN, start when urinary microalbuminemia begins **Interactions:** ↑ Effects w/ α-blockers, diuretics ↑ risk of hyperkalemia w/ K-sparing diuretics, trimethoprim, salt substitutes; ↑ risk of cough w/ capsaicin; ↑ effects of insulin, Li; ↓ effects w/ ASA, indomethacin, NSAIDs **Labs:** ↑ Serum K^+, creatinine, BUN **NIPE:** Maximum effect may take several weeks

Lithium Carbonate (Eskalith, Lithobid, others) Uses: *Manic episodes of bipolar illness* **Action:** Effects shift toward intraneuronal metabolism of catecholamines **Dose:** *Adults.* Acute mania: 600 mg PO tid or 900 mg SR bid. *Maint:* 300 mg PO tid–qid *Peds.* 6–12 y: 15–60 mg/kg/d in 3–4 ÷ doses; must be titrated; follow serum levels; ↓ in renal insufficiency, elderly **Caution:** [D, –] Many drug interactions **Contra:** Severe renal impairment or CV Dz, lactation **Sup-**

plied: Caps 150, 300, 600 mg; tabs 300 mg; SR tabs 300, 450 mg; syrup 300 mg/5 mL **SE:** Polyuria, polydipsia, nephrogenic DI, tremor; Na retention or diuretic use may potentiate toxicity; arrhythmias, dizziness **Notes:** See Table 2, page 265, for drug levels **Interactions:** ↑ Effects of TCA; ↑ effects w/ ACEIs, bumetanide, carbamazepine, ethacrynic acid, fluoxetine, furosemide, methyldopa, NSAIDs, phenytoin, phenothiazines, probenecid, tetracyclines, thiazide diuretics, dandelion, juniper; ↓ effects w/ acetazolamide, antacids, mannitol, theophyllines, urea, verapamil, caffeine **Labs:** False + urine glucose, ↑ serum glucose, creatinine kinase, TSH, I-131 uptake; ↓ uric acid, T_3, T_4 **NIPE:** Several weeks before full effects of med, ↑ fluid intake to 2–3 L/d

Lodoxamide (Alomide)
Uses: *Seasonal allergic conjunctivitis* **Action:** Stabilizes mast cells **Dose:** *Adults & Peds.* >2 y: 1–2 gtt in eye(s) qid ≤ 3 mo **Caution:** [B, ?] **Supplied:** Soln 0.1% **SE:** Ocular burning, stinging, HA

Lomefloxacin (Maxaquin)
Uses: *UTI, acute exacerbation of chronic bronchitis; prophylaxis in transurethral procedures* **Action:** Quinolone antibiotic; inhibits DNA gyrase. **Spectrum:** Good gram(–) activity including *H. influenzae* except *Stenotrophomonas maltophilia, Acinetobacter* sp, and some *P. aeruginosa* **Dose:** 400 mg/d PO; ↓ in renal insufficiency; ⊘ antacids **Caution:** [C, –] Interactions w/ cation-containing products **Contra:** Hypersensitivity to other quinolones, children < 18 y **Supplied:** Tabs 400 mg **SE:** Photosensitivity, Szs, HA, dizziness **Interactions:** ↑ Effects w/ cimetidine, probenecid; ↑ effects of cyclosporine, warfarin, caffeine; ↓ effects w/ antacids **Labs:** ↑ LFTs, ↓ K^+ **NIPE:** ↑ Risk of photosensitivity—use sunscreen, ↑ fluids to 2 L/d

Loperamide (Imodium)
Uses: *Diarrhea* **Action:** Slows intestinal motility **Dose:** *Adults.* Initially 4 mg PO, then 2 mg after each loose stool, up to 16 mg/d. *Peds.* 2–5 y, 13–20 kg: 1 mg PO tid. 6–8 y, 20–30 kg: 2 mg PO bid. 8–12 y, >30 kg: 2 mg PO tid **Caution:** [B, +] ⊘ use in acute diarrhea caused by *Salmonella, Shigella,* or *C. difficile* **Contra:** Pseudomembranous colitis, bloody diarrhea **Supplied:** Caps 2 mg; tabs 2 mg; liq 1 mg/5 mL (OTC) **SE:** Constipation, sedation, dizziness **Interactions:** ↑ Effects w/ antihistamines, CNS depressants, phenothiazines, TCAs, EtOH

Lopinavir/Ritonavir (Kaletra)
Uses: *HIV infection* **Action:** Protease inhibitor **Dose:** *Adults.* 3 caps or 5 mL PO bid. *Peds.* 7–15 kg: 12/3 mg/kg PO bid. 15–40 kg: 10/2.5 mg/kg PO bid. >40 kg: Adult dose (w/ food) **Caution:** [C, ?/–] Numerous drug interactions **Contra:** Concomitant drugs dependent on CYP3A or CYP2D6 **Supplied:** Caps 133.3 mg/33.3 mg (lopinavir/ritonavir), soln 400 mg/100 mg/5 mL **SE:** Soln has EtOH, ⊘ disulfiram and metronidazole; GI upset, asthenia, ↑ cholesterol and triglycerides, pancreatitis; protease metabolic syndrome **Interactions:** ↑ Effects w/ clarithromycin, erythromycin; ↑ effects of amiodarone, amprenavir, azole antifungals, bepridil, cisapride, cyclosporine, CCBs, ergot alkaloids, flecainide, flurazepam, HMG-CoA reductase inhibitors, indinavir, lidocaine, meperidine, midazolam, pimozide, propafenone, propoxyphene,

quinidine, rifabutin, saquinavir, sildenafil, tacrolimus, terfenadine, triazolam, zolpidem; ↓ effects w/ barbiturates, carbamazepine, dexamethasone, didanosine, efavirenz, nevirapine, phenytoin, rifabutin, rifampin, St. John's wort; ↓ effects of oral contraceptives, warfarin **NIPE:** Take w/ food, use barrier contraception

Loracarbef (Lorabid) Uses: *Upper and lower resp tract, skin, bone, urinary tract, abdomen, and gynecologic system bacterial infections* **Action:** 2nd-gen cephalosporin; inhibits cell wall synthesis. *Spectrum:* Weaker than 1st-gen against gram(+), enhanced activity against some gram(−) **Dose:** *Adults.* 200–400 mg PO bid. *Peds.* 7.5–15 mg/kg/d PO ÷ bid; on empty stomach; ↓ in severe renal insufficiency **Caution:** [B, +] **Supplied:** Caps 200, 400 mg; susp 125, 250 mg/5 mL **SE:** diarrhea **Interactions:** ↑ Effects w/ probenecid; ↑ effects of warfarin; ↑ nephrotoxicity w/ aminoglycosides, furosemide **NIPE:** Take w/o food

Loratadine (Claritin, Alavert) Uses: *Allergic rhinitis, chronic idiopathic urticaria* **Action:** Nonsedating antihistamine **Dose:** *Adults.* 10 mg/d PO *Peds.* 2–5 y: 5 mg PO qd. >6 y: Adult dose; take on an empty stomach; ↓ in hepatic insufficiency **Caution:** [B, +/−] **Contra:** Component hypersensitivity **Supplied:** Tabs 10 mg (OTC); rapidly disintegrating Reditabs 10 mg; syrup 1 mg/mL **SE:** HA, somnolence, xerostomia **Interactions:** ↑ Effects w/ CNS depressants, erythromycin, ketoconazole, MAOIs, protease inhibitors, procarbazine, EtOH **NIPE:** Take w/o food

Lorazepam (Ativan, others) [C-IV] Uses: *Anxiety and anxiety w/ depression; preop sedation; control of status epilepticus*; EtOH withdrawal; antiemetic **Action:** Benzodiazepine; antianxiety agent **Dose:** *Adults.* Anxiety: 1–10 mg/d PO in 2–3 ÷ doses. *Preop:* 0.05 mg/kg to 4 mg max IM 2 h before surgery. *Insomnia:* 2–4 mg PO hs. *Status epilepticus:* 4 mg/dose IV PRN q10–15 min; usual total dose 8 mg. *Antiemetic:* 0.5–2 mg IV or PO q4–6h PRN. *EtOH withdrawal:* 2–5 mg IV or 1–2 mg PO initial depending on severity; subsequent based on response **Peds.** Status epilepticus: 0.05 mg/kg/dose IV, repeat at 1–20 min intervals × 2 PRN. *Antiemetic, 2–15 y:* 0.05 mg/kg (to 2 mg/dose) prechemotherapy; ↓ in elderly; ⊘ administer IV >2 mg/min or 0.05 mg/kg/min **Caution:** [D, ?/−] **Contra:** Severe pain, severe hypotension, sleep apnea, narrow-angle glaucoma, hypersensitivity to propylene glycol or benzyl EtOH **Supplied:** Tabs 0.5, 1, 2 mg; soln, PO conc 2 mg/mL; inj 2, 4 mg/mL **SE:** Sedation, ataxia, tachycardia, constipation, resp depression **Notes:** Up to 10 min for effect if IV **Interactions:** ↑ Effects w/ cimetidine, disulfiram, probenecid, calendula, catnip, hops, lady's slipper, passionflower, kava kava, valerian; ↑ effects of phenytoin; ↑ CNS depression w/ anticonvulsants, antihistamines, CNS depressants, MAOIs, scopolamine, EtOH; ↓ effects w/ caffeine, tobacco; ↓ effects of levodopa **Labs:** ↑ LFTs **NIPE:** ⊘ DC abruptly

Losartan (Cozaar) Uses: *HTN,* CHF, DN **Action:** Angiotensin II antagonist **Dose:** 25–50 mg PO qd–bid; ↓ dose in elderly or hepatic impairment **Caution:** [C (1st tri), D 2nd and 3rd tri), ?/−] **Supplied:** Tabs 25, 50, 100 mg **SE:** ↓ BP in Pts on diuretics; GI upset, angioedema **Interactions:** ↑ Risk of hyperkalemia w/

K-sparing diuretics, K suppls, trimethoprim; ↑ effects of Li; ↓ effects w/ diltiazem, fluconazole, phenobarbital, rifampin **NIPE:** ⊘ PRG, breast-feeding

Lovastatin (Mevacor, Altocor)
Uses: *Hypercholesterolemia* **Action:** HMG-CoA reductase inhibitor **Dose:** 20 mg/d PO w/ PM meal; may ↑ at 4-wk intervals to 80 mg/d max; taken w/ meals; ⊘ grapefruit juice **Caution:** [X, –] ⊘ w/gemfibrozil. **Contra:** Active liver Dz **Supplied:** Tabs 10, 20, 40 mg **SE:** HA and GI intolerance common; Pt should promptly report any unexplained muscle pain, tenderness, or weakness (myopathy) **Notes:** Must maintain cholesterol-lowering diet; monitor LFT q12wk × 1 y, then q6mo **Interactions:** ↑ Effects w/ grapefruit juice; ↑ risk of severe myopathy w/ azole antifungals, cyclosporine, erythromycin, gemfibrozil, HMG-CoA inhibitors, niacin; ↑ effects of warfarin; ↓ effects w/ isradipine, pectin **Labs:** ↑ LFTs **NIPE:** ⊘ PRG, take drug in evening, periodic eye exams

Lymphocyte Immune Globulin [Antithymocyte Globulin, ATG] (Atgam)
Uses: *Allograft rejection in transplant Pts; aplastic anemia if not candidates for BMT* **Action:** ↓ Circulating T lymphocytes **Dose:** *Adults.* Prevent rejection: 15 mg/kg/day IV ×14 d, then qod ×7; initial w/in 24 h before/after transplant. *Treat rejection:* Same except use 10–15 mg/kg/day. *Peds.* 5–25 mg/kg/day IV. **Caution:** [C, ?] **Contra:** Hx Rxn to other equine γ-globulin prep, leukopenia, thrombocytopenia **Supplied:** Inj 50 mg/mL **SE:** DC w/ severe thrombocytopenia/leukopenia; rash, fever, chills, hypotension, HA, ↑ K+ **Notes:** *Test dose:* 0.1 mL 1:1000 dilution in NS **Interactions:** ↑ Immunosuppression w/ azathioprine, corticosteroids, immunosuppressants **Labs:** ↑ LFTs **NIPE:** Risk of febrile Rxn

Magaldrate (Riopan, Lowsium)
Uses: *Hyperacidity associated w/ peptic ulcer, gastritis, and hiatal hernia* **Action:** Low-Na antacid **Dose:** 5–10 mL PO between meals and hs **Caution:** [B, ?] **Contra:** Ulcerative colitis, diverticulitis, ileostomy/coleostomy, renal insufficiency due to Mg content **Supplied:** Susp (OTC) **SE:** GI upset **Notes:** <0.3 mg Na/tab or tsp **Interactions:** ↑ Effects of levodopa, quinidine; ↓ effects of allopurinol, anticoagulants, cefpodoxime, ciprofloxacin, clindamycin, digoxin, indomethacin, INH, ketoconazole, lincomycin, phenothiazines, quinolones, tetracyclines **NIPE:** ⊘ Other meds w/in 1–2 h

Magnesium Citrate (various) [OTC]
Uses: *Vigorous bowel prep*; constipation **Action:** Cathartic laxative **Dose:** *Adults.* 120–240 mL PO PRN. *Peds.* 0.5 mL/kg/dose, to a max of 200 mL PO; take w/ a beverage **Caution:** [B, +] **Contra:** Severe renal Dz, heart block, N/V, rectal bleeding **Supplied:** Effervescent soln (OTC) **SE:** Abdominal cramps, gas **Interactions:** ↓ Effects of anticoagulants, digoxin, fluoroquinolones, ketoconazole, nitrofurantoin, phenothiazines, tetracyclines **Labs:** ↑ Mg²⁺, ↓ protein, Ca²⁺, K+ **NIPE:** ⊘ Other meds w/in 1–2 h

Magnesium Hydroxide (Milk of Magnesia) [OTC]
Uses: *Constipation* **Action:** NS laxative **Dose:** *Adults.* 15–30 mL PO PRN. *Peds.* 0.5 mL/kg/dose PO PRN (follow dose w/ 8 oz of water) **Caution:** [B, +] **Contra:** Renal insufficiency or intestinal obstruction, ileostomy/colostomy **Supplied:** Tabs

311 mg; liq 400, 800 mg/5 mL (OTC) **SE:** Diarrhea, abdominal cramps **Interactions:** ↓ Effects of chlordiazepoxide, dicumarol, digoxin, indomethacin, INH, quinolones, tetracyclines **Labs:** ↑ Mg²⁺, ↓ protein, Ca²⁺, K⁺ **NIPE:** ⊘ Other meds w/in 1–2 h

Magnesium Oxide (Mag-Ox 400, others) **Uses:** *Replacement for low Mg levels* **Action:** Mg suppl **Dose:** 400–800 mg/d ÷ qd–qid w/ full glass of water **Caution:** [B, +] **Contra:** Ulcerative colitis, diverticulitis, ileostomy/colostomy, heart block, renal insufficiency **Supplied:** Caps 140 mg; tabs 400 mg (OTC) **SE:** Diarrhea, nausea **Interactions:** ↓ Effects of chlordiazepoxide, dicumarol, digoxin, indomethacin, INH, quinolones, tetracyclines **Labs:** ↑ Mg²⁺, ↓ protein, Ca²⁺, K⁺ **NIPE:** ⊘ Other meds w/in 1–2 h

Magnesium Sulfate (various) **Uses:** *Replacement for low Mg levels; preeclampsia and premature labor*; refractory hypokalemia and hypocalcemia **Action:** Mg suppl **Dose:** *Adults.* Suppl: 1–2 g IM or IV; repeat PRN. *Preeclampsia/premature labor:* 4 g load then 1–4 g/h IV inf. *Peds.* 25–50 mg/kg/dose IM or IV q4–6h for 3–4 doses; repeat if ↓ Mg persists; ↓ dose w/ low urine output or renal insufficiency **Caution:** [B, +] **Contra:** Heart block, renal failure **Supplied:** Inj 100, 125, 250, 500 mg/mL; PO soln 500 mg/mL; granules 40 mEq/5 g **SE:** CNS depression, diarrhea, flushing, heart block **Interactions:** ↑ CNS depression w/ antidepressants, antipsychotics, anxiolytics, barbiturates, hypnotics, narcotics; EtOH; ↑ neuromuscular blockade w/ aminoglycosides, atracurium, gallamine, pancuronium, tubocurarine, vecuronium **Labs:** ↑ Mg²⁺; ↓ protein, Ca²⁺, K⁺ **NIPE:** Check for absent patellar reflexes

Mannitol (various) **Uses:** *Cerebral edema, intraocular pressure, renal impairment, poisonings* **Action:** Osmotic diuretic **Dose:** *Diuresis: Adults.* 0.2 g/kg/dose IV over 3–5 min; if no diuresis w/in 2 h, DC. *Peds.* 0.75 g/kg/dose IV over 3–5 min; if no diuresis w/in 2 h, DC. *Cerebral edema: Adults & Peds.* 0.25 g/kg/dose IV push, repeated at 5-min intervals PRN; ↑ slowly to 1 g/kg/dose PRN for ↑ ICP **Caution:** [C, ?] w/ CHF or volume overload **Contra:** Anuria, dehydration, HF, PE **Supplied:** Inj 5, 10, 15, 20, 25% SE: Initial volume ↑ may exacerbate CHF; monitor for volume depletion, N/V/D **Interactions:** ↑ Effects of cardiac glycosides; ↓ effects of barbiturates, imipramine, Li, salicylates **Labs:** ↑ / ↓ Serum phosphate

Mechlorethamine (Mustargen) **WARNING:** Highly toxic agent, handle w/ care **Uses:** *Hodgkin's and NHL, cutaneous T-cell lymphoma (mycosis fungoides), lung CA, CML, malignant pleural effusions,* and CLL **Action:** Alkylating agent (bifunctional) **Dose:** 0.4 mg/kg single dose or 0.1 mg/kg/dose for 4 d; 6 mg/m² 1–2 ×/mo **Caution:** [D, ?] **Contra:** Presence of known infectious Dz **Supplied:** Inj 10 mg **SE:** Myelosuppression, thrombosis, or thrombophlebitis at inj site; tissue damage w/ extravasation (Na thiosulfate may be used topically to treat); N/V, skin rash, amenorrhea, and sterility (especially in men) and secondary leukemia in Pts treated for Hodgkin's Dz **Notes:** Highly volatile; administer w/in

30–60 min of prep **Interactions:** ↑ Risk of blood dyscrasias w/ amphotericin B; ↑ risk of bleeding w/ anticoagulants, NSAIDs, plt inhibitors, salicylates; ↑ myelosuppression w/ antineoplastic drugs, radiation therapy; ↓ effects of live virus vaccines **Labs:** ↑ Serum uric acid **NIPE:** ↑ Fluids to 2–3 L/d; ⊘ PRG, breast-feeding, vaccines, exposure to infection; ↑ risk of tinnitus

Meclizine (Antivert) Uses: *Motion sickness; vertigo* **Action:** Antiemetic, anticholinergic, and antihistaminic properties **Dose:** *Adults & Peds.* >12 y: 25 mg PO tid–qid PRN **Caution:** [B, ?] **Supplied:** Tabs 12.5, 25, 50 mg, chew tabs 25 mg; caps 25, 30 mg (OTC) **SE:** Drowsiness, xerostomia, and blurred vision common **Interactions:** ↑ Sedation w/ antihistamines, CNS depressants, neuroleptics, EtOH; ↑ anticholinergic effects w/ anticholinergics, atropine, disopyramide, haloperidol, phenothiazines, quinidine **NIPE:** Use prophylactically

Medroxyprogesterone (Provera, Depo-Provera) Uses: *Contraception; secondary amenorrhea; and abnormal uterine bleeding (AUB) caused by hormonal imbalance; endometrial CA* **Action:** Progestin suppl **Dose:** *Contraception:* 150 mg IM q3mo or 450 mg IM q4mo. *Secondary amenorrhea:* 5–10 mg/d PO for 5–10 d. *AUB:* 5–10 mg/d PO for 5–10 d beginning on the 16th or 21st d of menstrual cycle. *Endometrial CA:* 400–1000 mg/wk IM; ↓ in hepatic insufficiency **Caution:** [X, +] **Contra:** Hx of thromboembolic disorders, hepatic Dz, PRG **Supplied:** Tabs 2.5, 5, 10 mg; depot inj 100, 150, 400 mg/mL **SE:** Breakthrough bleeding, spotting, altered menstrual flow, anorexia, edema, thromboembolic complications, depression, weight gain **Notes:** Perform breast exam and Pap smear before therapy; as contraceptive obtain PRG test if last inj > 3 mo earlier **Interactions:** ↓ Effects w/ aminoglutethimide, phenytoin, carbamazepine, phenobarbital, rifampin, rifabutin **NIPE:** Sunlight exposure may cause melasma, if GI upset take w/ food

Megestrol Acetate (Megace) Uses: *Breast and endometrial CAs; appetite stimulant in CA and HIV-related cachexia* **Action:** Hormone; progesterone analogue **Dose:** *CA:* 40–320 mg/d PO in ÷ doses. *Appetite:* 800 mg/d PO ÷ **Caution:** [X, –] Thromboembolism **Contra:** PRG **Supplied:** Tabs 20, 40 mg; soln 40 mg/mL **SE:** May induce DVT; ⊘ DC therapy abruptly; edema, menstrual bleeding; photosensitivity, insomnia, rash, myelosuppression **Interactions:** ↑ Effects of warfarin **Labs:** ↑ LDH **NIPE:** ↑ Risk of photosensitivity—use sunscreen

Meloxicam (Mobic) Uses: *Osteoarthritis* **Action:** NSAID w/ ↑ COX-2 activity **Dose:** 7.5–15 mg/d PO; ↓ in renal insufficiency; take w/food **Caution:** [C, ?/–] Peptic ulcer, NSAID, or ASA sensitivity **Supplied:** Tabs 7.5 mg **SE:** HA, dizziness, GI upset, GI bleeding, edema **Interactions:** ↑ Effects of ASA, anticoagulants, corticosteroids, Li, EtOH, tobacco; ↓ effects w/ cholestyramine; ↓ effects of antihypertensives **Labs:** False + guaiac test, ↑ LFTs **NIPE:** Take w/ food, may take several days for full effect

Melphalan (L-PAM) (Alkeran) WARNING: Severe bone marrow depression, leukemogenic, and mutagenic Uses: *Multiple myeloma, ovarian CAs,* breast, testicular, and, melanoma; allogenic and ABMT in high doses **Action:** Alkylating agent (bifunctional) **Dose:** (Per protocols) 6 mg/d or 0.25 mg/kg/d for 4–7 d, repeated at 4–6-wk intervals, or 1 mg/kg single dose once q4–6wk; 0.15 mg/kg/d for 5 d q6wk. *High-dose high-risk multiple myeloma:* Single dose 140 mg/m². *ABMT:* 140–240 mg/m² IV; ↓ in renal insufficiency **Caution:** [D, ?] **Contra:** Hypersensitivity or resistance **Supplied:** Tabs 2 mg; inj 50, 100 mg **SE:** Myelosuppression (leukopenia and thrombocytopenia), secondary leukemia, alopecia, dermatitis, stomatitis, and pulmonary fibrosis; very rare hypersensitivity Rxns **Notes:** Take on empty stomach **Interactions:** ↑ Risk of nephrotoxicity w/ cisplatin, cyclosporine; ↓ effects w/ cimetidine, interferon alfa **Labs:** ↑ Uric acid, urine 5-HIAA **NIPE:** ↑ Fluids, ⊘ PRG, breast-feeding

Memantine (Namenda) Uses: Moderate/severe Alzheimer's **Action:** *N*-methyl-D-aspartate receptor antagonist **Dose:** Target 20 mg/d, start 5 mg/d, ↑ 5 mg/d to 20 mg/d, wait > 1 wk before ↑ dose; use ÷ doses above 5 mg/d **Caution:** [B, ?/–] Hepatic/mild–moderate renal impairment **Supplied:** Tabs 5, 10 mg **SE:** Dizziness **Notes:** Renal clearance ↓ by alkaline urine pH (↓ 80% at urine pH 8) **Interactions:** ↑ Effects with amantadine, carbonic anhydrase inhibitors, dextromethorphan, ketamine, sodium bicarbonate; ↑ effects with any drug, herb, food that alkalinizes urine **Labs:** Monitor BUN, SCr **NIPE:** Take w/o regard to food, EtOH ↑ adverse effects & ↓ effectiveness

Meningococcal Polysaccharide Vaccine (Menomune) Uses: *Immunize against *N. meningitidis* (meningococcus)*; recommended in some complement deficiency, asplenia, lab workers w/ exposure; college students by some professional groups **Action:** Live vaccine, active immunization **Dose:** *Adults & Peds.* >2 y: 0.5 mL SQ; ⊘ inject intradermally or IV; epinephrine (1:1000) must be available for anaphylactic/allergic Rxns **Caution:** [C, ?/–] **Contra:** Thimerosal sensitivity **Supplied:** Inj **SE:** Local inj site Rxns, HA **Notes:** Active against meningococcal serotypes A, C, Y, and W-135 but not group B **Interactions:** ↓ Effects w/ immunoglobulin if admin. w/in 1 mo **NIPE:** Pain & inflammation at inj site

Meperidine (Demerol) [C–II] Uses: *Moderate to severe pain* **Action:** Narcotic analgesic **Dose:** *Adults.* 50–150 mg PO or IM q3–4h PRN. *Peds.* 1–1.5 mg/kg/dose PO or IM q3–4h PRN, up to 100 mg/dose; ↓ in elderly and renal impairment **Caution:** [C/D (prolonged use or high doses at term, +] **Contra:** Recent or concomitant MAOIs, renal failure **Supplied:** Tabs 50, 100 mg; syrup 50 mg/mL; inj 10, 25, 50, 75, 100 mg/mL **SE:** Resp depression, Szs, sedation, constipation **Notes:** Analgesic effects potentiated w/ use of hydroxyzine; 75 mg IM = 10 mg of morphine IM; reduces Sz threshold **Interactions:** ↑ Effects w/ antihistamines, barbiturates, cimetidine, MAOIs, neuroleptics, selegiline, TCAs, St. John's wort, EtOH; ↑ effects of INH; ↓ effects w/ phenytoin **Labs:** ↑ Serum amylase, lipase

Meprobamate (Equinil, Miltown) [C–IV] Uses: *Short-term relief of anxiety* **Action:** Mild tranquilizer; antianxiety **Dose:** *Adults.* 400 mg PO tid–qid up to 2400 mg/d; SR 400–800 mg PO bid. *Peds. 6–12 y:* 100–200 mg bid–tid; SR 200 mg bid; ↓ in renal/liver insufficiency **Caution:** [D, +/–] **Contra:** Narrow-angle glaucoma, porphyria, PRG **Supplied:** Tabs 200, 400, 600 mg; SR caps 200, 400 mg **SE:** May cause drowsiness, syncope, tachycardia, edema **Interactions:** ↑ Effects w/ antihistamines, barbiturates, CNS depressants, narcotics, EtOH

Mercaptopurine [6-MP] (Purinethol) Uses: *Acute leukemias,* 2nd-line Rx of CML and NHL, maint ALL in children, immunosuppressant for autoimmune Dzs (Crohn's Dz) **Action:** Antimetabolite; mimics hypoxanthine **Dose:** 80–100 mg/m^2/d or 2.5–5 mg/kg/d; maint 1.5–2.5 mg/kg/d; concurrent allopurinol therapy requires a 67–75% dose reduction of 6-MP because of interference w/ metabolism by xanthine oxidase; ↓ in renal, hepatic insufficiency **Caution:** [D, ?] **Contra:** Severe hepatic Dz, bone marrow suppression, PRG **Supplied:** Tabs 50 mg **SE:** Mild hematologic toxicity; uncommon GI toxicity, except mucositis, stomatitis, and diarrhea; rash, fever, eosinophilia, jaundice, and hepatitis **Notes:** Use proper procedures for handling; take on empty stomach; ensure adequate hydration **Interactions:** ↑ Effects w/ allopurinol; ↑ risk of bone marrow suppression w/ trimethoprim-sulfamethoxazole; ↓ effects of warfarin **Labs:** False ↑ serum glucose, uric acid **NIPE:** ↑ Fluid intake to 2–3 L/d, may take 4+ wk for improvement

Meropenem (Merrem) Uses: *Intraabdominal infections, bacterial meningitis* **Action:** Carbapenem; inhibits cell wall synthesis, a β-lactam. *Spectrum:* Excellent gram(+) except MRSA and *E. faecium;* excellent gram(–) including extended-spectrum β-lactamase producers; good anaerobic **Dose:** *Adults.* 1 g IV q8h. *Peds.* 20–40 mg/kg IV q 8h; ↓ in renal insufficiency **Caution:** [B, ?] **Contra:** β-Lactam sensitivity **Supplied:** Inj 1 g/30 mL, 500 mg/20 mL **SE:** Less Sz potential than imipenem; diarrhea; thrombocytopenia **Notes:** Overuse can ↑ bacterial resistance **Interactions:** ↑ Effects w/ probenecid **Labs:** ↑ LFTs, BUN, creatinine, eosinophils ↓ Hmg, Hct, WBCs **NIPE:** Monitor for superinfection

Mesalamine (Rowasa, Asacol, Pentasa) Uses: *Mild to moderate distal ulcerative colitis, proctosigmoiditis, or proctitis* **Action:** Unknown; may topically inhibit prostaglandins **Dose:** *Retention enema:* qd hs or insert 1 supp bid. *PO:* 800–1000 mg PO 3–4×/d; ↓ initial dose in elderly **Caution:** [B, M] **Contra:** Salicylate sensitivity **Supplied:** Tabs 400 mg; caps 250 mg; supp 500 mg; rectal susp 4 g/60 mL **SE:** HA, malaise, abdominal pain, flatulence, rash, pancreatitis, pericarditis **Notes:** May discolor urine yellow-brown **Interactions:** ↓ Effect of digoxin **Labs:** ↑ LFTs, amylase, lipase

Mesna (Mesnex) Uses: *↓ Ifosfamide- and cyclophosphamide-induced hemorrhagic cystitis* **Action:** Antidote **Dose:** 20% of the ifosfamide dose (±) or cyclophosphamide dose IV 15 min prior to and 4 and 8 h after chemotherapy **Caution:** [B; ?/–] **Contra:** Thiol sensitivity **Supplied:** Inj 100 mg/mL; tablets 400 mg **SE:** Hypotension, allergic Rxns, HA, GI upset, taste perversion **Notes:** Hydration helps ↓ hemorrhagic cystitis **Interactions:** ↓ Effects of warfarin **Labs:** False + urine ketones

Mesoridazine (Serentil) WARNING: Can prolong QT interval in a dose-related fashion; torsades de points reported Uses: *Schizophrenia,* acute and chronic alcoholism, chronic brain syndrome Action: Phenothiazine antipsychotic Dose: Initial, 25–50 mg PO or IV tid; ↑ to 300–400 mg/d max Caution: [C, ?/–] Contra: Phenothiazine sensitivity, coadministration w/ drugs that cause QT_c prolongation, CNS depression Supplied: Tabs 10, 25, 50, 100 mg; PO conc 25 mg/mL; inj 25 mg/mL SE: Low incidence of EPS; hypotension, xerostomia, constipation, skin discoloration, tachycardia, lowered Sz threshold, blood dyscrasias, pigmentary retinopathy at high doses Interactions: ↑ Effects w/ antimalarials, BBs, chloroquine, TCAs, EtOH; ↑ effects of antidepressants, nitrates, antihypertensives; ↑ QT interval w/ amiodarone, azole antifungals, disopyramide, fluoxetine, macrolides, paroxetine, procainamide, quinidine, quinolones, TCAs, verapamil; ↓ effects w/ attapulgite, barbiturates, caffeine, tobacco; ↓ effects of barbiturates, guanethidine, guanadrel, levodopa, Li, sympathomimetics Labs: False + PRG test; ↑ serum glucose, cholesterol; ↓ uric acid NIPE: Photosensitivity—use sunscreen

Metaproterenol (Alupent, Metaprel) Uses: *Asthma and reversible bronchospasm* Action: Sympathomimetic bronchodilator Dose: Adults. Inhal: 1–3 inhal q3–4h, 12 inhal max/24 h; wait 2 min between inhal. PO: 20 mg q6–8h. Peds. Inhal: 0.5 mg/kg/dose, 15 mg/dose max inhaled q4–6h by neb or 1–2 puffs q4–6h. PO: 0.3–0.5 mg/kg/dose q6–8h Caution: [C, ?/–] Contra: Tachycardia, other arrhythmias Supplied: Aerosol 0.65 mg/inhal; soln for inhal 0.4, 0.6, 5%; tabs 10, 20 mg; syrup 10 mg/5 mL SE: Fewer β_1 effects than isoproterenol and longer acting; nervousness, tremor, tachycardia, HTN Interactions: ↑ Effects w/ sympathomimetic drugs, xanthines; ↑ risk of arrhythmias w/ cardiac glycosides, halothane, levodopa, theophylline, thyroid hormones; ↑ HTN w/ MAOIs; ↓ effects w/ BBs Labs: ↑ Serum K^+ NIPE: Separate additional aerosol use by 5 min

Metaxalone (Skelaxin) Uses: *Painful musculoskeletal conditions* Action: Centrally acting skeletal muscle relaxant Dose: 800 mg PO 3–4×/d Caution: [C, ?/–] Contra: Severe hepatic/renal impairment; caution in anemia Supplied: Tabs 400 mg SE: N/V, HA, drowsiness, hepatitis Interactions: ↑ Sedating effects w/ CNS depressants, EtOH Labs: False + urine glucose using Benedict's test

Metformin (Glucophage, Glucophage XR) WARNING: Associated w/ lactic acidosis Uses: *Type 2 DM* Action: ↓ Hepatic glucose production and intestinal absorption of glucose; improves insulin sensitivity Dose: Adults. Initial dose 500 mg PO bid; may ↑ 2550 mg/d max (administer w/ AM and PM meals; can convert total daily dose to qd dose of XR formulation). Peds. 10–16 y: 500 mg PO bid, ↑ by 500 mg weekly up to 2000 mg/d in ÷ doses; ⊘ use XR formulation in peds Caution: [B, +/–] Contra: ⊘ use if SCr >1.4 in females or >1.5 in males; contra in hypoxemic conditions, including acute CHF/sepsis; ⊘ EtOH; hold dose before and 48 h after ionic contrast Supplied: Tabs 500, 850, 1000 mg; XR tabs 500 mg SE: Anorexia, N/V, rash, lactic acidosis (rare, but serious) Interactions: ↑

Effects w/ amiloride, cimetidine, digoxin, furosemide, MAOIs, morphine, procainamide, quinidine, quinine, ranitidine, triamterene, trimethoprim, vancomycin; ↓ effects w/ corticosteroids, CCBs, diuretics, estrogens, INH, oral contraceptives, phenothiazines, phenytoin, sympathomimetics, thyroid drugs, tobacco **NIPE:** Take w/ food; ⊘ dehydration, EtOH

Methadone (Dolophine) [C-II]
Uses: *Severe pain; detoxification and maint of narcotic addiction* **Action:** Narcotic analgesic **Dose:** *Adults.* 2.5–10 mg IM q3–8h or 5–15 mg PO q8h; titrate as needed *Peds.*0.7 mg/kg/24 h PO or IM ÷ q8h; ↑ slowly to ⊘ resp depression; ↓ in renal Dz **Caution:** [B/D (prolonged use or high doses at term), + (w/ doses = 20 mg/24 h)], severe liver Dz **Supplied:** Tabs 5, 10, 40 mg; PO soln 5, 10 mg/5 mL; PO conc 10 mg/mL; inj 10 mg/mL **SE:** Resp depression, sedation, constipation, urinary retention, ventricular arrhythmias **Notes:** Equianalgesic w/ parenteral morphine; longer half-life; prolongs QT interval **Interactions:** ↑ Effects w/ cimetidine, CNS depressants, EtOH; ↑ effects of anticoagulants, EtOH, antihistamines, barbiturates, glutethimide, methocarbamol; ↓ effects w/ carbamazepine, nelfinavir, phenobarbital, phenytoin, primidone, rifampin, ritonavir **Labs:** ↑ Serum amylase, lipase

Methenamine (Hiprex, Urex, others)
Uses: *Suppression or elimination of bacteriuria associated w/ chronic/ recurrent UTI* **Action:** Converted to formaldehyde and ammonia in acidic urine; nonspecific bactericidal action **Dose:** *Adults.* Hippurate: 1 g bid. *Mandelate:* 1 g qid pc and hs *Peds 6–12 y.* Hippurate: 25–50 mg/kg/d ÷ bid. *Mandelate:* 50–75 mg/kg/d ÷ qid (take w/ food and ascorbic acid; adequate hydration) **Caution:** [C, +] **Contra:** Renal insufficiency, severe hepatic Dz, and severe dehydration; allergy to sulfonamides **Supplied:** *Methenamine hippurate* (Hiprex, Urex): 1-g tabs. *Methenamine mandelate:* 500-mg, 1-g EC tabs **SE:** Rash, GI upset, dysuria, ↑ LFTs **Interactions:** ↓ Effects w/ acetazolamide, antacids **Labs:** ↑ Serum catecholamines, urine glucose, urobilinogen; ↓ urine estriol, estrogens **NIPE:** ↑ Fluids to 2–3 L/d; take w/ food

Methimazole (Tapazole)
Uses: *Hyperthyroidism, thyrotoxicosis,* and prep for thyroid surgery or radiation **Action:** Blocks the formation of T_3 and T_4 **Dose:** *Adults.* Initial: 15–60 mg PO ÷ tid. *Maint:* 5–15 mg PO qd. *Peds.* Initial: 0.4–0.7 mg/kg/24 h PO ÷ tid. *Maint:* ⅓–⅔ of the initial dose PO qd; take w/ food **Caution:** [D, +/–] **Contra:** Breast-feeding **Supplied:** Tabs 5, 10 mg **SE:** GI upset, dizziness, blood dyscrasias **Notes:** Follow clinically and w/ TFT **Interactions:** ↑ Effects of digitalis glycosides, metoprolol, propranolol; ↓ effects of anticoagulants, theophylline; ↓ effects w/ amiodarone **Labs:** ↑ LFTs, PT **NIPE:** Take w/ food

Methocarbamol (Robaxin)
Uses: *Relief of discomfort associated w/ painful musculoskeletal conditions* **Action:** Centrally acting skeletal muscle relaxant **Dose:** *Adults.* 1.5 g PO qid for 2–3 d, then 1-g PO qid maint therapy; IV form rarely indicated. *Peds.* 15 mg/kg/dose, may repeat PRN (recommended for tetanus only) **Caution:** [C, +] **Contra:** Myasthenia gravis, renal impairment; cau-

tion in Sz disorders **Supplied:** Tabs 325, 500, 750 mg; inj 100 mg/mL **SE:** Can discolor urine; drowsiness, GI upset **Interactions:** ↑ Effects w/ CNS depressant, EtOH **Labs:** ↑ Urine 5-HIAA, urine vanillylmandelic acid **NIPE:** Monitor for blurred vision, nystagmus, diplopia

Methotrexate (Folex, Rheumatrex)
Uses: *ALL and AML (including leukemic meningitis), trophoblastic tumors (chorioepithelioma, choriocarcinoma, chorioadenoma destruens, hydatidiform mole), breast CA, Burkitt's lymphoma, mycosis fungoides, osteosarcoma, head and neck CA, Hodgkin's and NHL, lung CA; psoriasis; and RA* **Action:** Inhibits dihydrofolate reductase-mediated gen. of tetrahydrofolate **Dose:** *CA:* 7.5 mg/wk PO as a single dose or 2.5 mg q12h PO for 3 doses/wk; "high-dose" Rx requires leucovorin rescue to limit hematologic and mucosal toxicity; ↓ in renal/hepatic impairment **Caution:** [D, –] **Contra:** Severe renal/hepatic impairment, PRG/lactation **Supplied:** Tabs 2.5, 5, 7.5, 10, 15 mg; inj 2.5, 25 mg/mL; preservative-free inj 25 mg/mL **SE:** Myelosuppression, N/V/D, anorexia, mucositis, hepatotoxicity (transient and reversible; may progress to atrophy, necrosis, fibrosis, cirrhosis), rashes, dizziness, malaise, blurred vision, alopecia, photosensitivity, renal failure, pneumonitis, and, rarely, pulmonary fibrosis; chemical arachnoiditis and HA w/ IT delivery **Notes:** Monitor blood counts, LFTs, renal Fxn tests, CXR, and MTX levels **Interactions:** ↑ Effects w/ chloramphenicol, cyclosporine, etretinate, NSAIDs, phenylbutazone, phenytoin, penicillin, probenecid, salicylates, sulfonamides, sulfonylureas, EtOH; ↑ effects of cyclosporine, tetracycline, theophylline; ↓ effects w/ antimalarials, aminoglycosides, binding resins, cholestyramine, folic acid; ↓ effects of digoxin **Labs:** ↑ AST, ALT, alkaline phosphatase, bilirubin, cholesterol **NIPE:** ↑ Risk of photosensitivity—use sunscreen, ↑ fluids 2–3 L/d

Methyldopa (Aldomet)
Uses: *HTN* **Action:** Centrally acting antihypertensive **Dose:** *Adults.* 250–500 mg PO bid–tid (max 2–3 g/d) or 250 mg–1 g IV q6–8h. *Peds.* 10 mg/kg/24 h PO in 2–3 ÷ doses (max 40 mg/kg/24 h ÷ q6–12h) or 5–10 mg/kg/dose IV q6–8h to total dose of 20–40 mg/kg/24 h;↓ dose in renal insufficiency and in elderly **Caution:** [B (PO), C (IV), +] **Contra:** Liver Dz; MAOIs **Supplied:** Tabs 125, 250, 500 mg; PO susp 50 mg/mL; inj 50 mg/mL **SE:** Can discolor urine; initial transient sedation or drowsiness frequent; edema, hemolytic anemia; hepatic disorders **Interactions:** ↑ Effects w/ anesthetics, diuretics, levodopa, Li, methotrimeprazine, thioxanthenes, vasodilators, verapamil; ↑ effects of haloperidol, Li, tolbutamide; ↓ effects w/ amphetamines, Fe, phenothiazines, TCAs; ↓ effects of ephedrine **Labs:** Interference w/ SCr, glucose, AST, catecholamines; urine catecholamines, uric acid; false ↓ serum cholesterol, triglycerides **NIPE:** After 1–2 mo tolerance may develop

Methylergonovine (Methergine)
Uses: *Postpartum bleeding (uterine subinvolution)* **Action:** Ergotamine derivative **Dose:** 0.2 mg IM after delivery of placenta, may repeat at 264-h intervals or 0.2–0.4 mg PO q6–12h for 2–7 d **Caution:** [C, ?] **Contra:** HTN, PRG **Supplied:** Injectable forms; tabs 0.2 mg **SE:**

IV doses should be given over a period of >1 min w/ frequent BP monitoring; HTN, N/V **Interactions:** ↑ Vasoconstriction w/ ergot alkaloids, sympathomimetics, tobacco **NIPE:** ⊘ Smoking

Methylprednisolone (Solu-Medrol)   [See Steroids, Table 4, page 271]
Interactions: ↑ Effects w/ cyclosporine, clarithromycin, erythromycin, estrogens, ketoconazole, oral contraceptives, troleandomycin, grapefruit juice; ↑ effects of cyclosporine; ↓ effects w/ aminoglutethimide, barbiturates, carbamazepine, cholestyramine, colestipol, INH, phenytoin, phenobarbital, rifampin; ↓ effects of anticoagulants, hypoglycemics, INH, salicylates, vaccines **Labs:** ↓ Skin test Rxns; false ↑ serum cortisol, digoxin, theophylline, & urine glucose **NIPE:** ⊘ DC abruptly, ⊘ infections or vaccines

Metoclopramide (Reglan, Clopra, Octamide)   **Uses:** *Relief of diabetic gastroparesis, symptomatic GERD; chemotherapy-induced N/V, facilitate small-bowel intubation and radiologic evaluation of the upper GI tract,* stimulate gut in prolonged postop ileus **Action:** Stimulates motility of the upper GI tract; blocks dopamine in the chemoreceptor trigger zone **Dose:** *Adults.* Diabetic gastroparesis: 10 mg PO 30 min ac and hs for 2–8 wk PRN, or same dose given IV for 10 d, then switch to PO. *Reflux:* 10–15 mg PO 30 min ac and hs. *Antiemetic:* 1–3 mg/kg/dose IV 30 min before chemotherapy, then q2h for 2 doses, then q3h for 3 doses. *Peds.* Reflux: 0.1 mg/kg/dose PO qid. *Antiemetic:* 1–2 mg/kg/dose IV as for adults **Caution:** [B, –] Concomitant drugs w/ extrapyramidal ADRs **Contra:** Sz disorders, GI obstruction **Supplied:** Tabs 5, 10 mg; syrup 5 mg/5 mL; soln 10 mg/mL; inj 5 mg/mL **SE:** Dystonic Rxns common w/ high doses, treat w/ IV diphenhydramine; restlessness, drowsiness, diarrhea **Interactions:** ↑ Risk of serotonin syndrome w/ sertraline, venlafaxine; ↑ effects of acetaminophen, ASA, CNS depressants, cyclosporine, levodopa, Li, succinylcholine, tetracyclines, EtOH; ↓ effects w/ anticholinergics, narcotics; ↓ effects of cimetidine, digoxin **Labs:** ↑ Serum ALT, AST, amylase **NIPE:** Monitor for extrapyramidal effects

Metolazone (Mykrox, Zaroxolyn)   **Uses:** *Mild/moderate essential HTN and edema of renal Dz or cardiac failure* **Action:** Thiazide-like diuretic; inhibits Na reabsorption in the distal tubules **Dose:** *HTN:* 2.5–5 mg/d PO. *Edema:* 5–20 mg/d PO. *Peds.* 0.2–0.4 mg/kg/d PO ÷ q12h–qd **Caution:** [D, +] **Contra:** Thiazide or sulfonamide sensitivity, anuria **Supplied:** *Tabs:* Mykrox (rapid acting) 0.5 mg, Zaroxolyn 2.5, 5, 10 mg **SE:** Monitor fluid and electrolyte status during Rx; dizziness, hypotension, tachycardia, CP, photosensitivity; Mykrox and Zaroxolyn not bioequivalent **Interactions:** ↑ Effects w/ antihypertensives, barbiturates, narcotics, nitrates, EtOH, food; ↑ effects of digoxin, Li; ↑ hyperglycemia w/ BBs, diazoxide; ↑ hypokalemia w/ amphotericin B, corticosteroids, mezlocillin, piperacillin, ticarcillin; ↓ effects w/ cholestyramine, colestipol, hypoglycemics, insulin, NSAIDs, salicylates; ↓ effects of methenamine **Labs:** ↑ Serum and urine glucose, serum cholesterol, triglycerides, uric acid **NIPE:** ↑ Risk of photosensitivity—use sunscreen; ↑ risk of gout; monitor electrolytes

Metoprolol (Lopressor, Toprol XL)   **WARNING:** ⊘ acutely stop therapy as marked worsening of angina can result **Uses:** *HTN, angina, AMI, and CHF* **Action:** β-Adrenergic receptor blocker **Dose:** *Angina:* 50–100 mg PO bid. *HTN:* 100–450 mg/d PO. *AMI:* 5 mg IV ×3 doses, then 50 mg PO q6h ×48 h, then 100 mg PO bid. *CHF:* 12–25 mg/d PO ×2 wk, ↑ at 2-wk intervals to 200 mg/max, use low dose in Pts w/ greatest severity; ↓ in hepatic failure **Caution:** [C, +] Uncompensated CHF, bradycardia, heart block **Contra:** Arrhythmia w/tachycardia **Supplied:** Tabs 50, 100 mg; ER tabs 50, 100, 200 mg; inj 1 mg/mL **SE:** Drowsiness, insomnia, erectile dysfunction, bradycardia, bronchospasm **Interactions:** ↑ Effects w/ cimetidine, dihydropyridines, diltiazem, fluoxetine, hydralazine, methimazole, oral contraceptives, propylthiouracil, quinidine, quinolones; ↑ effects of hydralazine; ↑ bradycardia w/ digoxin, dipyridamole, verapamil; ↓ effects w/ barbiturates, NSAIDs, rifampin; ↓ effects of isoproterenol, theophylline **Labs:** ↑ BUN, SCr, LFTs, uric acid **NIPE:** Take w/ food, ⊘ DC abruptly—withdraw over 2 wk

Metronidazole (Flagyl, MetroGel)   **Uses:** *Bone/joint, endocarditis, intraabdominal, meningitis, and skin infections; amebiasis; trichomoniasis; bacterial vaginosis* **Action:** Interferes w/ DNA synthesis. *Spectrum:* Excellent coverage for anaerobic infections including *C. difficile*, also *H. pylori* in combination therapy **Dose:** *Adults.* Anaerobic infections: 500 mg IV q6–8h. *Amebic dysentery:* 750 mg/d PO for 5–10 d. *Trichomoniasis:* 250 mg PO tid for 7 d or 2 g PO ×1. *C. difficile infection:* 500 mg PO or IV q8h for 7–10 d (PO preferred; IV only if Pt NPO). *Vaginosis:* 1 applicatorful intravaginally bid or 500 mg PO bid for 7 d. *Acne rosacea/skin:* Apply bid. **Peds.** Anaerobic infections: 15 mg/kg/24 h PO or IV ÷ q6h. *Amebic dysentery:* 35–50 mg/kg/24 h PO in 3 ÷ doses for 5–10 d; ↓ in hepatic failure **Caution:** [B, M] ⊘ EtOH **Contra:** 1st tri of PRG **Supplied:** Tabs 250, 500 mg; XR tabs 750 mg; caps 375 mg; topical lotion and gel 0.75%; gel, vaginal 0.75% (5 g/applicator 37.5 mg in 70-g tube), cream 1% **SE:** May cause disulfiram-like Rxn; dizziness, HA, GI upset, anorexia, urine discoloration **Notes:** For Trichomoniasis, Rx Pt's partner; no aerobic bacteria activity; used in combination in serious mixed infections **Interactions:** ↑ Effects w/ cimetidine; ↑ effects of carbamazepine, fluorouracil, Li, warfarin; ↓ effects w/ barbiturates, cholestyramine, colestipol, phenytoin **Labs:** May cause ↓/zero values for LFTs, triglycerides, glucose **NIPE:** Take w/ food, possible metallic taste

Mexiletine (Mexitil)   **Uses:** *Suppression of symptomatic ventricular arrhythmias*; diabetic neuropathy **Action:** Class IB antiarrhythmic **Dose:** *Adults.* 200–300 mg PO q8h; 1200 mg/d max. *Peds.*2.5–5 mg/kg PO q 8h; drug interactions w/ hepatic enzyme inducers and suppressors requiring dosage changes (administer w/ food or antacids) **Caution:** [C, +] May worsen severe arrhythmias **Contra:** Cardiogenic shock or 2nd-/3rd-degree AV block w/o pacemaker **Supplied:** Caps 150, 200, 250 mg **SE:** Monitor LFTs; lightheadedness, dizziness, anxiety, incoordination, HA, GI upset, ataxia, hepatic damage, blood dyscrasias **Interactions:** ↑ Effects w/ fluvoxamine, quinidine, caffeine; ↑ effects of theophylline; ↓ effects w/ atropine, hydantoins, phenytoin, phenobarbital, rifampin, tobacco **Labs:** ↑ LFTs, + ANA

Mezlocillin (Mezlin) **Uses:** *Infections caused by susceptible gram(–) bacteria involving the skin, bone, resp tract, urinary tract, abdomen, and septicemia* **Action:** Bactericidal; inhibits cell wall synthesis. *Spectrum:* Gram(–) *Klebsiella, Proteus, E. coli, Enterobacter, P. aeruginosa,* and *Serratia* **Dose:** *Adults.* 3 g IV q4–6h. *Peds.* 200–300 mg/kg/d ÷ q4–6h; ↓ in renal/hepatic insufficiency **Caution:** [B, M] **Contra:** Penicillin sensitivity **Supplied:** Inj **SE:** GI upset, agranulocytosis, thrombocytopenia **Notes:** Often used w/ aminoglycoside **Interactions:** ↑ Effects w/ probenecid; ↓ effects of MRX **Labs:** ↑ LFTs, BUN, SCr; ↓ serum K+

Miconazole (Monistat, others) **Uses:** *Candidal infections, dermatomycoses (various tinea forms)* **Action:** Fungicide; alters permeability of the fungal cell membrane **Dose:** Apply to area bid for 2–4 wk. *Intravaginally:* 1 applicatorful or supp hs for 3 (4% or 200 mg) or 7 d (2% or 100 mg) **Caution:** [C, ?] Azole sensitivity **Supplied:** Topical cream 2%; lotion 2%; powder 2%; spray 2%; vaginal supp 100, 200 mg; vaginal cream 2%, 4% [OTC] **SE:** Vaginal burning, may potentiate warfarin **Interactions:** Antagonistic to amphotericin B in vivo **Interactions:** ↑ Effects of anticoagulants, cisapride, loratadine, phenytoin, quinidine; ↓ effects w/ amphotericin B; ↓ effects of amphotericin B **Labs:** ↑ Protein

Midazolam (Versed) [C-IV] **Uses:** *Preoperative sedation, conscious sedation for short procedures and mechanically ventilated Pts, induction of general anesthesia* **Action:** Short-acting benzodiazepine **Dose:** *Adults.* 1–5 mg IV or IM; titrate to effect. *Peds.* Preop: 0.25–1 mg/kg, 20 mg max PO. *Conscious sedation:* 0.08 mg/kg IM × 1. *General anesthesia:* 0.15 mg/kg IV, then 0.05 mg/kg/dose q2min for 1–3 doses PRN to induce anesthesia (↓ in eldcrly, w/ use of narcotics or CNS depressants) **Caution:** [D, +/–] CYP3A4 substrate, several drug interactions **Contra:** Narrow-angle glaucoma; use of amprenavir, nelfinavir, ritonavir **Supplied:** Inj 1, 5 mg/mL; syrup 2 mg/mL **SE:** Monitor for resp depression; hypotension in conscious sedation, nausea **Notes:** Reversal w/ flumazenil **Interactions:** ↑ Effects w/ azole antifungals, antihistamines, cimetidine, CCBs, CNS depressants, erythromycin, INH, phenytoin, protease inhibitors, grapefruit juice, EtOH; ↓ effects w/ rifampin, tobacco; ↓ effects of levodopa

Mifepristone [RU 486] (Mifeprex) **WARNING:** Pt counseling and information required **Uses:** *Termination of intrauterine pregnancies of <49 d* **Action:** Antiprogestin; ↑ prostaglandins, resulting in uterine contraction **Dose:** Administered w/ 3 office visits: day 1, three 200-mg tablets PO; day 3 if no abortion, two 200-mg misoprostol PO; on or about day 14, verify termination of PRG **Caution:** [X, –] **Contra:** Anticoagulation therapy, bleeding disorders **Supplied:** Tabs 200 mg **SE:** Abdominal pain and 1–2 wk of uterine bleeding **Notes:** Must be administered under physician's supervision **Interactions:** ↑ Effects w/ azole antifungals, erythromycin, grapefruit juice; ↓ effects w/ carbamazepine, dexamethasone, phenytoin, phenobarbital, rifampin, St. John's wort

Miglitol (Glyset) Uses: *Type 2 DM* Action: α-Glucosidase inhibitor; delays digestion of ingested carbohydrates Dose: Initial 25 mg PO tid; maint 50–100 mg tid (w/ 1st bite of each meal) Caution: [B, –] Contra: Obstructive or inflammatory GI disorders; ⊘ if SCr >2 Supplied: Tabs 25, 50, 100 mg SE: Used alone or in combination w/ sulfonylureas; flatulence, diarrhea, abdominal pain Interactions: ↑ Effects w/ celery, coriander, juniper berries, ginseng, garlic; ↓ effects w/ INH, niacin; ↓ effects of digoxin, propranolol, ranitidine

Milrinone (Primacor) Uses: *CHF* Action: + Inotrope and vasodilator; little chronotropic activity Dose: 50 μg/kg, then 0.375–0.75 μg/kg/min inf; ↓ dose in renal impairment Caution: [C, ?] Contra: Hypersensitivity to drug or amrinone Supplied: Inj 1 mg/mL SE: Arrhythmias, hypotension, HA Notes: Carefully monitor fluid/electrolyte status and BP/HR Interactions: ↑ Hypotension w/ disopyramide

Mineral Oil Uses: *Constipation* Action: Emollient laxative Dose: *Adults.* 5–45 mL PO PRN. *Peds.* >6 y: 5–20 mL PO bid Caution: [C, ?] N/V, difficulty swallowing, bedridden Pts Contra: Appendicitis, diverticulitis, ulcerative colitis Supplied: Liq [OTC] SE: Lipid pneumonia, anal incontinence, ↓ vitamin absorption Interactions: ↑ Effects w/ stool softeners; ↓ effects of cardiac glycosides, oral contraceptives, sulfonamides, warfarin

Minoxidil (Loniten, Rogaine) Uses: *Severe HTN; male and female pattern baldness* Action: Peripheral vasodilator; stimulates vertex hair growth Dose: *Adults.* PO: 2.5–10 mg PO bid–qid *Topical:* Apply bid to affected area. *Peds.* 0.2–1 mg/kg/24 h ÷ PO q12–24h; ↓ PO dose in elderly Caution: [C, +] Contra: Pheochromocytoma, hypersensitivity to components Supplied: Tabs 2.5, 5, 10 mg; topical soln (Rogaine) 2% SE: Pericardial effusion and volume overload may occur w/ PO use; hypertrichosis after chronic use; edema, ECG changes, weight gain Interactions: ↑ Hypotension w/ guanethidine Labs: ↑ Alkaline phosphatase, BUN, creatinine; ↓ Hmg, Hct

Mirtazapine (Remeron) WARNING: Closely monitor for worsening depression or emergence of suicidality, particularly in pediatric Pts Uses: *Depression* Action: Tetracyclic antidepressant Dose: 15 mg PO hs, up to 45 mg/d hs Caution: [C, ?] Contra: MAOIs w/in 14 d Supplied: Tabs 15, 30, 45 mg SE: Somnolence, ↑ cholesterol, constipation, xerostomia, weight gain, agranulocytosis Notes: ⊘ ↑ Dose at intervals of less than 1–2 wk Interactions: ↑ Effects w/ CNS depressants, fluvoxamine; ↑ risk of HTN crisis w/ MAOIs Labs: ↑ ALT, cholesterol, triglycerides

Misoprostol (Cytotec) Uses: *Prevention of NSAID-induced gastric ulcers*; induction of labor, incomplete and therapeutic abortion Action: Prostaglandin w/ both antisecretory and mucosal protective properties Dose: *Ulcer prevention:* 200 μg PO qid w/ meals; in females, start on 2nd or 3rd day of next normal menstrual period; 25–50 μg for induction of labor (term); 400 μg on day 3 of mifepristone for PRG termination (take w/ food) Caution: [X, –] Contra: PRG, component hypersensitivity **Supplied:** Tabs 100, 200 µg **SE:** Can cause miscarriage w/ potentially dangerous bleeding; HA, GI Sxs common (diarrhea, abdominal pain, constipation) **Interactions:** ↑ HA & GI symptoms w/ phenylbutazone

Mitomycin (Mutamycin) **Uses:** *Stomach, pancreas,* breast, colon CA; squamous cell carcinoma of the anus; non-small-cell lung, head, and neck, cervical, and breast CA; bladder CA (intravesically) **Action:** Alkylating agent; may also generate oxygen free radicals, induces DNA strand breaks **Dose:** 20 mg/m² q6–8wk or 10 mg/m² in combination w/ other myelosuppressive drugs; bladder CA 20–40 mg in 40 mL NS via a urethral catheter once/wk for 8 wk, followed by monthly Rxs for 1 y; ↓ dose in renal/hepatic impairment **Caution:** [D, –] **Contra:** Thrombocytopenia, leukopenia, coagulation disorders, SCr > 1.7 mg/dL **Supplied:** Inj **SE:** Myelosuppression (may persist up to 3–8 wk after dose and may be cumulative minimized by a lifetime dose <50–60 mg/m²), N/V, anorexia, stomatitis, and renal toxicity; microangiopathic hemolytic anemia (similar to hemolytic–uremic syndrome) w/ progressive renal failure; venoocclusive Dz of the liver, interstitial pneumonia, alopecia (rare); extravasation Rxns can be severe **Interactions:** ↑ Bronchospasm w/ vinca alkaloids; ↑ bone marrow suppression w/ antineoplastics

Mitotane (Lysodren) **Uses:** *Palliative Rx of inoperable adrenocortical carcinoma* **Action:** Unclear; induces mitochondrial injury in adrenocortical cells **Dose:** 8–10 g/d in 3–4 ÷ doses (begin at 2 g/d w/ glucocorticoid replacement); ↓ in hepatic insufficiency; adequate hydration necessary **Caution:** [C, ?] **Supplied:** Tabs 500 mg **SE:** Anorexia, N/V/D; acute adrenal insufficiency may be precipitated by physical stresses (shock, trauma, infection), Rx w/ steroids; allergic Rxns (rare), visual disturbances, hemorrhagic cystitis, albuminuria, hematuria, HTN or hypotension, minor aches, fever **Interactions:** ↑ Effects of CNS depressants, EtOH; ↓ effects of corticosteroids, phenytoin, phenobarbital, warfarin **Labs:** ↓ Protein-bound I **NIPE:** Full effects may take 2–3 mo

Mitoxantrone (Novantrone) **Uses:** *AML (w/ cytarabine), ALL, CML, CAP, MS,* breast CA, and NHL **Action:** DNA-intercalating agent; inhibitor of DNA topoisomerase II **Dose:** Per specific protocols; ↓ dose in hepatic failure, leukopenia, thrombocytopenia; maintain hydration **Caution:** [D, –] **Contra:** PRG **Supplied:** Inj 2 mg/mL **SE:** Myelosuppression, N/V, stomatitis, alopecia (infrequent), cardiotoxicity, urine discoloration **Interactions:** ↑ Bone marrow suppression w/ antineoplastics; ↓ effects of live virus vaccines **Labs:** ↑ AST, ALT, uric acid **NIPE:** ↑ fluids to 2–3 L/d, ⊘ vaccines, infection

Modafinil (Provigil) **Uses:** *Improve wakefulness in Pts w/ excessive daytime sleepiness associated w/ narcolepsy* **Action:** Possible mechanisms include altered dopamine and norepinephrine release, ↓ GABA-mediated neurotransmission **Dose:** 200 mg PO q AM **Caution:** [C, ?/–] ↑ effects of warfarin, diazepam, phenytoin; ↓ effects of oral contraceptives, cyclosporine, theophylline **Contra:** Component hypersensitivity **Supplied:** Tablets 100 mg, 200 mg **SE:** HA, N, D, paresthesias, rhinitis, agitation **Notes:** Consider lower doses in elderly Pts, reduce dose by 50% in Pts w/ hepatic impairment; use w/ caution in Pts w/ CV Dz **Interactions:** ↑ Effects of CNS stimulants, diazepam, phenytoin, propranolol, TCAs, warfarin; ↓ effect of cyclosporine, oral contraceptives, theophylline **NIPE:** Take w/o regard to food, monitor BP, use barrier contraception

Moexipril (Univasc) Uses: *HTN, post-MI,* DN Action: ACEI Dose:
7.5–30 mg in 1–2 ÷ doses 1 h ac Caution: [C (1st tri, D 2nd and 3rd tri), ?] Contra: ACEI sensitivity Supplied: Tabs 7.5, 15 mg; ↓ dose in renal impairment SE: Hypotension, edema, angioedema, HA, dizziness, cough Interactions: ↑ Effects with diuretics, antihypertensives, EtOH, probenecid, garlic; ↑ effects of insulin, Li; ↑ risk of hyperkalemia with K suppl, K-sparing diuretics; ↓ effects with antacids, ASA, NSAIDS, ephedra, yohimbe, ginseng Labs: ↑ BUN, creatinine, K⁺, ALT, AST, serum alkaline phosphatase; ↓ serum cholesterol; false + test for urine acetone NIPE: May alter sense of taste, may cause cough, ⊘ salt substitutes, ⊘ PRG, use barrier contraception.

Molindone (Moban) Uses: *Psychotic disorders* Action: Piperazine phenothiazine Dose: Adults. 50–75 mg/d, ↑ to 225 mg/d if necessary. Peds 3–5 y: 1–2.5 mg/d in 4 ÷ doses. 5–12 y: 0.5–1.0 mg/kg/d in 4 ÷ doses Caution: [C, ?] Narrow-angle glaucoma Contra: Drug or EtOH-induced CNS depression Supplied: Tabs 5, 10, 25, 50, 100 mg; conc 20 mg/mL SE: Hypotension, tachycardia, arrhythmias, EPS, Szs, constipation, xerostomia, blurred vision Interactions: ↑ Effects w/ antihypertensives; ↑ hyperkalemia w/ K-sparing diuretics, K suppls, salt substitutes, trimethoprim; ↑ effects of insulin, Li; ↓ effects w/ ASA, NSAIDs Labs: ↑ Serum K⁺, BUN, creatinine NIPE: Take w/o food, monitor for persistent cough

Montelukast (Singulair) Uses: *Prophylaxis and Rx of chronic asthma,
seasonal allergic rhinitis* Action: Leukotriene receptor antagonist Dose: Asthma: Adults & Peds. >15y: 10 mg/d PO taken in PM. Peds. 2–5 y: 4 mg/d PO taken in PM. 6–14 y: 5 mg/d PO in PM. Rhinitis: Adults & Peds. >15y: 10 mg qd Peds: 2–5 y: 4 mg qd. 6–14 y: 5 mg qd Caution: [B, M] Contra: Component hypersensitivity Supplied: Tabs 10 mg; chew tabs 4, 5 mg SE: HA, dizziness, fatigue, rash, GI upset, Churg–Strauss syndrome Notes: Not for acute asthma attacks Interactions: ↑ ↓ Effects w/ phenobarbital, rifampin Labs: ↑ AST, ALT

Morphine (Avinza XR, Duramorph, MS Contin, Kadian SR,
Oramorph SR, Roxanol) [C-II] Uses: *Relief of severe pain* Action: Narcotic analgesic Dose: Adults. PO: 5–30 mg q4h PRN; SR tabs 30–60 mg q8–12h (⊘ chew/crush). IV/IM: 2.5–15 mg q2–6h; supp 10–30 mg q4h. Peds.0.1–0.2 mg/kg/dose IM/IV q2–4h PRN to a max of 15 mg/dose Caution: [B (D if prolonged use or high doses at term), +/–] Contra: Severe asthma, resp depression, GI obstruction Supplied: Immediate-release tabs 10, 14, 20 mg; MS Contin CR tabs 15, 30, 60, 100, 200 mg; Oramorph SR CR tabs 15, 30, 60, 100 mg; Kadian SR caps 20, 30 50, 60, 100 mg; Avinza XR caps 30, 60, 90, 120 mg; soln 10, 20, 100 mg; supp 5, 10, 20 mg; inj 2, 4, 5, 8, 10, 15 mg/mL; Duramorph

preservative-free inj 0.5, 1 mg/mL; suppository 5, 10, 20, 30 mg **SE:** Narcotic SE (resp depression, sedation, constipation, N/V, pruritus) **Notes:** May require scheduled dosing to relieve severe chronic pain; MS Contin commonly used SR form (⊘ crush) **Interactions:** ↑ Effects w/ cimetidine, CNS depressants, dextroamphetamine, TCAs, EtOH, kava kava, valerian, St. John's wort; ↑ effects of warfarin; ↑ risk of HTN crisis w/ MAOIs; ↓ effects w/ opioids, phenothiazines **Labs:** ↑ Serum amylase, lipase

Moxifloxacin (Avelox)

Uses: *Acute sinusitis, acute bronchitis, skin/soft tissue infections, conjunctivitis, and community-acquired pneumonia* **Action:** Quinolone; inhibits DNA gyrase. *Spectrum:* Excellent gram(+) coverage except MRSA and *E. faecium;* good gram(–) coverage except *P. aeruginosa, S. maltophilia,* and *Acinetobacter* sp; good anaerobic coverage **Dose:** 400 mg/d PO (⊘ cation products, antacids) /IV qd. *Ophth:* 1 gt tid ×7d **Caution:** [C, ?/–] Quinolone sensitivity; interactions w/ Mg–, Ca–, Al–, and Fe-containing products and class IA and III antiarrhythmic agents **Contra:** Quinolone or component sensitivity **Supplied:** Tabs 400 mg, inj, ophth 0.5% **SE:** Dizziness, nausea, QT prolongation, Szs, photosensitivity, tendon rupture **Notes:** Take 4 h before or 8 h after antacids **Interactions:** ↑ Effects w/ probenecid; ↑ effects of diazepam, theophylline, caffeine, metoprolol, propranolol, phenytoin, warfarin; ↓ effects w/ antacids, didanosine, Fe salts, Mg, sucralfate, NaHCO₃, zinc **Labs:** ↑ LFTs, BUN, SCr, amylase, PT, triglycerides, cholesterol; ↓ Hmg, Hct **NIPE:** ⊘ Give to children <18 y; ↑ fluids to 2–3 L/d

Mupirocin (Bactroban)

Uses: *Impetigo; eradication of MRSA in nasal carriers* **Action:** Inhibits bacterial protein synthesis **Dose:** *Topical:* Apply small amount to affected area. *Nasal:* Apply bid in nostrils **Caution:** [B, ?] **Contra:** ⊘ Use concurrently w/ other nasal products **Supplied:** Oint 2%; cream 2% **SE:** Local irritation, rash **Interactions:** ↓ Bacterial action w/ chloramphenicol **NIPE:** ⊘ Use w/ other nasal drugs

Muromonab-CD3 (Orthoclone OKT3)

WARNING: Can cause anaphylaxis; monitor fluid status **Uses:** *Acute rejection following organ transplantation* **Action:** Blocks T-cell Fxn **Dose:** *Adults.* 5 mg/d IV for 10–14 d. *Peds.* 0.1 mg/kg/d for 10–14 d **Caution:** [C, ?/–] Murine sensitivity, fluid overload **Contra:** HF/fluid overload, Hx of Szs, PRG, uncontrolled HTN **Supplied:** Inj 5 mg/5 mL **SE:** Murine antibody; fever and chills after the 1st dose (premedicate w/ steroid/APAP/antihistamine); monitor closely for anaphylaxis or pulmonary edema **Notes:** Use 0.22- micron filter for administration **Interactions:** ↑ Effects w/ immunosuppressives; ↑ effects of live virus vaccines; ↑ risk of CNS effects & encephalopathy w/ indomethacin **Labs:** ↑ AST, ALT **NIPE:** ⊘ Immunizations, exposure to infection

Mycophenolate Mofetil (CellCept)

WARNING: ↑ Risk of infections, possible development of lymphoma **Uses:** *Prevent organ rejection after transplant* **Action:** Inhibits immunologically mediated inflammatory responses **Dose:** *Adults.*

1 g PO bid; **Peds.** BSA 1.2–1.5 m^2: 750 mg PO bid; *BSA >1.5 m^2*: 1 g PO bid; may taper up to 600 mg/m^2 PO bid; used w/ steroids and cyclosporine; ↓ in renal insufficiency or neutropenia. *IV:* Infuse over at least 2 hr. *PO:* Take on empty stomach, ⊘ open capsules **Caution:** [C, ?/–] **Contra:** Component hypersensitivity; IV use in polysorbate 80 allergy **Supplied:** Caps 250, 500 mg; inj 500 mg **SE:** N/V/D, pain, fever, HA, infection, HTN, anemia, leukopenia, edema **Interactions:** ↑ Effects w/ acyclovir, ganciclovir, probenecid; ↑ effects of acyclovir, ganciclovir; ↓ effects w/ antacids, cholestyramine, cyclosporine, Fe, food; ↓ effects of oral contraceptives, phenytoin, theophylline **Labs:** ↑ LFTs **NIPE:** Use barrier contraception during and 6 wk after drug therapy, ⊘ exposure to infection; take w/o food

Nabumetone (Relafen)
Uses: *Arthritis and pain* **Action:** NSAID; inhibits prostaglandins **Dose:** 1000–2000 mg/d ÷ qd–bid w/ food **Caution:** [C (D 3rd tri), +] **Contra:** Peptic ulcer, NSAID sensitivity, severe hepatic Dz **Supplied:** Tabs 500, 750 mg **SE:** Dizziness, rash, GI upset, edema, peptic ulcer **Interactions:** ↑ Effects w/ aminoglycosides; ↑ effects of anticoagulants, hypoglycemics, Li, MRX, thrombolytics; ↑ GI effects w/ ASA, corticosteroids, K suppls, NSAIDs, EtOH; ↓ effects of antihypertensives, diuretics **Labs:** ↑ LFTs, BUN, SCr; ↓ serum glucose, Hmg, Hct, plts **NIPE:** Photosensitivity—use sunscreen

Nadolol (Corgard)
Uses: *HTN and angina* **Action:** Competitively blocks β-adrenergic receptors, β$_1$, β$_2$ **Dose:** 40–80 mg/d; ↑ to 240 mg/d (angina) or 320 mg/d (HTN) may be needed; ↓ in renal insufficiency and elderly **Caution:** [C (1st tri; D if 2nd or 3rd tri), +] **Contra:** Uncompensated CHF, shock, heart block, asthma **Supplied:** Tabs 20, 40, 80, 120, 160 mg **SE:** Nightmares, paresthesias, hypotension, bradycardia, fatigue **Interactions:** ↑ Effects w/ antihypertensives, diuretics, nitrates, EtOH; ↑ effects of aminophylline, lidocaine; ↑ risk of HTN w/ clonidine, ephedrine, epinephrine, MAOIs, phenylephrine, pseudoephedrine; ↑ bradycardia w/ digitalis glycosides, ephedrine, epinephrine, phenylephrine, pseudoephedrine; ↓ effects w/ ampicillin, antacids, clonidine, NSAIDs, thyroid meds; ↓ effects of glucagon, theophylline **Labs:** ↑ K$^+$, cholesterol, triglycerides, BUN, uric acid **NIPE:** May ↑ cold sensitivity; ⊘ DC abruptly

Nafcillin (Nallpen)
Uses: *Infections caused by susceptible strains of Staphylococcus and Streptococcus* **Action:** Bactericidal; inhibits cell wall synthesis. *Spectrum:* Good gram(+) **Dose:** *Adults.* 1–2 g IV q4–6h. *Peds.* 50–200 mg/kg/d ÷ q4–6h **Caution:** [B, ?] Penicillin allergy **Supplied:** Inj **SE:** Interstitial nephritis, diarrhea, fever, nausea **Notes:** No adjustments for renal Fxn **Interactions:** ↑ Effects of MRX; ↓ effects w/ chloramphenicol, macrolides, tetracyclines; ↓ effects of cyclosporine, oral contraceptives, tacrolimus, warfarin **Labs:** ↑ Serum protein **NIPE:** Aminoglycosides not compatible, risk of drug inactivation w/ fruit juice/carbonated drinks; monitor for superinfection

Naftifine (Naftin)
Uses: *Tinea pedis, cruris, and corporis* **Action:** Antifungal antibiotic **Dose:** Apply bid **Caution:** [B, ?] **Contra:** Component sensitivity **Supplied:** 1% cream; gel **SE:** Local irritation

Nalbuphine (Nubain) **Uses:** *Moderate to severe pain; preop and obstetrical analgesia* **Action:** Narcotic agonist–antagonist; inhibits ascending pain pathways **Dose:** *Adults.* 10–20 mg IM or IV q4–6h PRN; max of 160 mg/d; single max dose, 20 mg. **Peds.** 0.2 mg/kg IV or IM to a max dose of 20 mg; ↓ in hepatic insufficiency **Caution:** [B (D if prolonged or high doses at term), ?] **Contra:** Sulfite sensitivity **Supplied:** Inj 10, 20 mg/mL **SE:** Causes CNS depression and drowsiness; caution in Pts receiving opiates **Interactions:** ↑ CNS depression w/ cimetidine, CNS depressants; EtOH ↑ effects of digitoxin, phenytoin, rifampin **Labs:** ↑ Serum amylase, lipase

Naloxone (Narcan) **Uses:** *Opioid addiction (diagnosis) and OD* **Action:** Competitive narcotic antagonist **Dose:** *Adults.* 0.4–2.0 mg IV, IM, or SQ q5min; max total dose, 10 mg. **Peds.** 0.01–1 mg/kg/dose IV, IM, or SQ; repeat IV q3min × 3 doses PRN **Caution:** [B, ?] May precipitate acute withdrawal in addicts **Supplied:** Inj 0.4, 1.0 mg/mL; neonatal inj 0.02 mg/mL **SE:** Hypotension, tachycardia, irritability, GI upset, pulmonary edema **Notes:** If no response after 10 mg, suspect nonnarcotic cause **Interactions:** ↓ Effects of opioids

Naltrexone (ReVia) **Uses:** *EtOH and narcotic addiction* **Action:** Competitively binds to opioid receptors **Dose:** 50 mg/d PO; ○ give until opioid-free for 7–10 d **Caution:** [C, M] **Contra:** Acute hepatitis, liver failure; opioid use **Supplied:** Tabs 50 mg **SE:** May cause hepatotoxicity; insomnia, GI upset, joint pain, HA, fatigue **Interactions:** ↑ Lethargy & somnolence w/ thioridazine; ↓ effects of opioids

Naphazoline and Antazoline (Albalon-A Ophthalmic, others), Naphazoline and Pheniramine Acetate (Naphcon A) **Uses:** *Relieve ocular redness and itching caused by allergy* **Action:** Vasoconstrictor and antihistamine **Dose:** 1–2 gtt up to 4×/d **Caution:** [C, +] **Contra:** Glaucoma, children <6 y, and w/ contact lenses **Supplied:** Soln 15 mL **SE:** CV stimulation, dizziness, local irritation **Interactions:** ↑ Risk of HTN crisis w/ MAOIs, TCAs

Naproxen (Aleve, Naprosyn, Anaprox) **Uses:** *Arthritis and pain* **Action:** NSAID; inhibits prostaglandins **Dose:** *Adults & Peds.* >12 y: 200–500 mg bid–tid to a max of 1500 mg/d; ↓ dose in hepatic impairment **Caution:** [B (D 3rd tri), +] **Contra:** NSAID sensitivity, peptic ulcer **Supplied:** Tabs 200, 250, 375, 500 mg; delayed-release (EC) tabs 375, 500 mg; susp 125 mg/5 mL **SE:** Dizziness, pruritus, GI upset, peptic ulcer, edema **Interactions:** ↑ Effects w/ aminoglycosides; ↑ effects of anticoagulants, hypoglycemics, Li, MRX, thrombolytics; ↑ GI effects w/ ASA, corticosteroids, K suppls, NSAIDs, EtOH; ↓ effects of antihypertensives, diuretics **Labs:** ↑ Urine 5-HIAA **NIPE:** Take w/ food

Naratriptan (Amerge) **Uses:** *Acute migraine attacks* **Action:** Serotonin 5-HT₁ receptor antagonist **Dose:** 1–2.5 mg PO once; repeat PRN in 4 h; ↓ dose in mild renal/hepatic insufficiency, take w/ fluids **Caution:** [C, M] **Contra:** Severe renal/hepatic impairment, ○ in angina, ischemic heart Dz, uncontrolled

HTN, cerebrovascular syndromes, and ergot use **Supplied:** Tabs 1, 2.5 mg **SE:** Dizziness, sedation, GI upset, paresthesias, ECG changes, coronary vasospasm, arrhythmias **Interactions:** ↑ Effects w/ MAOIs, SSRIs; ↑ effects of ergot drugs; ↓ effects w/ nicotine

Nateglinide (Starlix) **Uses:** * Type 2 DM* **Action:** ↑ pancreatic release of insulin **Dose:** 120 mg PO tid 1–30 min pc; ↓ to 60 mg tid if near target HbA$_{1c}$. (take 1 – 30 min ac) **Caution:** [C, –]. Caution w/ drugs metabolized by CYP2C9/3A4 **Contra:** Diabetic ketoacidosis, type 1 DM **Supplied:** Tabs 60, 120 mg **SE:** Hypoglycemia, URI; salicylates, nonselective BBs may enhance hypoglycemia **Interactions:** ↑ Effects w/ nonselective BBs, MAOIs, NSAIDs, salicylates, ↓ effects w/ corticosteroids, niacin, sympathomimetics, thiazide diuretics, thyroid meds **Labs:** ↑ Uric acid

Nedocromil (Tilade) **Uses:** *Mild–moderate asthma* **Action:** Antiinflammatory agent **Dose:** *Inhal:* 2 inhal 4×/d **Caution:** [B, ?/–] **Contra:** Component hypersensitivity **Supplied:** Met-dose inhaler **SE:** Chest pain, dizziness, dysphonia, rash, GI upset, infection **Notes:** Not for acute asthma attacks **NIPE:** May take 2–4 wk for full therapeutic effect

Nefazodone (Serzone) **WARNING:** Fatal hepatitis and liver failure possible, DC if LFT >3× ULN, ⊘ re-treat; closely monitor for worsening depression or emergence of suicidality, particularly in pediatric Pts **Uses:** *Depression* **Action:** Inhibits neuronal uptake of serotonin and norepinephrine **Dose:** Initially 100 mg PO bid; usual 300–600 mg/d in 2 ÷ doses **Caution:** [C, ?] **Contra:** MAOIs, pimozide, cisapride, carbamazepine **Supplied:** Tabs 100, 150, 200, 250 mg **SE:** Postural hypotension and allergic Rxns; HA, drowsiness, xerostomia, constipation, GI upset, liver failure **Notes:** Monitor LFTs, HR/BP **Interactions:** ↑ Effects w/ benzodiazepines, buspirone; ↑ effects of alprazolam, buspirone, carbamazepine, cyclosporine, digoxin, triazolam; ↑ risk of QT prolongation w/ astemizole, cisapride, pimozide; ↑ risk of serious and/or fatal Rxn w/ MAOIs; ↓ effects of propranolol **Labs:** ↑ LFTs, cholesterol; ↓ Hct **NIPE:** Take w/o food; may take 2–4 wk for full therapeutic effects

Nelfinavir (Viracept) **Uses:** *HIV infection* **Action:** Protease inhibitor; results in formation of immature, noninfectious virion **Dose:** *Adults.* 750 mg PO tid or 1250 mg PO bid. *Peds.* 20–30 mg/kg PO tid; take w/ food **Caution:** [B, ?] Many significant drug interactions **Contra:** Phenylketonuria, triazolam/midazolam use or any other drug highly dependent on CYP3A4 **Supplied:** Tabs 250 mg; PO powder **SE:** Food ↑ absorption; interacts w/ St. John's wort; dyslipidemia, lipodystrophy, diarrhea, rash **Interactions:** ↑ Effects w/ erythromycin, ketoconazole, indinavir, ritonavir; ↑ effects of barbiturates, carbamazepine, cisapride, ergot alkaloids, erythromycin, lovastatin, midazolam, phenytoin, saquinavir, simvastatin, triazolam; ↓ effects w/ barbiturates, carbamazepine, phenytoin, rifabutin, rifampin; ↓ effects of oral contraceptives **Labs:** ↑ LFTs **NIPE:** Take w/ food; use barrier contraception

Neomycin, Bacitracin, & Polymyxin B (Neosporin Ointment) (See Bacitracin, Neomycin, and Polymyxin B Topical)

Neomycin, Colistin, and Hydrocortisone (Cortisporin-TC Otic Drops); Neomycin, Colistin, Hydrocortisone, & Thonzonium (Cortisporin-TC Otic Suspension) Uses: *External otitis,* infections of mastoid/fenestration cavities **Action:** Antibiotic w/antiinflammatory **Dose:** *Adults.* 4–5 gtt in ear(s) tid–qid. *Peds.* 3–4 gtt in ear(s) tid–qid **Caution:** [C, ?] **Supplied:** Otic gtt and susp **SE:** Local irritation

Neomycin & Dexamethasone (AK-Neo-Dex Ophthalmic, NeoDecadron Ophthalmic) Uses: *Steroid-responsive inflammatory conditions of the cornea, conjunctiva, lid, and anterior segment* **Action:** Antibiotic w/ antiinflammatory corticosteroid **Dose:** 1–2 gtt in eye(s) q3–4h or thin coat tid–qid until response, then ↓ to qd **Caution:** [C, ?] **Supplied:** Cream neomycin 0.5%/dexamethasone 0.1%; oint neomycin 0.35%/dexamethasone 0.05%; soln neomycin 0.35%/dexamethasone 0.1% **SE:** local irritation **Notes:** Use under supervision of ophthalmologist

Neomycin & Polymyxin B (Neosporin Cream) [OTC] Uses: *Infection in minor cuts, scrapes, and burns* **Action:** Bactericidal **Dose:** Apply bid–qid **Caution:** [C, ?] **Contra:** component hypersensitivity **Supplied:** Cream neomycin 3.5 mg/polymyxin B 10,000 Units/g **SE:** Local irritation **Notes:** Different from Neosporin oint

Neomycin, Polymyxin B, & Dexamethasone (Maxitrol) Uses: *Steroid-responsive ocular conditions w/ bacterial infection* **Action:** Antibiotic w/ antiinflammatory corticosteroid **Dose:** 1–2 gtt in eye(s) q4–6h; apply oint in eye(s) 3–4×/d **Caution:** [C, ?] **Supplied:** Oint neomycin sulfate 3.5 mg/polymyxin B sulfate 10,000 Units/dexamethasone 0.1%/g; susp identical/5 mL **SE:** Local irritation **Notes:** Use under supervision of ophthalmologist

Neomycin-Polymyxin Bladder Irrigant [Neosporin GU Irrigant] Uses: *Continuous irrigant for prophylaxis against bacteriuria and gram(−) bacteremia associated w/ indwelling catheter use* **Action:** Bactericide **Dose:** 1 mL irrigant in 1 L of 0.9% NaCl; cont bladder irrigation w/ 1 L of soln/24 h **Caution:** [D] **Contra:** Component hypersensitivity **Supplied:** Soln neomycin sulfate 40 mg and polymyxin B 200,000 Units/mL; amp 1, 20 mL **SE:** Neomycin-induced ototoxicity or nephrotoxicity (rare) **Notes:** Potential for bacterial or fungal superinfection; not for inj

Neomycin, Polymyxin, & Hydrocortisone (Cortisporin Ophthalmic and Otic) Uses: *Ocular and otic bacterial infections* **Action:** Antibiotic and antiinflammatory **Dose:** *Otic:* 3–4 gtt in the ear(s) 3–4×/d. *Ophth:* Apply a thin layer to the eye(s) or 1 gt 1–4×/d **Caution:** [C, ?] **Supplied:** Otic susp; ophth soln; ophth oint **SE:** Local irritation

Neomycin, Polymyxin B, & Prednisolone (Poly-Pred Ophthalmic) Uses: *Steroid-responsive ocular conditions w/ bacterial infection*

Action: Antibiotic and antiinflammatory **Dose:** 1–2 gtt in eye(s) q4–6h; apply oint in eye(s) 3–4×/d **Caution:** [C, ?] **Supplied:** Susp neomycin 0.35%/polymyxin B 10,000 Units/prednisolone 0.5%/mL **SE:** Irritation **Notes:** Use under supervision of ophthalmologist

Neomycin Sulfate (Myciguent) [OTC] **Uses:** *Hepatic coma and pre-operative bowel prep* **Action:** Aminoglycoside, poorly absorbed PO; suppresses GI bacterial flora **Dose:** **Adults.** 3–12 g/24 h PO in 3–4 ÷ doses. **Peds.** 50–100 mg/kg/24 h PO in 3–4 ÷ doses **Caution:** [C, ?/–] Renal failure, neuromuscular disorders, hearing impairment **Contra:** Intestinal obstruction **Supplied:** Tabs 500 mg; PO soln 125 mg/5 mL **SE:** Hearing loss w/ long-term use; rash, N/V **Notes:** ⊘ use parenterally due to ↑ toxicity; part of the Condon bowel prep

Nesiritide (Natrecor) **Uses:** *Acutely decompensated CHF* **Action:** Human B-type natriuretic peptide **Dose:** 2 µg/kg IV bolus, then 0.01 µg/kg/min IV **Caution:** [C, ?/–] In Pts whom vasodilators are not appropriate **Contra:** SBP <90, cardiogenic shock **Supplied:** Vials 1.5 mg **SE:** Hypotension, HA, GI upset, arrhythmias, ↑ Cr **Notes:** Requires continuous BP monitoring **Interactions:** ↑ Hypotension w/ ACEIs, nitrates **Labs:** ↑ Creatinine

Nevirapine (Viramune) **WARNING:** Reports of fatal hepatotoxicity even after short-term use; severe life-threatening skin Rxns (Stevens–Johnson, toxic epidermal necrolysis, and hypersensitivity Rxns); monitor closely during 1st 8 wk of Rx **Uses:** *HIV infection* **Action:** Nonnucleoside RT inhibitor **Dose:** **Adults.** Initial 200 mg/d × 14 d, then 200 mg bid. **Peds.** <8 y: 4 mg/kg/d × 14 d, then 7 mg/kg bid. >8 y: 4 mg/kg/d × 14 d, then 4 mg/kg bid **Caution:** [C, +/–] OCP **Supplied:** Tabs 200 mg; susp 50 mg/5 mL **SE:** Life-threatening rash, HA, fever, diarrhea, neutropenia, hepatitis **Notes:** Give w/out regard to food **Interactions:** ↑ Effects w/ clarithromycin, erythromycin; ↓ effects w/ rifabutin, rifampin, St. John's wort; ↓ effects of clarithromycin, indinavir, ketoconazole, methadone, oral contraceptives, protease inhibitors, warfarin **NIPE:** Use barrier contraception

Niacin (Niaspan) **Uses:** *Adjunctive in significant hyperlipidemia* **Action:** Inhibits lipolysis; ↓ esterification of triglycerides; ↑ lipoprotein lipase activity **Dose:** 1–6 g ÷ doses/d; 9 g/d max **Caution:** [A (C if doses >RDA), +] **Contra:** Liver Dz, peptic ulcer, arterial hemorrhage **Supplied:** SR caps 125, 250, 300, 400, 500 mg; tabs 25, 50, 100, 250, 500 mg; SR tabs 150, 250, 500, 750 mg; elixir 50 mg/5 mL **SE:** Upper body and facial flushing and warmth following dose; may cause GI upset; HA, flatulence, paresthesias, liver damage, may exacerbate peptic ulcer, gout, or glucose control in DM. **Notes:** Administer w/ food; flushing may be ↓ by taking an ASA or NSAID 30–60 min prior to dose **Interactions:** ↑ Effects of antihypertensives, anticoagulants; ↓ effects of hypoglycemics, probenecid, sulfinpyrazone **Labs:** False ↑ urinary catecholamines, false + urine glucose, ↑ LFTs, uric acid **NIPE:** EtOH & hot beverages ↑ flushing

Nicardipine (Cardene) **Uses:** *Chronic stable angina and HTN*; prophylaxis of migraine **Action:** CCB **Dose:** **Adults.** PO: 20–40 mg PO tid. *SR:* 30–60 mg

PO bid. *IV:* 5 mg/h IV cont inf; ↑ by 2.5 mg/h q15min to max 15 mg/h. **Peds.** PO: 20–30 mg PO q 8h. *IV:* 0.5 – 5 µg/kg/min; ↓ in renal/hepatic impairment **Caution:** [C, ?/–] Heart block, CAD **Contra:** Cardiogenic shock **Supplied:** Caps 20, 30 mg; SR caps 30, 45, 60 mg; inj 2.5 mg/mL **SE:** Flushing, tachycardia, hypotension, edema, HA **Notes:** *PO-to-IV conversion:* 20 mg tid = 0.5 mg/h, 30 mg tid = 1.2 mg/h, 40 mg tid = 2.2 mg/h; take w/ food (not high fat) **Interactions:** ↑ Effects w/ azole antifungals, cimetidine, ranitidine, grapefruit juice; ↑ effects of cyclosporine, carbamazepine, prazosin, quinidine, tacrolimus; ↑ hypotension w/ antihypertensives, fentanyl, nitrates, quinidine, EtOH; ↑ dysrhythmias w/ digoxin, disopyramide, phenytoin; ↓ effects w/ NSAIDs, rifampin **Labs:** ↑ LFTs **NIPE:** ↑ Risk of photosensitivity—use sunscreen

Nicotine Gum (Nicorette) [OTC]
Uses: *Aid to smoking cessation for the relief of nicotine withdrawal* **Action:** Systemic delivery of nicotine **Dose:** Chew 9–12 pieces/d PRN; max 30 pieces/d **Caution:** [C, ?] **Contra:** Life-threatening arrhythmias, unstable angina **Supplied:** 2 mg, 4 mg/piece; mint, orange, original flavors **SE:** Tachycardia, HA, GI upset, hiccups **Notes:** Must stop smoking and perform behavior modification for max effect **Interactions:** ↑ Effects w/ cimetidine; ↑ effects of catecholamines, cortisol; ↑ hemodynamic & A-V blocking effects of adenosine; ↓ effects w/ coffee, cola **NIPE:** Chew 30 min for full dose of nicotine; ↓ absorption w/ coffee, soda, juices, wine w/in 15 min

Nicotine Nasal Spray (Nicotrol NS)
Uses: *Aid to smoking cessation for the relief of nicotine withdrawal* **Action:** Systemic delivery of nicotine **Dose:** 0.5 mg/actuation; 1–2 sprays/h, 10 sprays/h max **Caution:** [D, M] **Contra:** Life-threatening arrhythmias, unstable angina **Supplied:** Nasal inhaler 10 mg/mL **SE:** Local irritation, tachycardia, HA, taste perversion **Notes:** Must stop smoking and perform behavior modification for max effect **Interactions:** ↑ Effects w/ cimetidine, blue cohash; ↑ effects of catecholamines, cortisol; ↑ hemodynamic & A-V blocking effects of adenosine **NIPE:** ⊘ in Pts w/ chronic nasal disorders or severe reactive airway Dz; ↑ incidence of cough

Nicotine Transdermal (Habitrol, Nicoderm CQ [OTC], Nicotrol [OTC])
Uses: *Aid to smoking cessation for the relief of nicotine withdrawal* **Action:** Systemic delivery of nicotine **Dose:** Individualized; 1 patch (14–22 mg/d), and taper over 6 wk **Caution:** [D, M] **Contra:** Life-threatening arrhythmias, unstable angina **Supplied:** Habitrol and Nicoderm CQ 7, 14, 21 mg of nicotine/24 h; Nicotrol 5, 10, 15 mg/24 h **SE:** Insomnia, pruritus, erythema, local site Rxn, tachycardia **Notes:** Nicotrol worn for 16 h to mimic smoking patterns; others worn for 24 h; must stop smoking and perform behavior modification for max effect **Interactions:** ↑ Effects w/ cimetidine, blue cohash; ↑ effects of catecholamines, cortisol; ↑ hemodynamic & A-V blocking effects of adenosine; ↑ HTN w/ bupropion **NIPE:** Change application site daily

Nifedipine (Procardia, Procardia XL, Adalat, Adalat CC)
Uses: *Vasospastic or chronic stable angina and HTN*; tocolytic **Action:** CCB

Dose: *Adults.* SR tabs 30–90 mg/d. *Tocolysis:* 10–20 mg PO q4–6h. *Peds.*0.6–0.9 mg/kg/24 h ÷ tid–qid **Caution:** [C, +] Heart block, aortic stenosis **Contra:** Immediate-release prep for urgent or emergent HTN; acute MI **Supplied:** Caps 10, 20 mg; SR tabs 30, 60, 90 mg **SE:** HA common on initial Rx; reflex tachycardia may occur w/ regular release dosage forms; peripheral edema, hypotension, flushing, dizziness **Notes:** Adalat CC and Procardia XL not interchangeable; SL administration is neither safe nor effective and should be abandoned **Interactions:** ↑ Effects w/ antihypertensives, azole antifungals, cimetidine, cisapride, CCBs, diltiazem, famotidine, nitrates, quinidine, ranitidine, EtOH, grapefruit juice; ↑ effects of digitalis glycosides, phenytoin, vincristine; ↓ effects w/ barbiturates, nafcillin, NSAIDs, phenobarbital, rifampin, St. John's wort, tobacco; ↓ effects of quinidine **Labs:** ↑ LFTs **NIPE:** Take w/o regard to food; ↑ risk of photosensitivity—use sunscreen

Nilutamide (Nilandron) **WARNING:** Interstitial pneumonitis possible; most cases in 1st 3 mo; follow CXR before Rx **Uses:** *Combination w/ surgical castration for metastatic CAP* **Action:** Nonsteroidal antiandrogen **Dose:** 300 mg/d in ÷ doses for 30 d, then 150 mg/d **Caution:** [N/A] **Contra:** Severe hepatic impairment or resp insufficiency **Supplied:** Tabs 150 mg **SE:** Hot flashes, loss of libido, impotence, N/V/D, gynecomastia, hepatic dysfunction (follow LFTs), interstitial pneumonitis **Notes:** May cause a severe Rxn when taken w/ EtOH **Interactions:** ↑ Effects of phenytoin, theophylline, warfarin **Labs:** ↑ LFTs **NIPE:** Take w/o regard to food; visual adaptation may be delayed

Nimodipine (Nimotop) **Uses:** *Prevent vasospasm following subarachnoid hemorrhage* **Action:** CCB **Dose:** 60 mg PO q4h for 21 d; ↓ dose in hepatic failure **Caution:** [C, ?] **Contra:** Component hypersensitivity **Supplied:** Caps 30 mg **SE:** Hypotension, HA, constipation **Notes:** Caps may be administered via NG tube if caps cannot be swallowed whole **Interactions:** ↑ Effects w/ antihypertensives, cimetidine, nitrates, omeprazole, protease inhibitors, quinidine, valproic acid, EtOH, grapefruit juice; ↑ effects of phenytoin **Labs:** ↑ LFTs **NIPE:** ↑ Risk of photosensitivity—use sunscreen

Nisoldipine (Sular) **Uses:** *HTN* **Action:** CCB **Dose:** 10–60 mg/d PO; ⊘ take w/ grapefruit juice or high-fat meal; ↓ starting doses in elderly or hepatic impairment **Caution:** [C, ?] **Supplied:** ER tabs 10, 20, 30, 40 mg **SE:** Edema, HA, flushing **Interactions:** ↑ Effects w/ antihypertensives, azole antifungals, cimetidine, famotidine, nitrates, ranitidine, EtOH, high-fat foods; ↑ effects of tacrolimus; ↓ effects w/ NSAIDs, phenytoin, rifampin **Labs:** ↑ Serum creatine kinase, BUN, creatinine

Nitazoxanide (Alinia) **Uses:** * *Cryptosporidium-* or *Giardia*-induced diarrhea in Pts 1–11 y* **Action:** Antiprotozoal. **Spectrum:** *Cryptosporidium* or *Giardia* **Dose:** *Peds.* 12–47 mo: 5 mL (100 mg) PO q 12h × 3 d. *4–11 y:* 10 mL (200 mg) PO q 12h × 3 d; take w/ food **Caution:** [B, ?] **Contra:** **Supplied:** 100 mg/5 mL PO susp **SE:** Abdominal pain **Notes:** Susp contains sucrose; likely to interact w/highly protein-bound drugs

Nitrofurantoin (Macrodantin, Furadantin, Macrobid)
WARNING: Pulmonary Rxns possible **Uses:** *Prevention and Rx UTI* **Action:** Bacteriostatic; interferes w/ carbohydrate metabolism. *Spectrum:* Susceptible gram(−) and some gram(+) bacteria; *Pseudomonas, Serratia,* and most sp. *Proteus* generally resistant **Dose: Adults.** Suppression: 50–100 mg/d PO. *Rx:* 50–100 mg PO qid. **Peds.**4–7 mg/kg/24 h in 4 ÷ doses; take w/ food, milk, or antacid **Caution:** [B, +] ⊘ if CrCl <50 mL/min, PRG at term **Contra:** Renal failure, infants < 1 mo **Supplied:** Caps and tabs 50, 100 mg; SR caps 100 mg; susp 25 mg/5 mL **SE:** GI side effects common; dyspnea and a variety of acute and chronic pulmonary Rxns, peripheral neuropathy **Notes:** Macrocrystals (Macrodantin) cause less nausea than other forms of the drug **Interactions:** ↑ Effects w/ anticholinergics, probenecid, sulfinpyrazone; ↓ effects w/ antacids, quinolones **Labs:** False + urine glucose; false ↑ serum bilirubin, creatinine **NIPE:** Take w/ food; may discolor urine

Nitroglycerin (Nitrostat, Nitrolingual, Nitro-Bid Ointment, Nitro-Bid IV, Nitrodisc, Transderm-Nitro, others) **Uses:** *Angina pectoris, acute and prophylactic therapy, CHF, BP control* **Action:** Relaxation of vascular smooth muscle, dilates coronary arteries **Dose: Adults.** SL: 1 tab q5min SL PRN for 3 doses. *Translingual:* 1–2 met-doses sprayed onto mucosa q3–5min, max 3 doses. *PO:* 2.5–9 mg tid. *IV:* 5–20 µg/min, titrated to effect. *Topical:* Apply ½ in. of oint to the chest wall tid, wipe off at night. *TD:* 0.2–0.4 mg/h/patch qd. **Peds.**1 µg/kg/min IV, titrated to effect. **Caution:** [B, ?] Restrictive cardiomyopathy **Contra:** IV: Pericardial tamponade, constrictive pericarditis. PO: Concurrent use w/ sildenafil, tadalafil, vardenfil, head trauma, closed-angle glaucoma **Supplied:** SL tabs 0.3, 0.4, 0.6 mg; translingual spray 0.4 mg/dose; SR caps 2.5, 6.5, 9, 13 mg; SR tabs 2.6, 6.5, 9.0 mg; inj 0.5, 5, 10 mg/mL; oint 2%; TD patches 0.1, 0.2, 0.4, 0.6 mg/h; buccal CR 2, 3 mg **SE:** HA, hypotension, light-headedness, GI upset **Notes:** Tolerance to nitrates develops w/ chronic use after 1–2 wk; minimize by providing nitrate-free period each day, using shorter-acting nitrates tid, and removing long-acting patches and oint before hs to prevent development of tolerance **Interactions:** ↑ Hypotensive effects w/ antihypertensives, phenothiazines, sildenafil, EtOH; ↓ effects w/ ergot alkaloids; ↓ effects of SL tabs & spray w/ antihistamines, phenothiazines, TCAs **Labs:** False ↑ cholesterol, triglycerides **NIPE:** Replace SL tabs q6 mo & keep in original container

Nitroprusside (Nipride, Nitropress) **Uses:** *Hypertensive crisis, CHF, controlled hypotension periop (↓ bleeding).* *aortic dissection, pulmonary edema* **Action:** ↓ Systemic vascular resistance **Adult & Peds** 0.5–10 µg/kg/min IV inf, titrate to effect; usual dose 3 µg/kg/min **Caution:** [C, ?] ↓ cerebral perfusion **Contra:** High output failure, compensatory HTN **Supplied:** Inj 25 mg/mL **SE:** Excessive hypotensive effects, palpitations, HA **Notes:** Thiocyanate (metabolite), excreted by the kidney; thiocyanate toxicity at levels of 5–10 mg/dL, more likely when used for > 2–3 d; to treat aortic dissection, use BB concomitantly **Interactions:** ↑ Effects w/ antihypertensives, anesthetics, guanabenz, guanfacine, sildenafil; ↓ effects w/ estrogens, sympathomimetics **NIPE:** Discard colored soln other than light brown

Nizatidine (Axid)

Uses: *Duodenal ulcers, GERD, heartburn* **Action:** H_2-receptor antagonist **Dose:** *Adults.* Active ulcer: 150 mg PO bid or 300 mg PO hs; maint 150 mg PO hs. *GERD:* 300 mg PO bid; maint PO bid. *Heartburn:* 75 mg PO bid. *Peds.* GERD: 10 mg/kg PO bid in ÷ doses, 150 mg bid max ↓ dose in renal impairment **Caution:** [B, +] **Contra:** H_2 receptor antagonist sensitivity **Supplied:** Caps 75, 150, 300 mg **SE:** Dizziness, HA, constipation, diarrhea **Interactions:** ↑ Effects of glipizide, glyburide, nifedipine, nitrendipine, nisoldipine, salicylates, tolbutamide; ↓ effects w/ antacids, tomato/mixed veg juice; ↓ effects of azole anti-fungals, delavirdine, didanosine **Labs:** False + urobilinogen **NIPE:** Smoking ↑ gastric acid secretion

Norepinephrine (Levophed)

Uses: *Acute hypotension, cardiac arrest (adjunct)* **Action:** Peripheral vasoconstrictor acts on arterial/venous beds **Dose:** *Adults.* 8–12 µg/min IV, titrate. *Peds.* 0.05–0.1 mg/kg/min IV, titrate **Caution:** [C, ?] **Contra:** Hypotension due to hypovolemia **Supplied:** Inj 1 mg/mL **SE:** Brady-cardia, arrhythmia **Notes:** Correct volume depletion as much as possible before va-sopressors; interaction w/ TCAs leads to severe HTN; infuse into large vein to avoid extravasation; phentolamine 5–10 mg/10 mL NS injected locally for extravasa-tion **Interactions:** ↑ HTN w/ antihistamines, BBs, ergot alkaloids, guanethidine, MAOIs, methyldopa, oxytocic meds, TCAs; ↑ risk of arrhythmias w/ cyclo-propane, halothane

Norethindrone Acetate/Ethinyl Estradiol (FemHRT)

WARN-ING: Estrogens and progestins should not be used for the prevention of CV Dz; the WHI study reported ↑ risks of MI, breast CA, and DVT in postmenopausal women during 5 y of Rx w/ estrogens combined w/ medroxyprogesterone acetate relative to placebo **Uses:** *Rx of moderate to severe vasomotor Sxs associated w/ menopause; prevention of osteoporosis.* **Action:** Hormone replacement **Dose:** 1 tablet qd **Caution:** [X, –] **Contra:** PRG; Hx breast cancer; estrogen-dependent neoplasia; abnormal genital bleeding; Hx DVT, PE, or related disorders; recent (w/in past year) arterial thromboembolic Dz (CVA, MI) **Supplied:** 1 mg norethin-drone/5 µg ethinyl estradiol tablets **SE:** thrombosis, dizziness, HA, libido changes **Notes:** Use in women w/ intact uterus **Interactions:** ↑ Effects of caffeine; ↓ effects with barbiturates, carbamazepine, fosphenytoin, phenytoin, rifampin **Labs:** Effects hepatic Fxn tests and endocrine Fxn tests **NIPE:** ⊘ PRG, cigarette smoking

Norfloxacin (Noroxin)

Uses: *Complicated and uncomplicated UTI due to gram(–) bacteria, prostatitis, gonorrhea,* and *infectious diarrhea* **Action:** Quinolone, inhibits DNA gyrase. *Spectrum:* Susceptible *E. faecalis, E. coli, K. pneumoniae, P. mirabilis, P. aeruginosa, S. epidermidis, S. saprophyticus* **Dose:** 400 mg PO bid. *Gonorrhea:* 800 mg single dose. *Prostatitis:* 400 mg PO bid **Cau-tion:** [C, –] Tendinitis/tendon rupture, quinolone sensitivity, dose ↓ in renal impair-ment **Contra:** Hx of hypersensitivity or tendinitis w/ fluoroquinolones **Supplied:**

Tabs 400 mg **SE:** Photosensitivity, HA, GI **Notes:** Drug interactions w/ antacids, theophylline, and caffeine; good conc in the kidney and urine, poor blood levels; ⊘ use for urosepsis **Interactions:** ↑ Effects w/ probenecid; ↑ effects of diazepam, theophylline, caffeine, metoprolol, propranolol, phenytoin, warfarin; ↓ effects w/ antacids, didanosine, Fe salts, Mg, sucralfate, NaHCO₃, zinc; ↓ effects w/ food; **Labs:** ↑ LFTs, BUN, SCr **NIPE:** ⊘ Give to children <18 y; ↑ fluids to 2–3 L/d; may cause photosensitivity—use sunscreen

Norgestrel (Ovrette)   Uses: *Contraceptive* Action: Prevent follicular maturation and ovulation Dose: 1 tab/d; begin day 1 of menses Caution: [X, ?] Contra: Thromboembolic disorders, breast CA, PRG, severe hepatic Dz Supplied: Tabs 0.075 mg SE: Edema, breakthrough bleeding, thromboembolism Notes: Progestin-only products have higher risk of failure in prevention of PRG Interactions: ↓ Effects w/ barbiturates, carbamazepine, hydantoins, griseofulvin, penicillins, rifampin, tetracyclines, St. John's wort NIPE: Photosensitivity—use sunscreen; DC drug if suspect PRG—use barrier contraception until confirmed

Nortriptyline (Aventyl, Pamelor)   Uses: *Endogenous depression* Action: TCA; ↑ the synaptic CNS concs of serotonin and/or norepinephrine Dose: Adults. 25 mg PO tid–qid; doses >150 mg/d ⊘. Elderly. 10–25 mg hs. Peds. 6–7 y: 10 mg/d. 8–11 y: 10–20 mg/d. >11 y: 25–35 mg/d. ↓ Dose w/ hepatic insufficiency Caution: [D, +/–] Narrow-angle glaucoma, CV Dz Contra: TCA hypersensitivity, use w/ MAOI Supplied: Caps 10, 25, 50, 75 mg; soln 10 mg/5 mL SE: Anticholinergic side effects (blurred vision, urinary retention, xerostomia) Notes: Max effect seen after 2 wk Interactions: ↑ Effects w/ antihistamines, CNS depressants, cimetidine, fluoxetine, oral contraceptives, phenothiazines, quinidine, EtOH; ↑ effects of anticoagulants; ↑ risk of HTN w/ clonidine, levodopa, sympathomimetics; ↓ effects w/ barbiturates, carbamazepine, rifampin Labs: ↑ Serum bilirubin, alkaline phosphatase NIPE: Concurrent use w/ MAOIs have resulted in HTN, Szs, death; ↑ risk of photosensitivity—use sunscreen

Nystatin (Mycostatin)   Uses: *Mucocutaneous Candida infections (oral, skin, vaginal)* Action: Alters membrane permeability. Spectrum: Susceptible Candida sp Dose: Adults and children. PO: 400,000–600,000 Units PO "swish and swallow" qid. Vaginal: 1 tab vaginally hs for 2 wk. Topical: Apply bid–tid to affected area. Peds. Infants: 200,000 Units PO q6h. Caution: [B (C PO), +] Supplied: PO susp 100,000 Units/mL; PO tabs 500,000 Units; troches 200,000 Units; vaginal tabs 100,000 U; topical cream and oint 100,000 Units/g SE: GI upset, Stevens–Johnson syndrome Notes: Not absorbed PO; not effective for systemic infections NIPE: Store susp up to 10 d in refrigerator

Octreotide (Sandostatin, Sandostatin LAR)   Uses: *Suppresses/ inhibits severe diarrhea associated w/ carcinoid and neuroendocrine GI tumors (eg, VIPoma, ZE syndrome)*; bleeding esophageal varices Action: Long-acting peptide; mimics natural hormone somatostatin Dose: Adults. 100–600 µg/d SQ/IV in 2–4 ÷ doses; start 50 µg qd–bid. Sandostatin LAR (depot): 10–30 mg IM

q4wk *Peds.*1–10 µg/kg/24 h SQ in 2–4 ÷ doses. **Caution:** [B, +] Hepatic/renal impairment **Supplied:** Inj 0.05, 0.1, 0.2, 0.5, 1 mg/mL; 10, 20, 30 mg/5 mL depot **SE:** N/V, abdominal discomfort, flushing, edema, fatigue, cholelithiasis, hyper-/hypoglycemia, hepatitis **Interactions:** ↓ Effects of cyclosporine **Labs:** Small ↑ LFTs, ↓ serum thyroxine **NIPE:** May alter effects of hypoglycemics

Ofloxacin (Floxin, Ocuflox Ophthalmic)
Uses: *Lower resp tract, skin and skin structure, and UTI, prostatitis, uncomplicated gonorrhea, and *Chlamydia* infections; topical for bacterial conjunctivitis; otitis externa; if perforated ear drum >12 y* **Action:** Bactericide; inhibits DNA gyrase. *Spectrum:* S. pneumoniae, S. aureus, S. pyogenes, H. influenzae, P. mirabilis, N. gonorrhoeae, C. trachomatis, E. coli* **Dose:** *PO: Adults.* 200–400 mg PO bid or IV q12h. *Ophth: Adults & Peds.* >1 y: 1–2 gtt in eye(s) q2–4h for 2 d, then qid for 5 more d. *Otic: Adults & Peds.* >12 y: 10 gtt in ear(s) bid for 10 d. *Peds.* 1–12 y: 5 gtt in ear(s) bid for 10 d. ↓ in renal impairment; take on empty stomach **Caution:** [C, –] Interactions w/ antacids, sucralfate, and Al-, Ca-, Mg-, Fe-, or Zn-containing products (↓ absorption) **Contra:** Quinolone hypersensitivity **Supplied:** Tabs 200, 300, 400 mg; inj 20, 40 mg/mL; ophth and otic 0.3% **SE:** N/V/D, photosensitivity, insomnia, and HA **Notes:** Ophth form can be used in ears **Interactions:** ↑ Effects w/ cimetidine, probenecid, St. John's wort; ↑ effects of cyclosporine, procainamide, theophylline, warfarin, caffeine; ↓ effects w/ antacids, antineoplastics, Ca, didanosine, Fe, NaHCO₃, sucralfate, zinc **NIPE:** Take w/o food; use sunscreen; ↑ fluids to 2–3 L/d

Olanzapine (Zyprexa, Zyprexa Zydis)
Uses: *Bipolar mania, schizophrenia,* psychotic disorders **Action:** Dopamine and serotonin antagonist **Dose:** 5–10 mg/d, ↑ weekly PRN to 20 mg/d max **Caution:** [C, –] **Supplied:** Tabs 2.5, 5, 7.5, 10, 15, 20 mg; PO disintegrating tabs 5, 10, 15, 20 mg **SE:** HA, somnolence, orthostatic hypotension, tachycardia, dystonia, xerostomia, constipation **Notes:** Takes weeks to titrate to therapeutic dose; cigarette smoking ↓ levels **Interactions:** ↑ Effects w/ fluvoxamine, probenecid; ↑ sedation w/ CNS depressants, EtOH; ↑ Szs w/ anticholinergics, CNS depressants; ↓ hypotension w/ antihypertensives, diazepam; ↓ effects w/ activated charcoal, carbamazepine, omeprazole, rifampin, St. John's wort, tobacco; ↓ effects of dopamine agonists, levodopa **Labs:** ↑ LFTs **NIPE:** ↑ Risk of tardive dyskinesia, photosensitivity—use sunscreen, body temp impairment

Olopatadine (Patanol)
Uses: *Allergic conjunctivitis* **Action:** H₁-receptor antagonist **Dose:** 1–2 gtt in eye(s) bid q6–8h **Caution:** [C, ?] **Supplied:** Soln 0.1% 5 mL **SE:** Local irritation, HA, rhinitis **Notes:** ⊘ instill if wearing contact lenses

Olsalazine (Dipentum)
Uses: *Maint of remission of ulcerative colitis* **Action:** Topical antiinflammatory activity **Dose:** 500 mg PO bid; take w/ food **Caution:** [C, M] Salicylate sensitivity **Supplied:** Caps 250 mg **SE:** Diarrhea, HA, blood dyscrasias, hepatitis **Labs:** ↑ LFTs

Omalizumab (Xolair)
Uses: *Moderate to severe asthma in Pts, ≥12 y w/ reactivity to an allergen and whose Sxs are inadequately controlled w/ inhaled

steroids* **Action:** Anti-IgE antibody **Dose:** 150–375 mg SQ q2–4wk (dose/frequency determined by total serum IgE level and body weight—see package labeling) **Caution:** [B,?/–] **Contra:** Hx of component hypersensitivity **Supplied:** 150 mg in single-use 5-mL vial **SE:** Site Rxn, sinusitis, HA, anaphylaxis reported w/in 2 h of administration in 3 Pts **Notes:** Continue other asthma medications as indicated **Interactions:** No drug interaction studies done **NIPE:** ⊘ DC abruptly; not for acute bronchospasm; admin w/in 8 h of reconstitution and store in refrigerator

Omeprazole (Prilosec)

Uses: *Duodenal and gastric ulcers, ZE syndrome, GERD,* and *H. pylori* infections **Action:** Proton pump inhibitor **Dose:** 20–40 mg PO qd–bid **Caution:** [C, –] **Supplied:** Caps 10, 20, 40 mg **SE:** HA, diarrhea **Notes:** Combination (ie, antibiotic) therapy necessary for *H. pylori* infection **Interactions:** ↑ Effects of carbamazepine, diazepam, digoxin, glipizide, glyburide, nifedipine, nimodipine, nisoldipine, nitrendipine, phenytoin, tolbutamide, warfarin; ↓ effects w/ sucralfate; ↓ effects of ampicillin, cefpodoxime, cefuroxime, enoxacin, cyanocobalamin, ketoconazole **Labs:** ↑ LFTs; **NIPE:** Take w/o food

Ondansetron (Zofran)

Uses: *Prevent chemo-associated and postop N/V* **Action:** Serotonin receptor antagonist **Dose:** *Chemo: Adults & Peds.* 0.15 mg/kg/dose IV prior to chemo, then 4 and 8 h after 1st dose or 4–8 mg PO tid; give 1st dose 30 min prior to chemo. For chemo, administer on a schedule, not PRN. *Postop: Adults.* 4 mg IV immediately before induction of anesthesia or postop. *Peds.* <40 kg: 0.1 mg/kg. *>40 kg:* 4 mg IV ↓ dose w/ hepatic impairment **Caution:** [B, +/–] **Supplied:** Tabs 4, 8 mg; inj 2 mg/mL **SE:** Diarrhea, HA, constipation, dizziness **Interactions:** ↓ Effects w/ rifampin; **Labs:** ↑ Fibrinogen, AST, ALT, serum bilirubin, ↓ Hmg, serum albumin, transferrin, gamma globulin **NIPE:** Food ↑ absorption

Oprelvekin (Neumega)

Uses: *Prevent severe thrombocytopenia due to chemo* **Action:** Promotes proliferation and maturation of megakaryocytes (interleukin-11) **Dose:** *Adults.* 50 μg/kg/d SQ for 10–21 d. *Peds. >12 y: 75–100 μg/kg/d SQ for 10–21 d.* <12 y: Use only in clinical trials. **Caution:** [C, ?/–] **Supplied:** 5 mg powder for inj **SE:** Tachycardia, palpitations, arrhythmias, edema, HA, dizziness, insomnia, fatigue, fever, nausea, anemia, dyspnea **Interactions:** None noted **Labs:** ↓ Hmg, albumin **NIPE:** Monitor for peripheral edema; use med w/in 3 h of reconstitution

Oral Contraceptives, Biphasic, Monophasic, Triphasic, Progestin Only (see Table 7, page 276)

Uses: *Birth control and regulation of anovulatory bleeding* **Action:** *Birth control:* Suppresses LH surge, prevents ovulation; progestins thicken cervical mucus; inhibits fallopian tubule cilia, ↓ endometrial thickness to ↓ chances of fertilization. *Anovulatory bleeding:* Cyclic hormones mimic body's natural cycle and help regulate endometrial lining, resulting in regular bleeding q28d; may also reduce uterine bleeding and dysmenorrhea **Dose:** 28-d cycle pills taken qd; 21-d cycle pills taken qd, no pills taken during the last 7 d of the cycle (during menses) **Caution:** [X, +] Migraine, HTN, DM, sickle cell Dz, gallbladder Dz **Contra:** Undiagnosed abnormal vaginal bleeding, PRG, estrogen-dependent malignancy, hypercoagulation disorders, liver Dz, hemiplegic migraine, and smokers >35 y **Supplied:** 28-d cycle pills (21 hormonally active pills + 7 placebo/Fe suppl); 21-d cycle pills (21 hormonally active pills) **SE:** Intramenstrual bleeding, oligomenorrhea, amenorrhea, ↑ appetite/weight gain, loss of libido, fatigue, depression, mood swings, mastalgia, HA, melasma, ↑ vaginal discharge, acne/greasy skin, corneal edema, nausea **Notes:** Taken correctly, 99.9% effective for preventing PRG; not protective against STDs; encourage additional barrier contraceptive; long term, can ↓ risk of ectopic PRG, benign breast Dz, ovarian and uterine CA. *Rx for menstrual cycle control:* Start w/ a monophasic pill; pill must be taken for 3 mo before switching to another brand; if abnormal bleeding continues, change to pill w/ higher estrogen dose. *Rx for birth control:* Choose pill w/ most beneficial side effect profile for particular Pt; side effects numerous and due to Sxs of estrogen excess or progesterone deficiency; each pill's side effect profile is unique (found in package insert); tailor Rx to specific Pt

Orlistat (Xenical)
Uses: *Manage obesity in Pts w/ BMI ≥ 30 kg/m^2 or ≥ 27 kg/m^2 in presence of other risk factors; type 2 DM, dyslipidemia* **Action:** Reversible inhibitor of gastric and pancreatic lipases. **Dose:** 120 mg PO tid w/ a fat-containing meal **Caution:** [B, ?] May ↓ cyclosporine levels and ↓ daily dose requirements for warfarin **Contra:** Cholestatsis, chronic malabsorption **Supplied:** Capsules 120 mg **SE:** Abdominal pain/discomfort, fatty/oily stools, fecal urgency **Notes:** ⊘ Administer if meal contains no fat; GI effects ↑ w/ higher-fat meals; suppl w/ fat-soluble vitamins **Interactions:** ↑ Effects of pravastatin; ↓ effects of cyclosporine, fat-soluble vitamins **Labs:** Monitor warfarin, ↓ serum glucose, total cholesterol, LDL **NIPE:** ⊘ Administer if meal contains no fat; GI effects ↑ w/ higher-fat meals; supplement w/ fat-soluble vitamins

Orphenadrine (Norflex)
Uses: *Muscle spasms* **Action:** Central atropine-like effects cause indirect skeletal muscle relaxation, euphoria, and analgesia **Dose:** 100 mg PO bid, 60 mg IM/IV q12h **Caution:** [C, +] **Contra:** Glaucoma, GI obstruction, cardiospasm, MyG **Supplied:** Tabs 100 mg; SR tabs 100 mg; inj 30 mg/mL **SE:** Drowsiness, dizziness, blurred vision, flushing, tachycardia, constipation **Interactions:** ↑ CNS depression w/ anxiolytics, butorphanol, hypnotics, MAOIs, nalbuphine, opioids, pentazocine, phenothiazines, tramadol, TCAs, kava kava, valerian, EtOH; ↑ effects w/ anticholinergics **NIPE:** Impaired body temp regulation

Oseltamivir (Tamiflu)
Uses: *Prevention and Rx influenza A and B* **Action:** Inhibits viral neuraminidase **Dose:** *Adults.* 75 mg PO bid for 5 d. *Peds.* PO bid dosing: <14 kg: 30 mg. *16–23 kg:* 45 mg. *24–40 kg:* 60 mg; >*40 kg:* As adults; ↓ dose in renal impairment **Caution:** [C, ?/–] **Contra:** Component hypersensitivity **Supplied:** Caps 75 mg, powder 12 mg/mL **SE:** N/V, insomnia **Notes:** Initiate w/in 48 h of Sx onset or exposure **Interaction:** ↑ Effects w/ probenecid **NIPE:** Take w/o regard to food

Oxacillin (Bactocill, Prostaphlin) Uses: *Infections caused by suscep-tible strains of *S. aureus* and *Streptococcus** Action: Bactericidal; inhibits cell wall synthesis. Spectrum: Excellent gram(+), poor gram(−) Dose: *Adults.* 250–500 mg (1 g severe) IM/IV q4–6h. *Peds.* 150–200 mg/kg/d IV ÷ q4–6h; ↓ dose in signifi-cant renal Dz Caution: [B, M] Contra: Penicillin sensitivity Supplied: Inj; caps 250, 500 mg; soln 250 mg/5 mL SE: GI upset, interstitial nephritis, blood dyscrasias Interactions: ↑ Effects w/ disulfiram, probenecid; ↑ effects of antico-agulants, MRX; ↓ effects w/ chloramphenicol, tetracyclines, carbonated drinks, fruit juice, food; ↓ effects of oral contraceptives Labs: False + urine and serum protein NIPE: Take w/o food

Oxaprozin (Daypro) Uses: *Arthritis and pain* Action: NSAID; inhibits prostaglandins synthesis Dose: 600–1200 mg/d; ↓ dose in renal/hepatic impair-ment Caution: [C (D in 3rd tri or near term), ?] ASA/NSAID sensitivity, peptic ulcer, bleeding disorders Supplied: Caps 600 mg SE: CNS inhibition, sleep distur-bance, rash, GI upset, peptic ulcer, edema, renal failure Interactions: ↑ Effects of aminoglycosides, anticoagulants, ASA, diuretics, Li, MRX, ↓ effects of antihyper-tensives NIPE: ↑ Risk of photosensitivity—use sunscreen; take w/ food

Oxazepam (Serax) [C-IV] Uses: *Anxiety, acute EtOH withdrawal,* anxiety w/ depressive Sxs Action: Benzodiazepine Dose: *Adults.* 10–15 mg PO tid–qid; severe anxiety and EtOH withdrawal may require up to 30 mg qid. *Peds.* 1 mg/kg/d in ÷ doses Caution: [D, ?] Supplied: Caps 10, 15, 30 mg; tabs 15 mg SE: Sedation, ataxia, dizziness, rash, blood dyscrasias, dependence Notes: ⊘ Abrupt discontinuation; metabolite of diazepam (Valium) Interactions: ↑ CNS effects w/ anticonvulsants, antidepressants, antihistamines, barbiturates, MAOIs, opioids, phenothiaznes, kava kava, lemon balm, sassafras, valerian, EtOH; ↑ effects w/ cimetidine; ↓ effects w/ oral contraceptives, phenytoin, theophylline, tobacco; ↓ effects of levodopa Labs: False ↑ serum glucose NIPE: ⊘ DC abruptly

Oxcarbazepine (Trileptal) Uses: *Partial Szs,* bipolar disorders Ac-tion: Blocks voltage-sensitive Na⁺ channels, stabilization of hyperexcited neural membranes Dose: *Adults.* 300 mg PO bid, ↑ weekly to target maint 1200–2400 mg/d. *Peds.* 8–10 mg/kg bid, 500 mg/d max, ↑ weekly to target maint dose; ↓ in renal insufficiency Caution: [C, −] Cross-sensitivity to carbamazepine Contra: Sensitivity to components Supplied: Tabs 150, 300, 600 mg SE: Hyponatremia, HA, dizziness, fatigue, somnolence, GI upset, diplopia, mental conc difficulties Notes: ⊘ Abruptly DC, check Na⁺ if fatigue reported Interactions: ↑ Effects w/ benzodiazepines, EtOH; ↑ effects of phenobarbital, phenytoin; ↓ effects w/ barbi-turates, carbamazepine, phenobarbital, valproic acid, verapamil; ↓ effects of CCBs, oral contraceptives Labs: ↓ Thyroid levels, serum Na NIPE: Take w/o regard to food; use barrier contraception

Oxiconazole (Oxistat) Uses: *Tinea pedis, tinea cruris, and tinea cor-poris* Action: Antifungal antibiotic Spectrum: Most strains of *Epidermophyton floccosum, Trichophyton mentagrophytes, Trichophyton rubrum, Malassezia furfur*

Dose: Apply bid **Caution:** [B, M] **Contra:** Component hypersensitivity **Supplied:** Cream 1%; lotion **SE:** Local irritation

Oxybutynin (Ditropan, Ditropan XL)   Uses: *Symptomatic relief of urgency, nocturia, and incontinence associated w/ neurogenic or reflex neurogenic bladder* **Action:** Direct smooth muscle antispasmodic; ↑ bladder capacity **Dose:** *Adults & Peds.* > 5 y: 5 mg PO tid–qid; XL 5 mg PO qd; ↑ to 30 mg/d PO (5 and 10 mg/tab). *Peds.* 1–5 y: 0.2 mg/kg/dose bid–qid (syrup 5 mg/5 mL); ↓ dose in elderly; periodic drug holidays recommended **Caution:** [B, ? (use w/ caution)] **Contra:** Glaucoma, MyG, GI or GU obstruction, ulcerative colitis, megacolon **Supplied:** Tabs 5 mg; XL tabs 5, 10, 15 mg; syrup 5 mg/5 mL **SE:** Anticholinergic side effects; drowsiness, xerostomia, constipation, tachycardia**Interactions:** ↑ Effects w/ CNS depressants, EtOH; ↑ effects of atenolol, digoxin, nitrofurantoin; ↑ anticholinergic effects w/ antihistamines, anticholinergics; ↓ effects of haloperidol, levodopa **NIPE:** ↓ Temp regulation; ↑ photosensitivity—use sunscreen

Oxybutynin Transdermal System (Oxytrol)   Uses: *Rx of over-active bladder* **Action:** Direct smooth muscle antispasmodic; ↑ bladder capacity **Dose:** One 3.9 mg/d system apply 2×/wk to abdomen, hip, or buttock **Caution:** [B, ?/–] **Contra:** Urinary or gastric retention, uncontrolled narrow-angle glaucoma **Supplied:** 3.9 mg/d transdermal system **SE:** Anticholinergic effects, itching/red-ness at application site **Notes:** ⊘ Reapplication to the same site w/in 7 d **Interactions:** ↑ Effects w/ anticholinergics **NIPE:** Metabolized by the cytochrome P450 CYP3A4 enzyme system

Oxycodone [Dihydrohydroxycodeinone] (OxyContin, OxyIR, Roxicodone) [C-II]   WARNING: Swallow whole, ⊘ crush; high abuse potential **Uses:** *Moderate/severe pain, usually in combination w/ nonnarcotic analgesics* **Action:** Narcotic analgesic **Dose:** *Adults.* 5 mg PO q6h PRN. *Peds.* 6–12 y: 1.25 mg PO q6h PRN. *>12 y:* 2.5 mg q6h PRN. ↓ In severe liver Dz **Caution:** [B (D if prolonged use or near term), M] **Contra:** Hypersensitivity, resp depression **Supplied:** Immediate-release caps (OxyIR) 5 mg; tabs (Percolone) 5 mg; CR (OxyContin) 10, 20, 40, 80 mg; liq 5 mg/5 mL; soln conc 20 mg/mL **SE:** Hypotension, sedation, dizziness, GI upset, constipation, risk of abuse **Notes:** OxyContin used for chronic CA pain; may be sought after as drug of abuse **Interactions:** ↑ CNS & resp. depression w/ amitriptylline, barbiturates, cimetidine, clomipramine, MAOIs, nortriptylline, protease inhibitors, TCAs **Labs:** False ↑ serum amylase, lipase **NIPE:** Take w/ food

Oxycodone & Acetaminophen (Percocet, Tylox) [C-II]   Uses: *Moderate to severe pain* **Action:** Narcotic analgesic **Dose:** *Adults.* 1–2 tabs/caps PO q4–6h PRN (acetaminophen max dose 4 g/d). *Peds* Oxycodone 0.05–0.15 mg/kg/dose q 4–6h PRN, up to 5 mg/dose **Caution:** [B (D if prolonged use or near term), M] **Contra:** Hypersensitivity, resp depression **Supplied:** Percocet tabs, mg oxycodone/mg APAP: 2.5/325, 5/325, 7.5/325, 10/325, 7.5/500, 10/650; Tylox caps 5 mg oxycodone, 500 mg APAP; soln 5 mg oxycodone and 325 mg APAP/5

mL **SE:** Hypotension, sedation, dizziness, GI upset, constipation **Interactions:** ↑ CNS & resp depression w/ amitriptylline, barbiturates, cimetidine, clomipramine, MAOIs, nortriptylline, protease inhibitors, TCAs **Labs:** False ↑ serum amylase, lipase **NIPE:** Take w/ food

Oxycodone & Aspirin (Percodan, Percodan-Demi) [C-II]
Uses: *Moderate–moderately severe pain* **Action:** Narcotic analgesic w/ NSAID **Dose:** *Adults.* 1–2 tabs/caps PO q4–6h PRN. *Peds.*Oxycodone 0.05–0.15 mg/kg/dose q 4–6h PRN, up to 5 mg/dose; ↓ dose in severe hepatic failure **Caution:** [B (D if prolonged use or near term), M] Peptic ulcer **Contra:** Component hypersensitivity **Supplied:** Percodan 4.5 mg oxycodone hydrochloride, 0.38 mg oxycodone terephthalate, 325 mg ASA; Percodan-Demi 2.25 mg oxycodone hydrochloride, 0.19 mg oxycodone terephthalate, 325 mg ASA **SE:** Sedation, dizziness, GI upset, constipation **Interactions:** ↑ CNS & resp. depression w/ amitriptylline, barbiturates, cimetidine, clomipramine, MAOIs, nortriptylline, protease inhibitors, TCAs; ↑ effects of anticoagulants **Labs:** False ↑ serum amylase, lipase **NIPE:** Take w/ food

Oxymorphone (Numorphan) [C-II]
Uses: *Moderate to severe pain, sedative* **Action:** Narcotic analgesic **Dose:** 0.5 mg IM, SQ, IV initially, 1–1.5 mg q4–6h PRN. *PR:* 5 mg q4–6h PRN **Caution:** [B, ?] **Contra:** ↑ ICP, severe resp depression **Supplied:** Inj 1, 1.5 mg/mL; supp 5 mg **SE:** Hypotension, sedation, GI upset, constipation, histamine release **Notes:** Chemically related to hydromorphone **Interactions:** ↑ Effects w/ CNS depressants, cimetidine, neuroleptics, EtOH; ↓ effects w/ phenothiazines **Labs:** False ↑ amylase, lipase

Oxytocin (Pitocin)
Uses: *Induction of labor and control of postpartum hemorrhage*; promote milk letdown in lactating women **Action:** Stimulate muscular contractions of the uterus and milk flow during nursing **Dose:** 0.001–0.002 Units/min IV inf; titrate 0.02 Units/min max. *Breast-feeding:* 1 spray in both nostrils 2–3 min before feeding **Caution:** [Uncategorized, no anomalies expected, +/–] **Contra:** Where vaginal delivery is not favorable, fetal distress **Supplied:** Inj 10 Units/mL; nasal soln 40 Units/mL **SE:** Uterine rupture and fetal death; arrhythmias, anaphylaxis, water intoxication **Notes:** Monitor vital signs; nasal form for breast-feeding only **Interactions:** ↑ Pressor effects w/ sympathomimetics

Paclitaxel (Taxol)
Uses: *Ovarian and breast CA* **Action:** Mitotic spindle poison promotes microtubule assembly and stabilization against depolymerization **Dose:** See specific protocols; use glass or polyolefin containers using polyethylene-lined nitroglycerin tubing sets; PVC inf sets result in leaching of plasticizer; ↓ dose in hepatic failure; maintain hydration **Caution:** [D, –] **Contra:** Neutropenia <1500 WBC/mm^3; solid tumors **Supplied:** Inj 6 mg/mL **SE:** Myelosuppression, peripheral neuropathy, transient ileus, myalgia, bradycardia, hypotension, mucositis, N/V/D, fever, rash, HA, and phlebitis; hematologic toxicity schedule-dependent; leukopenia dose-limiting by 24-h inf; neurotoxicity dose-limiting by short (1–3 h) inf **Notes:** Hypersensitivity Rxns (dyspnea, hypotension, urticaria, rash)

usually w/in 10 min of starting inf; minimize w/corticosteroid, antihistamine (H$_1$- and H$_2$-antagonist) pretreatment. **Interactions:** ↑ Effects w/ BBs, cyclosporine, dexamethasone, diazepam, digoxin, etoposide, ketoconazole, midazolam, quinidine, teniposide, troleandomycin, verapamil, vincristine; ↑ risk of bleeding w/ anticoagulants, plt inhibitors, thrombolytics; ↑ myelosuppression when cisplatin is admin before paclitaxel; ↓ effects w/ carbamazepine, phenobarbital; ↓ effects of live virus vaccines **Labs:** ↑ ALT, AST, serum bilirubin, alkaline phosphatase **NIPE:** ⊘ PRG, breast-feeding, live virus vaccines; use barrier contraception

Palivizumab (Synagis) **Uses:** *Prevent RSV infection* **Action:** Monoclonal antibody **Dose:** *Peds.* 15 mg/kg IM monthly, typically Nov–Apr **Caution:** [C, ?] Caution in renal or hepatic dysfunction **Contra:** Hypersensitivity **Supplied:** Vials 50, 100 mg **SE:** URI, rhinitis, cough, ↑ LFT, local irritation **NIPE:** Use drug w/in 6 h after reconstitution; ⊘ inj in gluteal site; for prophylaxis

Palonosetron (Aloxi) **WARNING:** May prolong QT$_c$ interval **Uses:** *Prevention of acute and delayed N/V w/ moderately and highly emetogenic cancer chemo* **Action:** 5HT3 serotonin receptor antagonist **Dose:** 0.25 mg IV 30 min prior to chemo; ⊘ repeat w/in 7 d **Caution:** [B, ?] **Contra:** Component hypersensitivity **Supplied:** 0.25 mg/5 mL vial **SE:** HA, constipation, dizziness, abdominal pain, anxiety **Interactions:** Potential for drug interactions low

Pamidronate (Aredia) **Uses:** *Hypercalcemia of malignancy and Paget's Dz; palliation of symptomatic bone mets* **Action:** Inhibits normal and abnormal bone resorption **Dose:** *Hypercalcemia:* 60 mg IV over 4 h or 90 mg IV over 24 h. *Paget's:* 30 mg/d IV slow inf for 3 d **Caution:** [C, ?/–] **Contra:** PRG **Supplied:** Powder for inj 30, 60, 90 mg **SE:** Fever, tissue irritation at inj site, uveitis, fluid overload, HTN, abdominal pain, N/V, constipation, UTI, bone pain, hypokalemia, hypocalcemia, hypomagnesemia, hypophosphatemia **Interactions:** ↓ Serum Ca levels w/ foscarnet; ↓ effects w/ Ca, vitamin D **NIPE:** ⊘ Ingest food w/ Ca or vitamins w/ minerals before or 2–3 h after admin of drug

Pancrelipase (Pancrease, Cotazym, Creon, Ultrase) **Uses:** *Exocrine pancreatic secretion deficiency (CF, chronic pancreatitis, other pancreatic insufficiency) and for steatorrhea of malabsorption syndrome* **Action:** Pancreatic enzyme suppl **Dose:** 1–3 caps (tabs) w/meals and snacks; dosage ↑ to 8 caps (tabs); ⊘ crush or chew EC products; dosage is dependent on digestive requirements of Pt; ⊘ antacids **Caution:** [C, ?/–] **Contra:** Hypersensitivity to pork products **Supplied:** Caps, tabs **SE:** N/V, abdominal cramps **Notes:** Each Pt should receive individualized enzymatic therapy **Interactions:** ↓ Effects w/ antacids w/ Ca or Mg; ↓ effects of Fe **Labs:** ↑ Serum and urine uric acid **NIPE:** Take w/ food; stress adherence to diet (usually low-fat, high-protein, high-calorie)

Pancuronium (Pavulon) **Uses:** *Paralysis of Pts on mechanical ventilation* **Action:** Nondepolarizing neuromuscular blocker **Dose:** *Adults.* 2–4 mg IV q2–4h PRN. *Peds.* 0.02–0.1 mg/kg/dose q2–4h PRN; ↓ dose for renal/hepatic impairment; intubate Pt and keep on controlled ventilation; use adequate sedation or analgesia **Caution:** [C, ?/–] **Contra:** Component or bromide sensitivity **Supplied:** Inj 1, 2 mg/mL **SE:** Tachycardia, HTN, pruritus, other histamine Rxns **Interactions:** ↑ Effects w/ aminoglycosides, bacitracin, clindamycin, enflurane, K-depleting diuretics, isoflurane, lidocaine, Li, metocurine, quinine, sodium colistimethate, succinylcholine, tetracycline, trimethaphan, tubocurarine, verapamil; ↓ effects w/ carbamazepine, phenytoin, theophylline

Pantoprazole (Protonix) Uses: *GERD, erosive gastritis,* ZE syndrome, PUD **Action:** Proton pump inhibitor **Dose:** 40 mg/d PO; ⊘ crush or chew tabs; 40 mg IV/d (not >3 mg/min and use Protonix filter) **Caution:** [B, ?/–] **Supplied:** Tabs 40 mg; inj **SE:** Chest pain, anxiety, GI upset, ↑ levels on LFTs

Paregoric [Camphorated Tincture of Opium] [C-III] Uses: *Diarrhea,* pain, and neonatal opiate withdrawal syndrome **Action:** Narcotic **Dose:** *Adults.* 5–10 mL PO qd–qid PRN. *Peds.*0.25–0.5 mL/kg qd–qid. *Neonatal withdrawal syndrome*: 3–6 gtt PO q3–6 h PRN to relieve Sxs for 3–5 d, then taper over 2–4 wk **Caution:** [B (D if prolonged use or high dose near term, +] **Contra:** Tincture (children); convulsive disorder **Supplied:** Liq 2 mg morphine = 20 mg opium/5 mL **SE:** Hypotension, sedation, constipation **Notes:** Contains anhydrous morphine from opium; short-term use only **Interactions:** ↓ Effects of ampicillin esters, azole antifungals, Fe salts **Labs:** ↑ LFTs, SCr **NIPE:** Take w/o regard to food

Paroxetine (Paxil, Paxil CR) **WARNING:** Closely monitor for worsening depression or emergence of suicidality, particularly in pediatric Pts Uses: *Depression, OCD, panic disorder, social anxiety disorder,* PMDD **Action:** SSRI **Dose:** 10–60 mg PO single daily dose in AM; CR 25 mg/d PO; ↑ 12.5 mg/wk (max range 26–62.5 mg/d) **Caution:** [B, ?/] **Contra:** MAOI **Supplied:** Tabs 10, 20, 30, 40 mg; susp 10 mg/5 mL; CR 12.5, 25 mg **SE:** Sexual dysfunction, HA, somnolence, dizziness, GI upset, diarrhea, xerostomia, tachycardia **Interactions:** ↑ Effects w/ cimetidine; ↑ effects of BBs, dexfenfluramine, dextromethorphan, fenfluramine, haloperidol, MAOIs, theophylline, thioridazine, TCAs, warfarin, St. John's wort, EtOH; ↓ effects w/ cyproheptadine, phenobarbital, phenytoin; ↓ effects of digoxin, phenytoin **Labs:** ↑ LFTs **NIPE:** Take w/o regard to food, may take up to 4 wk for full effect

Pegfilgrastim (Neulasta) Uses: *↓ Frequency of infection in Pts w/ nonmyeloid malignancies receiving myelosuppressive anticancer drugs that cause febrile neutropenia* **Action:** Colony-stimulating factor **Dose:** *Adults.* 6 mg SQ × 1/chemo cycle. *Peds.* 100 μg/kg SQ × 1/chemo cycle **Caution:** [C, M] in sickle cell **Contra:** Hypersensitivity to drugs used to treat *E. coli* or to filgrastim **Supplied:** *Syringes:* 6 mg/0.6 mL **SE:** HA, fever, weakness, fatigue, dizziness, insomnia, edema, N/V/D, stomatitis, anorexia, constipation, taste perversion, dyspepsia, abdominal pain, granulocytopenia, neutropenic fever, ↑ LFT, uric acid, arthralgia, myalgia, bone pain, ARDS, alopecia, splenic rupture, aggravation of sickle cell Dz **Notes:** Never give between 14 d before and 24 h after dose of cytotoxic chemo **In-**

teractions: ↑ Effects w/ Li **Labs:** ↑ Alkaline phosphatase, LDH, uric acid **NIPE:** ⊘ Exposure to infection

Peg Interferon Alfa-2a (Pegasys) Uses: *Chronic hepatitis C w/ compensated liver Dz* **Action:** Biologic response modifier **Dose:** 180 μg (1 mL) SQ qwk × 48 wk; ↓ in renal impairment **Caution:** [C, /?–] **Contra:** Autoimmune hepatitis, decompensated liver Dz **Supplied:** 180 μg/mL inj **SE:** Depression, insomnia, suicidal behavior, GI upset, neutropenia and thrombocytopenia, alopecia, pruritus **Notes:** May aggravate neuropsychiatric, autoimmune, ischemic, and infectious disorders **NIPE:** ⊘ Exposure to infection, use barrier contraception

Peg Interferon Alfa-2b (PEG-Intron) Uses: *Rx hepatitis C* **Action:** Immune modulation **Dose:** 1 μg/kg/wk SQ; 1.5 μg/kg/wk combined w/ribavirin **Caution:** [C, ?/–] w/psychiatric Hx **Contra:** Autoimmune hepatitis, decompensated liver Dz, hemoglobinopathy **Supplied:** Vials 50, 80, 120, 150 μg/0.5 mL **SE:** Depression, insomnia, suicidal behavior, GI upset, neutropenia and thrombocytopenia, alopecia, pruritus **Notes:** ↓ Flu-like Sxs by giving hs or w/APAP; follow CBC and plts **Interactions:** ↑ Myelosuppression w/ antineoplastics; ↑ effects of doxorubicin, theophylline; ↑ neurotoxicity w/ vinblastine **Labs:** ↑ ALT, ↓ neutrophils, plts **NIPE:** Maintain hydration; use barrier contraception

Pemetrexed (Alimta) Uses: *W/ cisplatin in nonresectable mesothelioma* **Action:** Antifolate antineoplastic **Dose:** 500 mg/m² IV over 10 min day 1 of each 21-d cycle; 30 min after, 75 mg/m² cisplatin IV over 2 h; ↓ dose based on hematologic or neural toxicity **Caution:** [D, –] Renal/hepatic/BM impairment **Contra:** Component sensitivity **Supplied:** 500-mg vial **SE:** Neutropenia, leukopenia, thrombocytopenia, N/V/D, anorexia, stomatitis, renal failure, neuropathy, fever, fatigue, mood changes, dyspnea, anaphylactic Rxns **Notes:** ⊘ NSAIDs, follow CBC and plts

Pemirolast (Alamast) Uses: *Allergic conjunctivitis* **Action:** Mast cell stabilizer **Dose:** 1–2 gtt in each eye qid **Caution:** [C, ?/–] **Supplied:** 1 mg/mL **SE:** HA, rhinitis, cold/flu symptoms, local irritation **Notes:** Wait 10 min before inserting contact lenses

Penbutolol (Levatol) Uses: *HTN* **Action:** β-Adrenergic receptor blocker, β₁, β₂ **Dose:** 20–40 mg/d; ↓ in hepatic insufficiency **Caution:** [C (1st tri; D if 2nd/3rd tri), M] **Contra:** Asthma, cardiogenic shock, cardiac failure, heart block, bradycardia **Supplied:** Tabs 20 mg **SE:** Flushing, hypotension, fatigue, hyperglycemia, GI upset, sexual dysfunction, bronchospasm **Interactions:** ↑ Effects w/ CCBs, fluoroquinolones; ↑ bradycardia w/ adenosine, amiodarone, digitalis, dipyridamole, epinephrine, neuroleptics, phenylephrine, physostigmine, tacrine; ↑ effects of lidocaine, verapamil; ↓ effects w/ antacids, NSAIDs; ↓ effects of insulin, hypoglycemics, theophylline **Labs:** ↑ Serum glucose, BUN, K⁺, lipoprotein, triglycerides, uric acid **NIPE:** ↑ Cold sensitivity

Penciclovir (Denavir) Uses: *Herpes simplex (herpes labialis/cold sores)* **Action:** Competitive inhibitor of DNA polymerase **Dose:** Apply at 1st sign of lesions, then q2h for 4 d **Caution:** [B, ?/–] **Contra:** Hypersensitivity **Supplied:** Cream 1% [OTC] **SE:** Erythema, HA **Notes:** ⊘ apply to mucous membranes

Penicillin G, Aqueous (Potassium or Sodium) (Pfizerpen, Pentids)

Uses: *Bacteremia, endocarditis, pericarditis, resp tract infections, meningitis, neurosyphilis, skin/skin structure infections* **Action:** Bactericide; inhibits cell wall synthesis. *Spectrum:* Most gram(+) (not staphylococci), streptococci, *N. meningitidis*, syphilis, clostridia, and anaerobes (not *Bacteroides*) **Dose:** *Adults.* 400,000–800,000 Units PO qid; IV doses vary depending on indications; range 0.6–24 MU/d in ÷ doses q4h. *Peds.* Newborns <1 wk: 25,000–50,000 Units/kg/dose IV q12h. *Infants 1 wk–<1 mo:* 25,000–50,000 Units/kg/dose IV q6h. *Children:* 100,000–300,000 Units/kg/24h IV ÷ q4h; ↓ in renal impairment **Caution:** [B, M] **Contra:** Hypersensitivity **Supplied:** Tabs 200,000, 250,000, 400,000, 800,000 Units; susp 200,000, 400,000 Units/5 mL; powder for inj **SE:** Hypersensitivity Rxns; interstitial nephritis, diarrhea, Szs **Notes:** Contains 1.7 mEq of K⁺/MU **Interactions:** ↑ Effects w/ probenecid; ↑ effects of MRX; ↑ risk of bleeding w/ anticoagulants; ↓ effects w/ chloramphenicol, macrolides, tetracyclines; ↓ effects of oral contraceptives **Labs:** ↑ LFTs, ↓ serum albumin, folate **NIPE:** Monitor for superinfection; use barrier contraception

Penicillin G Benzathine (Bicillin)

Uses: *Single-dose regimen for streptococcal pharyngitis, rheumatic fever, glomerulonephritis prophylaxis, and syphilis* **Action:** Bactericide; inhibits cell wall synthesis. *Spectrum:* See Penicillin G **Dose:** *Adults.* 1.2–2.4 MU deep IM inj q2–4wk. *Peds.* 50,000 Units/kg/dose, 2.4 MU/dose max; deep IM inj q2–4 wk **Caution:** [B, M] **Contra:** Hypersensitivity **Supplied:** Inj 300,000, 600,000 Units/mL; Bicillin L-A contains the benzathine salt only; Bicillin C-R contains a combination of benzathine and procaine (300,000 Units procaine w/ 300,000 Units benzathine/mL or 900,000 Units benzathine w/ 300,000 Units procaine/2 mL) **SE:** Pain at inj site, acute interstitial nephritis, anaphylaxis **Notes:** Sustained action w/detectable levels up to 4 wk; drug of choice for Rx of noncongenital syphilis **Interactions:** See Penicillin G

Penicillin G Procaine (Wycillin, others)

Uses: *Resp tract infections, scarlet fever, skin and soft tissue infections, syphilis* **Action:** Bactericide; inhibits cell wall synthesis. *Spectrum:* Penicillin G-sensitive organisms that respond to low, persistent serum levels **Dose:** *Adults.* 0.6–4.8 MU/d in ÷ doses q12–24h; give probenecid at least 30 min prior to penicillin to prolong action. *Peds.* 25,000–50,000 Units/kg/d IM ÷ qd–bid **Caution:** [B, M] **Contra:** Hypersensitivity **Supplied:** Inj 300,000, 500,000, 600,000 Units/mL **SE:** Pain at inj site, interstitial nephritis, anaphylaxis **Notes:** Long-acting parenteral penicillin; blood levels up to 15 h **Interactions:** See Penicillin G, Aqueous

Penicillin V (Pen-Vee K, Veetids, others)

Uses: Susceptible streptococci infections, otitis media, URIs, skin/soft tissue infections (penicillin-sensitive staph) **Action:** Bactericidal; inhibits cell wall synthesis. *Spectrum:* Most gram(+), including streptococci **Dose:** *Adults.* 250–500 mg PO q6h, q8h, q12h.

Peds. 25–50 mg/kg/25h PO in 4 doses; ↓ in renal Dz; take on empty stomach **Caution:** [B, M] **Contra:** Hypersensitivity **Supplied:** Tabs 125, 250, 500 mg; susp 125, 250 mg/5 mL **SE:** GI upset, interstitial nephritis, anaphylaxis, convulsions **Notes:** Well-tolerated PO penicillin; 250 mg = 400,000 Units of penicillin G **Interactions:** See Penicillin G, Aqueous

Pentamidine (Pentam 300, NebuPent)

Uses: *Rx and prevention of PCP* **Action:** Inhibits DNA, RNA, phospholipid, and protein synthesis **Dose:** *Rx: Adults & Peds.* 4 mg/kg/24 h IV qd for 14–21 d. *Prevention: Adults & Peds.* >5 y: 300 mg once q4wk, administered via Respirgard II neb; IV requires ↓ dose in renal impairment **Caution:** [C, ?] **Contra:** Component hypersensitivity **Supplied:** Inj 300 mg/vial; aerosol 300 mg **SE:** Associated w/ pancreatic islet cell necrosis leading to hyperglycemia; CP, fatigue, dizziness, rash, GI upset, pancreatitis, renal impairment, blood dyscrasias **Notes:** Follow CBC (leukopenia and thrombocytopenia); monitor glucose and pancreatic Fxn monthly for the 1st 3 mo; monitor for hypotension following IV administration **Interactions:** ↑ Nephrotoxic effects w/ aminoglycosides, amphotericin B, capreomycin, cidofovir, cisplatin, cyclosporine, colistin, ganciclovir, methoxyflurane, polymyxin B, vancomycin; ↑ bone marrow suppression w/ antineoplastics, radiation therapy **Labs:** ↑ LFTs, serum K+ **NIPE:** Reconstitute w/ sterile H_2O only, inhalation may cause metallic taste; ↑ fluids to 2–3 L/d

Pentazocine (Talwin) [C-IV]

Uses: *Moderate to severe pain* **Action:** Partial narcotic agonist–antagonist **Dose:** *Adults.* 30 mg IM or IV; 50–100 mg PO q3–4h PRN. *Peds.* 5–8 y: 15 mg IM q4h PRN. *8–14 y:* 30 mg IM q4h PRN; ↓ dose in renal/hepatic impairment **Caution:** [C (1st tri, D if prolonged use or high doses near term), +/–] **Contra:** Hypersensitivity **Supplied:** Tabs 50 mg (+ naloxone 0.5 mg); inj 30 mg/mL **SE:** Associated w/ considerable dysphoria; drowsiness, GI upset, xerostomia. *Szs* **Notes:** 30–60 mg IM equianalgesic to 10 mg of morphine IM **Interactions:** ↑ CNS depression w/ antihistamines, barbiturates, hypnotics, phenothiazines, EtOH; ↑ effects w/ cimetidine; ↑ effects of digitoxin, phenytoin, rifampin; ↓ effects of opioids **Labs:** ↑ Serum amylase, lipase **NIPE:** May cause withdrawal in Pts using opioids

Pentobarbital (Nembutal, others) [C-II]

Uses: *Insomnia, convulsions,* and induced coma following severe head injury **Action:** Barbiturate **Dose:** *Adults.* Sedative: 20–40 mg PO or PR q6–12h. *Hypnotic:* 100–200 mg PO or PR hs PRN. *Induced coma:* Load 5–10 mg/kg IV, then maint 1–3 mg/kg/h IV cont inf to keep the serum level between 20 and 50 mg/mL. *Peds.* Hypnotic: 2–6 mg/kg/dose PO hs PRN. *Induced coma:* See adult dosage **Caution:** [D, +/–] Significant hepatic impairment **Contra:** Hypersensitivity **Supplied:** Caps 50, 100 mg; elixir 18.2 mg/5 mL (= 20 mg pentobarbital); supp 30, 60, 120, 200 mg; inj 50 mg/mL **SE:** Can cause resp depression, hypotension when used aggressively IV for cerebral edema; bradycardia, hypotension, sedation, lethargy, hangover, rash, Stevens–Johnson syndrome, blood dyscrasias, resp depression **Notes:** Tolerance to sedative–hypnotic effect acquired w/in 1–2 wk **Interactions:** ↑ Effects w/ chloramphenicol, MAOIs, narcotic analgesics, kava kava, valerian, EtOH; ↓ effects of BBs, CCBs, corticosteroids, cyclosporine, digitoxin, disopyramide, doxycycline, estrogen, griseofulvin, neuroleptics, oral anticoagulants, oral contraceptives, propafenone, quinidine, tacrolimus, theophylline, TCAs **Labs:** ↑ Ammonia; ↓ bilirubin

Pentosan Polysulfate Sodium (Elmiron)   Uses: *Relief of pain/discomfort associated w/ interstitial cystitis* **Action:** Acts as buffer on bladder wall **Dose:** 100 mg PO tid on empty stomach w/ water 1 h ac or 2 h pc **Caution:** [B, ?/–] **Contra:** Hypersensitivity **Supplied:** Caps 100 mg **SE:** Alopecia, N/D, HA, ↑ LFTs, anticoagulant effects, thrombocytopenia **Notes:** Reassess Pts after 3 mo **Interactions:** Risk of ↑ anticoagulation w/ anticoagulants, ASA, thrombolytics

Pentoxifylline (Trental)   Uses: *Symptomatic management of peripheral vascular Dz* **Action:** Lowers blood cell viscosity by restoring erythrocyte flexibility **Dose:** *Adults.* 400 mg PO tid pc; treat for at least 8 wk to see full effect; ↓ to bid if GI or CNS effects occur **Caution:** [C, +/–] **Contra:** Cerebral or retinal hemorrhage **Supplied:** Tabs 400 mg **SE:** Dizziness, HA, GI upset **Interactions:** ↑ Effects w/ cimetidine, fluoroquinolones, H₂ antagonists, warfarin; ↑ effects of antihypertensives, theophylline **Labs:** ↓ Serum Ca²⁺, Mg²⁺ **NIPE:** Take w/ food

Pergolide (Permax)   Uses: *Parkinson's Dz* **Action:** Centrally active dopamine receptor agonist **Dose:** Initially, 0.05 mg PO tid, titrated q2–3d to desired effect; usual maint 2–3 mg/d in ÷ doses **Caution:** [B, ?/–] **Contra:** Ergot sensitivity **Supplied:** Tabs 0.05, 0.25, 1.0 mg **SE:** Dizziness, somnolence, confusion, nausea, constipation, dyskinesia, rhinitis, MI **Notes:** May cause hypotension during initiation of therapy **Interactions:** ↑ Risk of dyskinesia w/ levodopa; ↑ hypotension w/ antihypertensives; ↓ effects w/ antipsychotics, butyrophenones, haloperidol, metoclopramide, phenothiazines, thioxanthenes **Labs:** ↓ Prolactin **NIPE:** Take w/ food

Perindopril Erbumine (Aceon)   Uses: *HTN,* CHF, DN, post-MI **Action:** ACEI **Dose:** 4–8 mg/d; ⊘ taking w/ food; ↓ in elderly/renal impairment **Caution:** [C (1st tri, D 2nd and 3rd tri), ?/–] ACE-inhibitor–induced angioedema, **Contra:** Bilateral renal artery stenosis, primary hyperaldosteronism **Supplied:** Tabs 2, 4, 8 mg **SE:** HA, hypotension, dizziness, GI upset, cough **Notes:** Can use w/ diuretics **Interactions:** ↑ Effects w/ antihypertensives, diuretics; ↑ effects of cyclosporine, insulin, Li, sulfonylureas, tacrolimus; ↓ effects w/ NSAIDs **Labs:** ↑ Serum K⁺, LFTs, uric acid, cholesterol, creatinine **NIPE:** ↓ Effects if taken w/ food; risk of persistent cough

Permethrin (Nix, Elimite)   Uses: *Eradication of lice and scabies* **Action:** Pediculicide **Dose:** Adults & Peds. Saturate hair and scalp; allow 10 min before rinsing **Caution:** [B, ?/–] **Contra:** Hypersensitivity **Supplied:** Topical liq 1%; cream 5% **SE:** Local irritation **Notes:** Disinfect clothing, bedding, combs/brushes **NIPE:** Drug remains on hair up to 2 wk, reapply in 1 wk if live lice

Perphenazine (Trilafon) **Uses:** *Psychotic disorders, severe nausea,* intractable hiccups **Action:** Phenothiazine; blocks brain dopaminergic receptors **Dose:** *Antipsychotic:* 4–16 mg PO tid; max 64 mg/d. *Hiccups:* 5 mg IM q6h PRN or 1 mg IV at intervals not <1–2 mg/min, 5 mg max. *Peds.* 1–6 y: 4–6 mg/d PO in ÷ doses. *6–12 y:* 6 mg/d PO in ÷ doses. >12 y: 4–16 mg PO 2–4 ×/d; ↓ in hepatic insufficiency **Caution:** [C, ?/–] Narrow-angle glaucoma, severe hyper-/hypotension **Contra:** Phenothiazine sensitivity, bone marrow depression, severe liver or cardiac Dz **Supplied:** Tabs 2, 4, 8, 16 mg; PO conc 16 mg/5 mL; inj 5 mg/mL **SE:** Hypotension, tachycardia, bradycardia, EPS, drowsiness, Szs, photosensitivity, skin discoloration, blood dyscrasias, constipation **Interactions:** ↑ Effects w/ antidepressants; ↑ effects of anticholinergics, antidepressants, propranolol, phenytoin; ↑ CNS effects w/ CNS depressants, EtOH; ↓ effects w/ antacids, Li, phenobarbital, caffeine, tobacco; ↓ effects of levodopa, Li **Labs:** ↑ Serum cholesterol, glucose, ↓ uric acid, false + urine PRG test **NIPE:** Take oral dose w/ food; risk of photosensitivity—use sunscreen

Phenazopyridine (Pyridium, others) **Uses:** *Lower urinary tract irritation* **Action:** Local anesthetic on urinary tract mucosa **Dose:** *Adults.* 100–200 mg PO tid. *Peds.* 6–12 y: 12 mg/kg/24 h PO in 3 ÷ doses; ↓ in renal insufficiency **Caution:** [B, ?] Hepatic Dz **Contra:** Renal failure **Supplied:** Tabs 100, 200 mg **SE:** GI disturbances; causes red-orange urine color, which can stain clothing; HA, dizziness, acute renal failure, methemoglobinemia **Labs:** Interferes w/ urinary tests for glucose, ketones, bilirubin, protein, steroids **NIPE:** Urine may turn red; take pc

Phenelzine (Nardil) **Uses:** *Depression* **Action:** MAOI **Dose:** 15 mg tid. *Elderly:* 15–60 mg/d in ÷ doses **Caution:** [C, –] Interactions w/ SSRI, ergots, triptans **Contra:.** CHF, Hx liver Dz **Supplied:** Tabs 15 mg **SE:** May cause postural hypotension; edema, dizziness, sedation, rash, sexual dysfunction, xerostomia, constipation, urinary retention **Notes:** May take 2–4 wk to see effect; ⊘ tyramine-containing foods **Interactions:** ↑ HTN Rxn w/ amphetamines, fluoxetine, levodopa, metaraminol, phenylephrine, phenylpropanolamine, pseudoephedrine, reserpine, sertraline, tyramine, EtOH, foods w/ tyramine, caffeine, tryptophan; ↑ effects of barbiturates, narcotics, sedatives, sumatriptan, TCAs, ephedra, ginseng **Labs:** ↓ Glucose, false + ↑ in bilirubin & uric acid

Phenobarbital [C-IV] **Uses:** *Sz disorders,* insomnia, and anxiety **Action:** Barbiturate **Dose:** *Adults.* Sedative–hypnotic: 30–120 mg PO or IM PRN. *Anticonvulsant:* Load 10–12 mg/kg in 3 ÷ doses, then 1–3 mg/kg/24 h PO, IM, or IV. *Peds.* Sedative–hypnotic: 2–3 mg/kg/24 h PO or IM hs PRN. *Anticonvulsant:* Load 15–20 mg/kg ÷ in 2 equal doses 4 h apart, then 3–5 mg/kg/24h PO ÷ in 2–3 doses. **Caution:** [D, M] **Contra:** Porphyria, liver dysfunction **Supplied:** Tabs 8, 15, 16, 30, 32, 60, 65, 100 mg; elixir 15, 20 mg/5 mL; inj 30, 60, 65, 130 mg/mL **SE:** Bradycardia, hypotension, hangover, Stevens–Johnson syndrome, blood dyscrasias, resp depression **Notes:** Tolerance develops to sedation; paradoxic hyperactivity seen in pediatric Pts; long half-life allows single daily dosing (see Table

2, page 265) **Interactions:** ↑ CNS depression w/ CNS depressants, anesthetics, antianxiety meds, antihistamines, narcotic analgesics, EtOH, Indian snakeroot, kava kava; ↑ effects w/ chloramphenicol, MAOIs, procarbazine, valproic acid; ↓ effects w/ rifampin; ↓ effects of anticoagulants, BBs, carbamazepine, clozapine, corticosteroids, doxorubicin, doxycycline, estrogens, felodipine, griseofulvin, haloperidol, methadone, metronidazole, oral contraceptives, phenothiazines, quinidine, TCAs, theophylline, verapamil **Labs:** ↑ LFTs, creatinine, ↑ or ↓ bilirubin **NIPE:** May take 2–3 wk for full effects, ⊘ DC abruptly

Phenylephrine (Neo-Synephrine)   Uses: *Vascular failure in shock, hypersensitivity, or drug-induced hypotension; nasal congestion*; mydriatic **Action:** α-Adrenergic agonist **Dose: Adults.** Mild/moderate hypotension: 2–5 mg IM or SQ elevates BP for 2 h; 0.1–0.5 mg IV elevates BP for 15 min. *Severe hypotension/shock:* Cont inf at 100–180 mg/min; after BP stabilized, maint rate of 40–60 mg/min. *Nasal congestion:* 1–2 sprays/nostril PRN. *Ophth:* 1 gtt 15–30 min before exam. **Peds.** Hypotension: 5–20 µg/kg/dose IV q10–15 min or 0.1–0.5 mg/kg/min IV inf, titrate to effect. *Nasal congestion:* 1 spray/nostril q3–4h PRN **Caution:** [C, +/–] HTN, acute pancreatitis, hepatitis, coronary Dz, narrow-angle glaucoma, hyperthyroidism **Contra:** Bradycardia, arrhythmias **Supplied:** Inj 10 mg/mL; nasal soln 0.125, 0.16, 0.25, 0.5, 1%; ophth soln 0.12, 2.5, 10% **SE:** Arrhythmias, HTN, peripheral vasoconstriction activity potentiated by oxytocin, MAOIs, and TCAs; HA, weakness, necrosis, ↓ renal perfusion **Notes:** Promptly restore blood volume if loss has occurred; use large veins for inf to avoid extravasation; phentolamine 10 mg in 10–15 mL of NS for local inj as antidote for extravasation **Interactions:** ↑ HTN w/ BBs, MAOIs; ↑ pressor response w/ guanethidine, methyldopa, reserpine, TCAs

Phenytoin (Dilantin)   Uses: *Sz disorders* Action: Inhibits Sz spread in the motor cortex **Dose:** *Load: Adults & Peds.* 15–20 mg/kg IV, max inf rate 25 mg/min or PO in 400-mg doses at 4-h intervals. *Maint: Adults.* Initially, 200 mg PO or IV bid or 300 mg hs; then follow serum levels. *Peds.* 4–7 mg/kg/24h PO or IV + qd–bid; ⊘ PO susp if possible due to erratic absorption **Caution:** [D, +] **Contra:** Heart block, sinus bradycardia **Supplied:** Caps 30, 100 mg; chew tabs 50 mg; PO susp 30, 125 mg/5 mL; inj 50 mg/mL **SE:** Nystagmus and ataxia early signs of toxicity; gum hyperplasia w/ long-term use. *IV:* Hypotension, bradycardia, arrhythmias, phlebitis; peripheral neuropathy, rash, blood dyscrasias, Stevens–Johnson syndrome **Notes:** Follow levels (see Table 2, page 265); phenytoin is bound to albumin, and levels reflect bound and free phenytoin; in the presence of ↓ albumin and azotemia, low phenytoin levels may be therapeutic (normal free levels); changes in dosage (↑ or ↓) should not be carried out at intervals shorter than 7–10 d **Interactions:** ↑ Effects w/ amiodarone, allopurinol, chloramphenicol, disulfiram, INH, omeprazole, sulfonamides, quinolones, trimethoprim, ↑ effects of Li; ↓ effects w/ cimetidine, cisplatin, diazoxide, folate, pyridoxine, rifampin; ↓ effects of

azole antifungals, benzodiazepines, carbamazepine, corticosteroids, cyclosporine, digitalis glycosides, doxycycline, furosemide, levodopa, oral contraceptives, quinidine, tacrolimus, theophylline, thyroid meds, valproic acid **Labs:** ↑ Serum cholesterol, glucose, alkaline phosphatase **NIPE:** Take w/ food; may alter urine color; use barrier contraception; ⊘ DC abruptly

Physostigmine (Antilirium) Uses: *Antidote for TCA, atropine, and scopolamine OD; glaucoma* **Action:** Reversible cholinesterase inhibitor **Dose:** *Adults.* 2 mg IV or IM q 20 min. *Peds.* 0.01–0.03 mg/kg/dose IV q15–30 min up to total of 2 mg if needed **Caution:** [C, ?] **Contra:** GI or GU obstruction, CV Dz **Supplied:** Inj 1 mg/mL; ophth oint 0.25% **SE:** Rapid IV admin associated w/ convulsions; cholinergic side effects; asystole sweating, salivation, lacrimation, GI upset, changes in heart rate **Notes:** Excessive readministration of physostigmine can result in cholinergic crisis; cholinergic crisis reversed w/ atropine **Interactions:** ↑ Resp depression w/ succinylcholine, ↑ effects w/ cholinergics, jaborandi tree, pill-bearing spurge **Labs:** ↑ ALT, AST, serum amylase

Phytonadione [Vitamin K] (AquaMEPHYTON, others) Uses: *Coagulation disorders caused by faulty formation of factors II, VII, IX, and X*; hyperalimentation **Action:** Cofactor for the production of factors II, VII, IX, and X **Dose:** *Adults and Children.* Anticoagulant-induced prothrombin deficiency: 1–10 mg PO or IV slowly. *Hyperalimentation:* 10 mg IM or IV qwk. *Infants.* 0.5–1 mg/dose IM, SQ, or PO **Caution:** [C, +] **Contra:** Hypersensitivity **Supplied:** Tabs 5 mg; inj 2, 10 mg/mL **SE:** Anaphylaxis can result from IV dosage; administer IV slowly; GI upset (PO), inj site Rxns **Notes:** W/ parenteral Rx, the 1st change in prothrombin usually seen in 12–24 h **Interactions:** ↓ Effects w/ antibiotics, cholestyramine, colestipol, salicylates, sucralfate; ↓ effects of oral anticoagulants **Labs:** Falsely ↑ urine steroids

Pimecrolimus (Elidel) Uses: *Atopic dermatitis* **Action:** T-lymphocyte inhibition **Dose:** Apply bid for at least 1 wk following resolution **Caution:** [C, ?/–] Caution w/ local infection, lymphadenopathy **Contra:** Hypersensitivity **Supplied:** Ointment 0.03%, 0.1%; 30-g, 60-g tubes **SE:** Phototoxicity, local irritation/burning, flu-like Sxs **Notes:** apply to dry skin only; wash hands after use

Pindolol (Visken) Uses: *HTN* **Action:** β-Adrenergic receptor blocker, β_1, β_2, ISA **Dose:** 5–10 mg bid, 60 mg/d max; ↓ in hepatic/renal failure **Caution:** [B (1st tri; D if 2nd or 3rd tri), +/–] **Contra:** Uncompensated CHF, cardiogenic shock, bradycardia, heart block, asthma, COPD **Supplied:** Tabs 5, 10 mg **SE:** Insomnia, dizziness, fatigue, edema, GI upset, dyspnea; fluid retention may exacerbate CHF **Interactions:** ↑ Effects w/ amiodarone, antihypertensives, diuretics; ↓ effects w/ NSAIDs; ↓ effect of hypoglycemics **Labs:** ↑ LFTs, uric acid **NIPE:** ⊘ DC abruptly; ↑ cold sensitivity

Pioglitazone (Actos) Uses: *Type 2 DM* **Action:** ↑ Insulin sensitivity **Dose:** 15–45 mg/d **Caution:** [C, –] **Contra:** Hepatic impairment **Supplied:** Tabs

15, 30, 45 mg **SE:** Weight gain, URI, HA, hypoglycemia, edema **Interactions:** ↑ Effects w/ ketoconazole; ↓ effects of oral contraceptives **Labs:** ↑ LFTs, ↓ Hmg, Hct **NIPE:** Take w/o regard to food; use barrier contraception

Piperacillin (Pipracil) Uses: *Infections of skin, bone, resp tract, urinary tract, and abdomen, and septicemia* **Action:** 4th-gen PCN; bactericidal; inhibits cell wall synthesis. *Spectrum:* Primarily gram(+) better *Enterococcus, H. influenza*, not staph; gram(–) *E. coli, Proteus, Shigella, Pseudomonas*, not β-lactamase-producing **Dose: Adults.** 3 g IV q4–6h. **Peds.** 200–300 mg/kg/d IV ÷ q4–6h; ↓ dose in renal failure **Caution:** [B, M] Penicillin sensitivity **Supplied:** Inj **SE:** ↓ Plt aggregation, interstitial nephritis, renal failure, anaphylaxis, hemolytic anemia **Notes:** Often used in combination w/ aminoglycoside **Interactions:** ↑ Effects w/ probenecid; ↑ effects of anticoagulants, MRX; ↓ effects w/ macrolides, tetracyclines; ↓ effects of oral contraceptives **Labs:** ↑ LFTs, BUN, creatinine, + direct Coombs' test, ↓ K⁺ **NIPE:** Inactivation of aminoglycosides if drugs given together—admin at least 1 h apart

Piperacillin–Tazobactam (Zosyn) Uses: *Infections involving skin, bone, resp tract, urinary tract, and abdomen, and septicemia* **Action:** PCN plus β-lactamase inhibitor; bactericidal; inhibits cell wall synthesis. *Spectrum:* Good gram(+), excellent gram(–); covers β-lactamase producers **Dose: Adults.** 3.375–4.5 g IV q6h; ↓ dose in renal failure **Caution:** [B, M] Penicillin or β-lactam sensitivity **Supplied:** Inj **SE:** Diarrhea, HA, insomnia, GI upset, serum sickness-like Rxn, pseudomembranous colitis **Notes:** Often used in combination w/ aminoglycoside. See Piperacillin Interactions; **Additional Labs:** ↓ Hmg, Hct, protein, albumin

Pirbuterol (Maxair) Uses: *Prevention and Rx of reversible bronchospasm* **Action:** β₂-Adrenergic agonist **Dose:** 2 inhal q4–6h; max 12 inhal/d **Caution:** [C, ?/–] **Supplied:** Aerosol 0.2 mg/actuation; Autohaler dry powder 0.2 mg/actuation **SE:** Nervousness, restlessness, trembling, HA, taste changes, tachycardia **Interactions:** ↑ Effects w/ epinephrine, sympathomimetics; ↑ vascular effects w/ MAOIs, TCAs; ↓ effects w/ BBs **NIPE:** Rinse mouth after use; shake well before use

Piroxicam (Feldene) Uses: *Arthritis and pain* **Action:** NSAID; inhibits prostaglandins **Dose:** 10–20 mg/d **Caution:** [B (1st tri; D if 3rd tri or near term), +] GI bleeding **Contra:** ASA or NSAID sensitivity **Supplied:** Caps 10, 20 mg **SE:** Dizziness, rash, GI upset, edema, acute renal failure, peptic ulcer **Interactions:** ↑ Effects w/ probenecid; ↑ effects of aminoglycosides, anticoagulants, hypoglycemics, Li, MRX; ↑ risk of bleeding w/ ASA, corticosteroids, NSAIDs, feverfew, garlic, ginger, ginkgo biloba, EtOH; ↓ effect w/ ASA, antacids, cholestyamine; ↓ effect of BBs, diuretics **Labs:** ↑ BUN, LFTs, serum Cl, serum Na, PT **NIPE:** Take w/ food, full effect after 2 wk admin; ↑ risk of photosensitivity—use sunscreen

Plasma Protein Fraction (Plasmanate, others) Uses: *Shock and hypotension* **Action:** Plasma volume expander **Dose:** Initial, 250–500 mL IV (not >10 mL/min); subsequent inf depends on clinical response. **Peds.** 10–15

mL/kg/dose IV; subsequent inf depends on clinical response **Caution:** [C, +] **Contra:** Renal insufficiency, CHF **Supplied:** Inj 5% **SE:** Hypotension associated w/ rapid inf; hypocoagulability, metabolic acidosis, PE **Notes:** 130–160 mEq Na/L; not substitute for RBC

Pneumococcal 7-Valent Conjugate Vaccine (Prevnar) **Uses:** *Immunization against pneumococcal infections in infants and children* **Action:** Active immunization **Dose:** 0.5 mL IM/dose; series of 3 doses; 1st dose at 2 mo of age w/ subsequent doses q2mo **Caution:** [C, +] Thrombocytopenia **Contra:** Diphtheria toxoid sensitivity, febrile illness **Supplied:** Inj **SE:** Local Rxns, arthralgia, fever, myalgia

Pneumococcal Vaccine, Polyvalent (Pneumovax-23) **Uses:** *Immunization against pneumococcal infections in Pts predisposed or at high risk (all people ≥65 y of age)* **Action:** Active immunization **Dose:** 0.5 mL IM. **Caution:** [C, ?] **Contra:** ⊘ vaccinate during immunosuppressive therapy **Supplied:** Inj 25 mg each of polysaccharide isolates per 0.5-mL dose **SE:** Fever, inj site Rxn, hemolytic anemia, thrombocytopenia, anaphylaxis **Interactions:** ↓ Effects w/ corticosteroids, immunosuppressants

Podophyllin (Podocon-25, Condylox Gel 0.5%, Condylox) **Uses:** *Topical therapy of benign growths (genital and perianal warts [condylomata acuminata],* papillomas, fibromas) **Action:** Direct antimitotic effect; exact mechanism unknown **Dose:** *Condylox gel and Condylox:* Apply 3 consecutive d/wk for 4 wk. *Podocon-25:* Use sparingly on the lesion, leave on for 1–4 h, then thoroughly wash off **Caution:** [C, ?] Immunosuppression **Contra:** DM, bleeding lesions **Supplied:** Podocon-25 (w/benzoin) 15-mL bottles; Condylox gel 0.5% 35 g clear gel; Condylox soln 0.5% 35 g clear **SE:** Local Rxns, significant absorption; anemias, tachycardia, paresthesias, GI upset, renal/hepatic damage **Notes:** Podocon-25 applied only by the clinician; ⊘ dispense

Polyethylene Glycol [PEG]–Electrolyte Solution (GoLYTELY, CoLyte) **Uses:** *Bowel prep prior to examination or surgery* **Action:** Osmotic cathartic **Dose:** *Adults.* Following 3–4-h fast, drink 240 mL of soln q10min until 4 L consumed. *Peds.* 25–40 mL/kg/h for 4–10 h **Caution:** [C, ?] **Contra:** GI obstruction, bowel perforation, megacolon, ulcerative colitis **Supplied:** Powder for reconstitution to 4 L **SE:** Cramping or nausea, bloating **Notes:** 1st BM should occur in approximately 1 h

Polyethylene Glycol [PEG] 3350 (MiraLax) **Uses:** *Occasional constipation* **Action:** Osmotic laxative **Dose:** 17 g powder (1 heaping tablespoon) in 8 oz (1 cup) of water and drink; max 14 d **Caution:** [C, ?] R/o bowel obstruction before use **Contra:** GI obstruction, allergy to PEG **Supplied:** Powder for reconstitution; bottle cap holds 17 g **SE:** Upset stomach, bloating, cramping, gas, severe diarrhea, hives **Notes:** Can add to water, juice, soda, coffee, or tea

Polymyxin B & Hydrocortisone (Otobiotic Otic) **Uses:** *Superficial bacterial infections of external ear canal* **Action:** Antibiotic antiinflammatory combination **Dose:** 4 gtt in ear(s) tid–qid **Caution:** [B, ?] **Supplied:** Soln polymyxin B 10,000 Units/hydrocortisone 0.5%/mL **SE:** Local irritation **Notes:** Useful in neomycin allergy

Potassium Citrate (Urocit-K) **Uses:** *Alkalinize urine, prevention of urinary stones (uric acid, Ca stones if hypocitraturic)* **Action:** Urinary alkalinizer **Dose:** 10–20 mEq PO tid w/ meals, max 100 mEq/d **Caution:** [A, +] **Contra:** Severe renal impairment, dehydration, hyperkalemia, peptic ulcer; use of K-sparing diuretics or salt substitutes **Supplied:** 540-, 1080-mg tabs **SE:** GI upset, hypocalcemia, hyperkalemia, metabolic alkalosis **Notes:** Tabs 540 mg = 5 mEq, 1080 mg = 10 mEq **Interactions:** ↑ Risk of hyperkalemia w/ACEIs, K-sparing diuretics

Potassium Citrate & Citric Acid (Polycitra-K) **Uses:** *Alkalinize urine, prevent urinary stones (uric acid, Ca stones if hypocitraturic)* **Action:** Urinary alkalinizer **Dose:** 10–20 mEq PO tid w/ meals, max 100 mEq/d **Caution:** [A, +] **Contra:** Severe renal impairment, dehydration, hyperkalemia, peptic ulcer; use of K-sparing diuretics or salt substitutes **Supplied:** Soln 10 mEq/5 mL; powder 30 mEq/packet **SE:** GI upset, hypocalcemia, hyperkalemia, metabolic alkalosis **Interactions:** ↑ Risk of hyperkalemia w/ACEIs, K-sparing diuretics

Potassium Iodide [Lugol's Solution] (SSKI, Thyro-Block) **Uses:** *Thyroid storm,* reduction of vascularity before thyroid surgery, block thyroid uptake of radioactive isotopes of I, thin bronchial secretions **Action:** I suppl **Dose:** *Adults & Peds.* >2 y: Preop thyroidectomy: 50–250 mg PO tid (2–6 gtt strong I soln); administer 10 d preop. *Peds.* 1 y: Thyroid crisis: 300 mg (6 gtt SSKI q8h). *Peds. <1 y:* ½ adult dose **Caution:** [D, +] Hyperkalemia, tuberculosis, PE, bronchitis, renal impairment **Contra:** I sensitivity **Supplied:** Tabs 130 mg; soln (SSKI) 1 g/mL; Lugol's soln, strong I 100 mg/mL; syrup 325 mg/5 mL **SE:** Fever, HA, urticaria, angioedema, goiter, GI upset, eosinophilia **Interactions:** ↑ Risk of hypothyroidism w/ antithyroid drugs and Li; ↑ risk of hyperkalemia w/ACEIs, K-sparing diuretics, K suppls **Labs:** May alter TFTs **NIPE:** Take pc w/ food or milk

Potassium Supplements (Kaon, Kaochlor, K-Lor, Slow-K, Micro-K, Klorvess, others) **Uses:** *Prevention or Rx of hypokalemia* (eg, diuretic use) **Action:** K suppl **Dose:** *Adults.* 20–100 mEq/d PO ÷ qd–bid; IV 10–20 mEq/h, max 40 mEq/h and 150 mEq/d (monitor K⁺ levels frequently w/high-dose IV). *Peds.* Calculate K deficit; 1–3 mEq/kg/d PO ÷ qd–qid; IV max dose 0.5–1 mEq/kg/h **Caution:** [A, +] Renal insufficiency, use w/inSAIDs and ACEIs **Contra:** Hyperkalemia **Supplied:** PO forms (see Table 8, page 280); injectable forms **SE:** Can cause GI irritation; bradycardia, hyperkalemia, heart block **Notes:** Mix powder and liquid w/ beverage (unsalted tomato juice, etc); follow serum K⁺; Cl⁻ salt recommended in coexisting alkalosis; for coexisting acidosis use acetate, bicarbonate, citrate, or gluconate salt **Interactions:** ↑ Effects w/ ACEI, K-sparing diuretics, salt substitutes **NIPE:** Take w/ food

Pramipexole (Mirapex) **Uses:** *Parkinson's Dz* **Action:** Dopamine agonist **Dose:** 1.5–4.5 mg/d, initial 0.375 mg/d in 3 ÷ doses; titrate slowly **Caution:**

[C, ?/–] **Contra:** Component hypersensitivity **Supplied:** Tabs 0.125, 0.25, 1, 1.5 mg **SE:** Postural hypotension, asthenia, somnolence, abnormal dreams, GI upset, EPS **Interactions:** ↑ Effects w/ cimetidine, diltiazem, quinidine, quinine, ranitidine, triamterene, verapamil; ↑ effects of levodopa; ↑ CNS depression w/ CNS depressants, EtOH; ↓ effects w/ antipsychotics, butyrophenones, metoclopramide, phenothiazines, thioxanthenes **NIPE:** May take w/ food; ⊘ DC abruptly

Pramoxine (Anusol Ointment, Proctofoam-NS, others)

Uses: *Relief of pain and itching from hemorrhoids and anorectal surgery*; topical for burns and dermatosis **Action:** Topical anesthetic **Dose:** Apply cream, oint, gel, or spray freely to anal area q3h **Caution:** [C, ?] **Supplied:** [OTC] All 1%; foam (Proctofoam-NS), cream, oint, lotion, gel, pads, spray **SE:** Contact dermatitis **NIPE:** ⊘ Use on large areas

Pramoxine + Hydrocortisone (Enzone, Proctofoam-HC)

Uses: *Relief of pain and itching from hemorrhoids* **Action:** Topical anesthetic, antiinflammatory **Dose:** Apply freely to anal area tid–qid **Caution:** [C, ?/–] **Supplied:** Cream pramoxine 1% acetate 0.5/1%; foam pramoxine 1% hydrocortisone 1%; lotion pramoxine 1% hydrocortisone 0.25/1/2.5%, pramoxine 2.5% and hydrocortisone 1% **SE:** Contact dermatitis **NIPE:** ⊘ Use on large areas

Pravastatin (Pravachol)

Uses: ↓ Cholesterol **Action:** HMG-CoA reductase inhibitor **Dose:** 10–40 mg PO hs; ↓ dose in significant renal/hepatic insufficiency **Caution:** [X, –] **Contra:** Liver Dz or persistent LFT ↑ **Supplied:** Tabs 10, 20, 40 mg **SE:** Use caution w/ concurrent gemfibrozil; HA, GI upset, hepatitis, myopathy, renal failure **Interactions:** ↑ Risk of myopathy & rhabdomyolysis w/ clarithromycin, clofibrate, cyclosporine, danazol, erythromycin, fluoxetine, gemfibrozil, niacin, nefazodone, troleandomycin; ↑ effects w/ azole antifungals, cimetidine, grapefruit juice; ↓ effects w/ cholestyramine, isradipine **Labs:** ↑ LFTs **NIPE:** ⊘ PRG, breast-feeding; take w/o regard to food; full effect may take up to 4 wks; ↑ risk of photosensitivity—use sunscreen

Prazosin (Minipress)

Uses: *HTN* **Action:** Peripherally acting α-adrenergic blocker **Dose:** *Adults.* 1 mg PO tid; can ↑ to max daily dose of up to 20 mg/d. *Peds.* 5–25 µg/kg/dose q6h, up to 25 µg/kg/dose **Caution:** [C, ?] **Contra:** Component hypersensitivity **Supplied:** Caps 1, 2, 5 mg **SE:** Dizziness, edema, palpitations, fatigue, GI upset **Notes:** Can cause orthostatic hypotension, take the 1st dose hs; tolerance develops to this effect; tachyphylaxis may result **Interactions:** ↑ Hypotension w/ antihypertensives, diuretics, nitrates, EtOH; ↓ effects w/ NSAIDs, butcher's broom **Labs:** ↑ Serum Na levels, vanillylmandelic acid level; alters test for pheochromocytoma **NIPE:** ⊘ DC abruptly

Prednisolone

[See Table 4, page 271] **Interactions:** ↑ Effects w/ clarithromycin, erythromycin, estrogen, ketoconazole, oral contraceptives, troleandomycin; ↓ effects w/ antacids, aminoglutethimide, barbiturates, cholestyramine, colestipol, phenytoin, rifampin; ↓ effects of anticoagulants, hypoglycemics, INH, salicylates, vaccine toxoids **Labs:** False – skin allergy tests; false ↑ cortisol, digoxin, theophylline **NIPE:** ⊘ Use live virus vaccines, ⊘ DC abruptly; take w/ food.

Prednisone [See Table 4, page 271] **Interactions:** ↑ Effects w/ clarithromycin, cyclosporine, erythromycin, estrogen, ketoconazole, oral contraceptives, troleandomycin; ↓ effects w/ antacids, aminoglutethimide, barbiturates, carbamazepine, cholestyramine, colestipol, phenytoin, rifampin; ↓ effects of anticoagulants, hypoglycemics, INH, salicylates, vaccine toxoids **Labs:** False − skin allergy tests, false ↑ cortisol, digoxin, theophylline **NIPE:** Take w/ food; ⊘ use live virus vaccine, ⊘ DC abruptly, infection may be masked

Probenecid (Benemid, others) **Uses:** *Prevent gout and hyperuricemia; prolongs serum levels of penicillins or cephalosporins* **Action:** Renal tubular blocking agent **Dose:** *Adults.* Gout: 250 mg bid for 1 wk, then 0.5 g PO bid; can ↑ by 500 mg/mo up to 2–3 g/d. *Antibiotic effect:* 1–2 g PO 30 min before antibiotic dose. *Peds.* >2 y: 25 mg/kg, then 40 mg/kg/d PO ÷ qid **Caution:** [B, ?] **Contra:** High-dose ASA, moderate–severe renal impairment, age <2 y **Supplied:** Tabs 500 mg **SE:** HA, GI upset, rash, pruritus, dizziness, blood dyscrasias **Notes:** ⊘ Use during acute gout attack **Interactions:** ↑ Effects of acyclovir, allopurinol; ↑ effects of benzodiazepines, cephalosporins, ciprofloxacin, clofibrate, dapsone, dyphylline, MRX, NSAIDs, olanzapine, rifampin, sulfonamides, sulfonylureas zidovudine; ↓ effects w/ niacin, EtOH; ↓ effects of penicillamine **Labs:** False + urine glucose; false ↑ level of theophylline **NIPE:** Take w/ food, ↑ fluids to 2–3 L/d; ⊘ ASA, NSAIDs, salicylates

Procainamide (Pronestyl, Procan) **Uses:** *Supraventricular and ventricular arrhythmias* **Action:** Class 1A antiarrhythmic; depresses the excitability of cardiac muscle to electrical stimulation and slows conduction in the atrium, bundle of His, ventricle **Dose:** *Adults.* Recurrent VF/VT: 20 mg/min IV (max total 17 mg/kg). *Maint:* 1–4 mg/min. *Stable wide-complex tachycardia of unknown origin, AF w/ rapid rate in WPW:* 20 mg/min IV until arrhythmia suppression, hypotension, QRS widens >50%, then 1–4 mg/min. *Chronic dosing:* 50 mg/kg/d PO in ÷ doses q4–6h. *Peds.* Chronic maint: 15–50 mg/kg/24 h PO ÷ q3–6h; ↓ in renal/hepatic impairment **Caution:** [C, +] **Contra:** Complete heart block. 2nd- or 3rd-degree heart block w/o pacemaker, torsades de pointes, SLE **Supplied:** Tabs and caps 250, 375, 500 mg; SR tabs 250, 500, 750, 1000 mg; inj 100, 500 mg/mL **SE:** Can cause hypotension and a lupus-like syndrome; GI upset, taste perversion, arrhythmias, tachycardia, heart block, angioneuropathic edema **Notes:** Follow levels (see Table 2, page 265) **Interactions:** ↑ Effects w/ acetazolamide, amiodarone, cimetidine, ranitidine, trimethoprim; ↑ effects of anticholinergics, antihypertensives; ↓ effects w/ procaine, EtOH **Labs:** ↑ LFTs, + Coombs' test **NIPE:** Take w/ food if GI upset, ⊘ crush SR tab

Procarbazine (Matulane) **WARNING:** Highly toxic; handle w/ care **Uses:** *Hodgkin's Dz,* NHL, brain tumors **Action:** Alkylating agent; inhibits DNA and RNA synthesis **Dose:** Refer to specific protocol **Caution:** [D, ?] W/

EtOH ingestion **Contra:** Inadequate bone marrow reserve **Supplied:** Caps 50 mg **SE:** Myelosuppression, hemolytic Rxns (w/ G6PD deficiency), N/V/D; disulfiram-like Rxn; cutaneous Rxns; constitutional Sxs, myalgia, and arthralgia; CNS effects, azoospermia, and cessation of menses **Interactions:** ↑ CNS depression w/ antihistamines, antihypertensives, barbiturates, CNS depressants, narcotics, phenothiazines; ↑ effects of hypoglycemics; ↑ risk of HTN w/ guanethidine, levodopa, MAOIs, methyldopa, sympathomimetics, TCAs, tyramine-containing foods; ↓ effects of digoxin **NIPE:** Disulfiram-like Rxn w/ EtOH; ↑ fluids to 2–3 L/d; ↑ risk of photosensitivity—use sunscreen; ⊘ exposure to infection

Prochlorperazine (Compazine)

Uses: *N/V, agitation, and psychotic disorders* **Action:** Phenothiazine; blocks postsynaptic dopaminergic CNS receptors **Dose:** *Adults.* Antiemetic: 5–10 mg PO tid–qid or 25 mg PR bid or 5–10 mg deep IM q4–6h. *Antipsychotic:* 10–20 mg IM acutely or 5–10 mg PO tid–qid for maint; ↑ doses may be required for antipsychotic effect. *Peds.* 0.1–0.15 mg/kg/dose IM q4–6h or 0.4 mg/kg/24 h PO ÷ tid–qid **Caution:** [C, +/–] Narrow-angle glaucoma, severe liver/cardiac Dz **Contra:** Phenothiazine sensitivity, bone marrow suppression **Supplied:** Tabs 5, 10, 25 mg; SR caps 10, 15, 30 mg; syrup 5 mg/5 mL; supp 2.5, 5, 25 mg; inj 5 mg/mL **SE:** EPS common; treat w/ diphenhydramine **Interactions:** ↑ Effects w/ chloroquine, indomethacin, narcotics, procarbazine, SSRIs, pyrimethamine; ↑ effects of antidepressants, BBs, EtOH; ↓ effects w/ antacids, anticholinergics, barbiturates, tobacco; ↓ effects of guanethidine, levodopa, Li **Labs:** False + urine bilirubin, amylase, phenylketonuria, ↑ serum prolactin **NIPE:** ⊘ DC abruptly; ↑ risk of photosensitivity—use sunscreen; urine may turn pink/red

Promethazine (Phenergan)

Uses: *N/V, motion sickness* **Action:** Phenothiazine; blocks postsynaptic mesolimbic dopaminergic receptors in the brain **Dose:** *Adults.* 12.5–50 mg PO, PR, or IM bid–qid PRN. *Peds.* 0.1–0.5 mg/kg/dose PO or IM q2–6h PRN **Caution:** [C, +/–] **Contra:** Component hypersensitivity, narrow-angle glaucoma **Supplied:** Tabs 12.5, 25, 50 mg; syrup 6.25 mg/5 mL, 25 mg/5 mL; supp 12.5, 25, 50 mg; inj 25, 50 mg/mL **SE:** Drowsiness, tardive dyskinesia, EPS, lowered Sz threshold, hypotension, GI upset, blood dyscrasias, photosensitivity **Interactions:** ↑ Effects w/ CNS depressants, MAOIs, EtOH; ↑ effects of antihypertensives; ↓ effects w/ anticholinergics, barbiturates, tobacco; ↓ effect of levodopa **NIPE:** Effects skin allergy tests; use sunscreen for photosensitivity

Propafenone (Rythmol)

Uses: *Life-threatening ventricular arrhythmias and AF* **Action:** Class IC antiarrhythmic; blocks the fast inward Na current in heart muscle and Purkinje fibers, and slows the rate of ↑ of phase 0 of the action potential **Dose:** *Adults.* 150–300 mg PO q8h. *Peds.* 8–10 mg/kg/d ÷ in 3–4 doses; may ↑ 2 mg/kg/d, to max of 20 mg/kg/d **Caution:** [C, ?] Amprenavir or ritonavir use **Contra:** Uncontrolled CHF, bronchospasm, cardiogenic shock, conduction disorders **Supplied:** Tabs 150, 225, 300 mg **SE:** Dizziness, unusual taste, 1st-degree heart block, arrhythmias, prolongation of QRS and QT intervals; fatigue, GI upset, blood dyscrasias **Interactions:** ↑ Effects w/ cimetidine, quinidine; ↑ effects of anticoagulants, BBs, digitalis glycosides, theophylline; ↓ effects w/ rifampin, phenobarbital, rifabutin **Labs:** ↑ ANA titers **NIPE:** Take w/o regard to food

Propantheline (Pro-Banthine) **Uses:** *PUD,* symptomatic Rx of small intestine hypermotility, spastic colon, ureteral spasm, bladder spasm, pylorospasm **Action:** Antimuscarinic agent **Dose:** *Adults.* 15 mg PO ac and 30 mg PO hs; ↓ dose in elderly. *Peds.* 2–3 mg/kg/24h PO ÷ tid–qid **Caution:** [C, ?] **Contra:** Narrow-angle glaucoma, ulcerative colitis, toxic megacolon, GI or GU obstruction **Supplied:** Tabs 7.5, 15 mg **SE:** Anticholinergic side effects (xerostomia and blurred vision common) **Interactions:** ↑ Anticholinergic effects w/ antihistamines, antidepressants, atropine, haloperidol, phenothiazines, quinidine, TCAs; ↑ effects of atenolol, digoxin; ↓ effects w/ antacids **NIPE:** May cause heat intolerance, ↑ risk of photosensitivity—use sunscreen

Propofol (Diprivan) **Uses:** *Induction or maint of anesthesia; continuous sedation in intubated Pts* **Action:** Sedative–hypnotic; mechanism unknown **Dose:** *Adults.* 2–2.5 mg/kg induction, then 0.1–0.2 mg/kg/min inf. *ICU sedation:* 5–50 µg/kg/min cont inf; ↓ dose in elderly, debilitated, or ASA II or IV Pts. *Peds. Anesthesia:* 2.5–3.5 mg/kg induction; then 125–300 µg/kg/min **Caution:** [B, +] **Contra:** When general anesthesia is contraindicated **Supplied:** Inj 10 mg/mL **SE:** May ↑ triglycerides w/ extended dosing; hypotension, pain at inj site, apnea, anaphylaxis **Notes:** 1 mL of propofol contains 0.1 g fat **Interactions:** ↑ Effects w/ antihistamines, opioids, hypnotics, EtOH **Labs:** ↓ Serum cortisol levels

Propoxyphene (Darvon); Propoxyphene & Acetaminophen (Darvocet); & Propoxyphene & Aspirin (Darvon Compound-65, Darvon-N + Aspirin) [C-IV] **Uses:** *Mild–moderate pain* **Action:** Narcotic analgesic **Dose:** 1–2 PO q4h PRN; ↓ in hepatic impairment, elderly **Caution:** [C (D if prolonged use), M] Hepatic impairment (APAP), peptic ulcer (ASA); severe renal impairment **Contra:** Hypersensitivity **Supplied:** *Darvon:* Propoxyphene HCl caps 65 mg. *Darvon-N:* Propoxyphene napsylate 100-mg tabs. *Darvocet-N:* Propoxyphene napsylate 50 mg/APAP 325 mg. *Darvocet-N 100:* Propoxyphene napsylate 100 mg/APAP 650 mg. *Darvon Compound-65:* Propoxyphene HCl caps 65-mg/ASA 389 mg/caffeine 32 mg. *Darvon-N w/ ASA:* Propoxyphene napsylate 100 mg/ASA 325 mg **SE:** OD can be lethal; hypotension, dizziness, sedation, GI upset, ↑ levels on LFTs **Interactions:** ↑ CNS depression w/ antidepressants, antihistamines, barbiturates, glutethimide, methocarbamol, protease inhibitors, EtOH, St. John's wort; ↑ effects of BBs, carbamazepine, MAOIs, phenobarbital, TCAs, warfarin; ↓ effects w/ tobacco **Labs:** ↑ LFTs, serum amylase, lipase **NIPE:** Take w/ food if GI upset

Propranolol (Inderal) **Uses:** *HTN, angina, MI, hyperthyroidism, essential tremor, hypertropic subaortic stenosis, pheochromocytoma; prevents migraines and atrial arrhythmias* **Action:** β-Adrenergic receptor blocker, β₁, β₂; only BB to block conversion of T_4 to T_3 **Dose:** *Adults.* Angina: 80–320 mg/d PO ÷ bid–qid or 80–160 mg/d SR. *Arrhythmia:* 10–80 mg PO tid–qid or 1 mg IV slowly, repeat q5min up to 5 mg. *HTN:* 40 mg PO bid or 60–80 mg/d SR. ↑ weekly to max 640 mg/d. *Hypertrophic subaortic stenosis:* 20–40 mg PO tid–qid. *MI:* 180–240 mg PO ÷ tid–qid. *Migraine prophylaxis:* 80 mg/d ÷ qid–tid, ↑ weekly to max 160–240 mg/d ÷ tid–qid; wean off if no response in 6 wk. *Pheochromocytoma:* 30–60 mg/d ÷ tid–qid. *Thyrotoxicosis:* 1–3 mg IV single dose; 10–40 mg PO q6h. *Tremor:* 40 mg PO bid, ↑ as needed to max 320 mg/d. **Peds.** Arrhythmia: 0.5–1.0 mg/kg/d ÷ tid–qid, ↑ as needed q3–7d to max 60 mg/d; 0.01–0.1 mg/kg IV over 10 min, max dose 1 mg. *HTN:* 0.5–1.0 mg/kg ÷ bid–qid, ↑ as needed q3–7d to 2 mg/kg/d max; ↓ dose in renal impairment **Caution:** [C (1st tri, D if 2nd or 3rd tri), +] **Contra:** Uncompensated CHF, cardiogenic shock, bradycardia, heart block, PE, severe resp Dz **Supplied:** Tabs 10, 20, 40, 60, 80 mg; SR caps 60, 80, 120, 160 mg; oral soln 4, 8, 80 mg/mL; inj 1 mg/mL **SE:** Bradycardia, hypotension, fatigue, GI upset, erectile dysfunction, hypoglycemia **Interactions:** ↑ Effects w/ antihypertensives, cimetidine, fluvoxamine, flecainide, hydralazine, methimazole, neuroleptics, nitrates, propylthiouracil, quinidine, quinolones, theophylline, EtOH; ↑ effects of digitalis, glycosides, hypoglycemics, hydralazine, lidocaine, neuroleptics, rizatriptan; ↓ effects w/ NSAIDs, phenobarbital, phenytoin, rifampin, tobacco **Labs:** ↑ LFTs, BUN, K⁺, serum lipoprotein, triglycerides, uric acid; ↑ or ↓ serum glucose **NIPE:** ⊘ DC abruptly; ↑ cold sensitivity

Propylthiouracil [PTU] Uses: *Hyperthyroidism* Action: Inhibits production of T_3 and T_4 and conversion of T_4 to T_3 **Dose:** *Adults.* Initial: 100 mg PO q8h (may need up to 1200 mg/d); after Pt euthyroid (6–8 wk), taper dose by ½ q4–6wk to maint. 50–150 mg/24 h; can usually be DC in 2–3 y; ↓ dose in elderly **Peds.** Initial: 5–7 mg/kg/24 h PO ÷ q8h. *Maint:* ¼–⅔ of initial dose **Caution:** [D, –] **Contra:** Hypersensitivity **Supplied:** Tabs 50 mg **SE:** Monitor Pt clinically; monitor TFT, fever, rash, leukopenia, dizziness, GI upset, taste perversion, SLE-like syndrome **Interactions:** ↑ Effects w/ iodinated glycerol, Li, KI, NaI **Labs:** ↑ LFTs, PT; ↑ effects of anticoagulants **NIPE:** Take w/ food for GI upset; omit dietary sources of I; full effects take 6–12 wk

Protamine (generic) Uses: *Reversal of heparin effect* Action: Neutralizes heparin by forming a stable complex **Dose:** Based on amount of heparin reversal desired; give IV slowly; 1 mg reverses approximately 100 Units of heparin given in the preceding 3–4 h, 50 mg max dose **Caution:** [C, ?] **Contra:** Hypersensitivity **Supplied:** Inj 10 mg/mL **SE:** Follow coagulation studies; may have anticoagulant effect if given w/out heparin; hypotension, bradycardia, dyspnea, hemorrhage

Pseudoephedrine (Sudafed, Novafed, Afrinol, others) Uses: *Decongestant* Action: Stimulates α-adrenergic receptors, resulting in vasoconstriction **Dose:** *Adults.* 30–60 mg PO q6–8h; SR caps 120 mg PO q12h. *Peds.* 4 mg/kg/24 h PO ÷ qid; ↓ dose in renal insufficiency **Caution:** [C, +] **Contra:**

Poorly controlled HTN or CAD Dz and in MAOIs **Supplied:** Tabs 30, 60 mg; caps 60 mg; SR tabs 120, 240 mg; SR caps 120 mg; liq 7.5 mg/0.8 mL, 15, 30 mg/5 mL **SE:** HTN, insomnia, tachycardia, arrhythmias, nervousness, tremor **Notes:** Ingredient in many cough and cold preps **Interactions:** ↑ Risk of HTN crisis w/ MAOIs; ↑ effects w/ BBs, sympathomimetics; ↓ effects w/ TCAs; ↓ effect of methyldopa, reserpine

Psyllium (Metamucil, Serutan, Effer-Syllium)   **Uses:** *Constipation and diverticular Dz of the colon* **Action:** Bulk laxative **Dose:** 1 tsp (7 g) in a glass of water qd–tid **Caution:** [B, ?] Psyllium in effervescent (Effer-Syllium) form usually contains K⁺; use caution in Pts w/ renal failure; phenylketonuria (in products w/ aspartame) **Contra:** ⊘ use if suspected bowel obstruction **Supplied:** Granules 4, 25 g/tsp; powder 3.5 g/packet **SE:** Diarrhea, abdominal cramps, bowel obstruction, constipation, bronchospasm **Interactions:** ↓ Effects of digitalis glycosides, K-sparing diuretics, nitrofurantoin, salicylates, tetracyclines, warfarin **NIPE:** Psyllium dust inhalation may cause wheezing, runny nose, watery eyes

Pyrazinamide (generic)   **Uses:** *Active TB in combination w/ other agents* **Action:** Bacteriostatic; mechanism unknown **Dose:** *Adults.* 15–30 mg/kg/24 h PO ÷ tid–qid; max 2 g/d. *Peds.* 15–30 mg/kg/d PO ÷ qd–bid; dosage regimen differs for directly observed therapy; ↓ dose for renal/hepatic impairment **Caution:** [C, +/–] **Contra:** Severe hepatic damage, acute gout **Supplied:** Tabs 500 mg **SE:** Hepatotoxicity, malaise, GI upset, arthralgia, myalgia, gout, photosensitivity **Notes:** Use in combination w/ other anti-TB drugs; consult *MMWR* for the latest TB recommendations; dosage regimen differs for directly observed therapy **Interactions:** ↓ Effects of cyclosporine, tacrolimus **Labs:** False + urine ketones **NIPE:** ↑ Risk of photosensitivity—use sunscreen; ↑ fluids to 2 L/d

Pyridoxine [Vitamin B₆]   **Uses:** *Rx and prevention of vitamin B₆ deficiency* **Action:** Suppl of vitamin B₆ **Dose:** *Adults.* Deficiency: 10–20 mg/d PO. *Drug-induced neuritis:* 100–200 mg/d; 25–100 mg/d prophylaxis. *Peds.* 5–25 mg/d × 3 wk **Caution:** [A (C if doses exceed RDA), +] **Contra:** Component hypersensitivity **Supplied:** Tabs 25, 50, 100 mg; inj 100 mg/mL **SE:** Allergic Rxns, HA, nausea **Interactions:** ↓ Pyridoxine needs w/ chloramphenicol, cycloserine, hydralazine, immunosuppressant drugs, INH, oral contraceptives, penicillamine, high-protein diet; ↓ effects of levodopa, phenobarbital, phenytoin **Labs:** False ↑ urobilinogen **NIPE:** Lactation suppressed w/ pyridoxine

Quazepam (Doral) [C-IV]   **Uses:** *Insomnia* **Action:** Benzodiazepine **Dose:** 7.5–15 mg PO hs PRN; ↓ dose in the elderly, hepatic failure **Caution:** [X, ?/–] Narrow-angle glaucoma **Contra:** PRG, sleep apnea **Supplied:** Tabs 7.5, 15 mg **SE:** Sedation, hangover, somnolence, resp depression **Notes:** ⊘ DC abruptly **Interactions:** ↑ Effects w/ azole antifungals, cimetidine, digoxin, disulfiram, INH, levodopa, macrolides, neuroleptics, phenytoin, quinolones, SSRIs, verapamil, grapefruit juice, EtOH; ↓ effects w/ carbamazepine, rifampin, rifabutin, tobacco **NIPE:** ⊘ Breastfeed, PRG, DC abruptly; use barrier contraception

Quetiapine (Seroquel) Uses: *Acute exacerbations of schizophrenia* Action: Serotonin and dopamine antagonism Dose: 150–750 mg/d; initiate at 25–100 mg bid–tid; slowly ↑ dose; ↓ dose for hepatic and geriatric Pts Caution: [C, –] Contra: Component hypersensitivity Supplied: Tabs 25, 100, 200 mg SE: Multiple reports of confusion w/ nefazodone; HA, somnolence, weight gain, orthostatic hypotension, dizziness, cataracts, neuroleptic malignant syndrome, tardive dyskinesia, QT prolongation Interactions: ↑ Effects w/ azole antifungals, cimetidine, macrolides, EtOH; ↑ effects of antihypertensives, lorazepam; ↓ effects w/ barbiturates, carbamazepine, glucocorticoids, phenytoin, rifampin, thioridazine; ↓ effects of dopamine antagonists, levodopa Labs: ↑ LFTs, cholesterol, triglycerides NIPE: ↑ risk of cataract formation, tardive dyskinesia; take w/o regard to food; ↓ body temp regulation

Quinapril (Accupril) WARNING: ACEIs used during the 2nd and 3rd tri of PRG can cause injury and even death to the developing fetus Uses: *HTN, CHF, DN, post-MI* Action: ACEI Dose: 10–80 mg PO qd single dose; ↓ in renal impairment Caution: [D, +] Contra: ACEI sensitivity or angioedema Supplied: Tabs 5, 10, 20, 40 mg SE: Dizziness, HA, hypotension, ↓ renal Fxn, angioedema, taste perversion, cough Interactions: ↑ Effects w/ diuretics, antihypertensives; ↑ effects of insulin, Li; ↓ effects w/ ASA, NSAIDs; ↓ effects of quinolones, tetracyclines Labs: ↑ BUN, SCr NIPE: ↓ Absorption w/ high-fat foods; ↑ risk of cough

Quinidine (Quinidex, Quinaglute) Uses: *Prevention of tachydysrhythmias, malaria* Action: Class 1A antiarrhythmic; ↑ the refractory period in atrial and ventricular muscle, in SA and AV conduction systems, and the Purkinje fibers Dose: Adults. Conversion of AF or flutter: Use after digitalization, 200 mg q2–3h for 8 doses; then ↑ daily dose to a max of 3–4 g or until normal rhythm. Peds. 15–60 mg/kg/24 h PO in 4–5 ÷ doses; ↓ dose in renal impairment Caution: [C, +] Ritonavir use Contra: Digitalis toxicity and AV block; conduction disorders Supplied: Sulfate: Tabs 200, 300 mg; SR tabs 300 mg. Gluconate: SR tabs 324 mg; inj 80 mg/mL SE: Extreme hypotension may be seen w/ IV administration; syncope, QT prolongation, GI upset, arrhythmias, fatigue, cinchonism (tinnitus, hearing loss, delirium, visual changes), fever, hemolytic anemia, thrombocytopenia, rash Notes: Follow serum levels (see Table 2, page 265); sulfate salt is 83% quinidine; gluconate salt is 62% quinidine; must use in combination w/ drug that slows AV conduction (eg, digoxin, diltiazem, BB) Interactions: ↑ Effects w/ acetazolamide, antacids, amiodarone, azole antifungals, cimetidine, K, macrolides, NaHCO₃, thiazide diuretics, lily-of-the-valley, pheasant's eye herb, scopolia root, squill; ↑ effects of anticoagulants, dextromethorphan, digitalis glycosides, disopyramide, haloperidol, metoprolol, nifedipine, procainamide, propafenone, propranolol, TCAs, verapamil; ↓ effects w/ barbiturates, disopyramide, nifedipine, phenobarbital, phenytoin, rifampin, sucralfate NIPE: Take w/ food, ↑ risk of photosensitivity—use sunscreen

Quinupristin–Dalfopristin (Synercid) Uses: *Infections caused by vancomycin-resistant E. faecium and other gram(+) organisms* Action: Inhibits both the early and late phases of protein synthesis at the ribosomes. *Spectrum:* Susceptible infections due to vancomycin-resistant *Enterococcus faecium*, methicillin-susceptible *Staphylococcus aureus*, and *Streptococcus pyogenes*; *not* active against *Enterococcus faecalis* **Dose: Adults & Peds** 7.5 mg/kg IV q8–12h (use central line if possible); not compatible w/ NS or heparin; flush IV lines w/ dextrose; ↓ in hepatic failure **Caution:** [B, M] **Contra:** Hypersensitivity **Supplied:** Inj 500 mg (150 mg quinupristin/350 mg dalfopristin) **SE:** Hyperbilirubinemia, inf site Rxns and pain, arthralgia, myalgia **Notes:** Multiple drug interactions (eg, cyclosporine) **Interactions:** ↑ Effects of CCBs, carbamazepine, cyclosporine, diazepam, disopyramide, docetaxel, lovastatin, methylprednisolone, midazolam, paclitaxel, protease inhibitors, quinidine, tacrolimus, vinblastine **Labs:** ↑ LFTs, BUN, creatinine, Hct; ↑ or ↓ serum glucose, K+

Rabeprazole (Aciphex)
Uses: *PUD, GERD, ZE* **Action:** Proton pump inhibitor **Dose:** 20 mg/d; may be ↑ to 60 mg/d; ⊘ crush tabs **Caution:** [B, ?/–] **Supplied:** Tabs 60 mg **SE:** HA, fatigue, GI upset **Interactions:** ↑ Effects of cyclosporine, digoxin; ↓ effects of ketoconazole **Labs:** ↑ LFTs, TSH **NIPE:** Take w/o regard to food; ↑ risk of photosensitivity—use sunscreen

Raloxifene (Evista)
Uses: *Prevention of osteoporosis* **Action:** Partial antagonist of estrogen that behaves like estrogen **Dose:** 60 mg/d **Caution: Contra:** Thromboembolism, PRG **Supplied:** Tabs 60 mg **SE:** Chest pain, insomnia, rash, hot flashes, GI upset, hepatic dysfunction **Interactions:** ↓ Effects w/ ampicillin, cholestyramine **NIPE:** ⊘ PRG, breast-feeding; take w/o regard to food; ↑ risk of venous thromboembolic effects

Ramipril (Altace)
WARNING: ACEIs used during the 2nd and 3rd tri of PRG can cause injury and even death to the developing fetus **Uses:** *HTN, CHF, DN, post-MI* **Action:** ACEI **Dose:** 2.5–20 mg/d PO ÷ qd–bid; ↓ in renal failure **Caution:** [D, +] **Contra:** ACE-inhibitor-induced angioedema **Supplied:** Caps 1.25, 2.5, 5, 10 mg **SE:** Cough, HA, dizziness, hypotension, renal impairment, angioedema **Notes:** May use in combination w/ diuretics **Interactions:** ↑ Effects w/ α-adrenergic blockers, loop diuretics; ↑ effects of insulin, Li; ↑ risk of hyperkalemia w/ K+, K-sparing diuretics, K salt substitutes, trimethoprim; ↓ effects w/ ASA, NSAIDs, food; **Labs:** ↑ BUN, creatinine, K+, ↓ Hmg, Hct, cholesterol **NIPE:** ↑ Risk of photosensitivity—use sunscreen; ↑ risk of cough esp w/ capsaicin; take w/o food

Ranitidine Hydrochloride (Zantac)
Uses: *Duodenal ulcer, active benign ulcers, hypersecretory conditions, and GERD* **Action:** H_2-receptor antagonist **Dose: Adults.** *Ulcer:* 150 mg PO bid, 300 mg PO hs, or 50 mg IV q6–8h; or 400 mg IV/d cont inf, then maint of 150 mg PO hs. *Hypersecretion:* 150 mg PO bid, up to 600 mg/d. *GERD:* 300 mg PO bid; maint 300 mg PO hs. **Peds.** 0.75–1.5 mg/kg/dose IV q6–8h or 1.25–2.5 mg/kg/dose PO q12h; ↓ dose in renal failure **Caution:** [B, +] **Contra:** Component hypersensitivity **Supplied:** Tabs 75, 150, 300 mg; syrup 15 mg/mL; inj 25 mg/mL **SE:** Dizziness, sedation, rash, GI upset **Notes:**

PO and parenteral doses differ **Interactions:** ↑ Effects of glipizide, glyburide, lidocaine, nifedipine, nitrendipine, nisoldipine, procainamide, TCAs, theophylline, tolbutamide, warfarin; ↓ effects w/ antacids, tobacco; ↓ effects of cefuroxime, cefpodoxime, diazepam, enoxacin, ketoconazole, itraconazole, oxaprozin **Labs:** ↑ SCr, LFTs, false + urine protein **NIPE:** ASA, NSAIDs, EtOH, caffeine ↑ stomach acid production

Rasburicase (Elitek)
Uses: *Elevated plasma uric acid due to tumor lysis (peds)* **Action:** Catalyzes uric acid **Dose:** *Peds.* 0.15 or 0.20 mg/kg IV over 30 min, qd × 5 **Caution:** [C, ?/–] Falsely ↓ uric acid values **Contra:** Anaphylaxis, screen for G6PD deficiency to ⊘ hemolysis, methemoglobinemia **Supplied:** 1.5 mg inj **SE:** Fever, neutropenia, GI upset, HA, rash

Repaglinide (Prandin)
Uses: *Type 2 DM* **Action:** Stimulates insulin release from pancreas **Dose:** 0.5–4 mg ac, start 1–2 mg, ↑ to 16 mg/d max; take pc **Caution:** [C, ?/–] **Contra:** DKA, type 1 DM **Supplied:** Tabs 0.5, 1, 2 mg **SE:** HA, hyper-/hypoglycemia, GI upset **Interactions:** ↑ Effects w/ ASA, BBs, chloramphenicol, erythromycin, ketoconazole, miconazole, MAOIs, NSAIDs, probenecid, sulfa drugs, warfarin, celery, coriander, dandelion root, fenugreek, garlic, ginseng, juniper berries; ↓ effects w/ barbiturates, carbamazepine, CCBs, corticosteroids, diuretics, estrogens, INH, oral contraceptives, phenytoin, phenothiazines, rifampin, sympathomimetics, thiazide diuretics, thyroid drugs **NIPE:** Take 15 min before meal; skip drug if meal skipped

Reteplase (Retavase)
Uses: *Post-AMI* **Action:** Thrombolytic agent **Dose:** 10 Units IV over 2 min, 2nd dose in 30 min 10 Units IV over 2 min **Caution:** [C, ?/–] **Contra:** Internal bleeding, spinal surgery or trauma, Hx CNS vascular malformations, uncontrolled hypotension, sensitivity to thrombolytics **Supplied:** Inj 10.8 Units/2 mL **SE:** Bleeding, allergic Rxns **Interactions:** ↑ Risk of bleeding w/ ASA, abciximab, dipyridamole, heparin, NSAIDs, oral anticoagulants, vitamin K antagonists **Labs:** ↓ Fibrinogen, plasminogen **NIPE:** Monitor ECG during Rx for ↑ risk of reperfusion arrhythmias

Ribavirin (Virazole)
Uses: *RSV infection in infants and hepatitis C (in combination w/ interferon alfa-2b)* **Action:** Unknown **Dose:** *RSV:* 6 g in 300 mL sterile water inhaled over 12–18 h. *Hep C:* 600 mg PO bid in combination w/ interferon alfa-2b (see Rebetron) **Caution:** [X, ?] **Contra:** PRG, autoimmune hepatitis, CrCl <50 mL/min **Supplied:** Powder for aerosol 6 g; caps 200 mg **SE:** May accumulate on soft contact lenses; fatigue, HA, GI upset, anemia, myalgia, alopecia, bronchospasm **Notes:** Aerosolized by a SPAG; monitor Hbg/Hct frequently; PRG test monthly **Interactions:** ↓ Effects w/ Al, Mg, simethicone; ↓ effect of zidovudine **Labs:** ↑ Bilirubin, uric acid; ↓ Hmg **NIPE:** ⊘ PRG, breast-feeding; ↑ risk of photosensitivity—use sunscreen; take w/o regard to food

Rifabutin (Mycobutin)
Uses: *Prevention of MAC infection in AIDS Pts w/ a CD4 count <100* **Action:** Inhibits DNA-dependent RNA polymerase activity **Dose:** *Adults.* 150–300 mg/d PO. *Peds.* 1 y: 15–25 mg/kg/d PO. *2–10 y:* 4.4–18.8

mg/kg/d PO. *14–16 y:* 2.8–5.4 mg/kg/d PO **Caution:** [B; ?/–] WBC <1000/mm³ or plts <50,000/mm³; ritonavir **Contra:** Hypersensitivity **Supplied:** Caps 150 mg **SE:** Discolored urine, rash, neutropenia, leukopenia, myalgia, ↑ LFTs **Notes:** Adverse effects/drug interactions similar to rifampin **Interactions:** ↑ Effects w/ ritonavir; ↓ effects of anticoagulants, anticonvulsants, barbiturates, benzodiazepines, BBs, clofibrate, corticosteroids, cyclosporine, dapsone, delavirdine, digoxin, eprosartan, fluconazole, hypoglycemics, ketoconazole, nifedipine, oral contraceptives, propafenone, protease inhibitors, quinidine, tacrolimus, theophylline **Labs:** ↑ ALT, AST, alkaline phosphatase **NIPE:** Urine and body fluids may turn reddish brown in color, discoloration of soft contact lenses, use barrier contraception, take w/o food

Rifampin (Rifadin)
Uses: *TB and Rx and prophylaxis of *N. meningitidis,* *H. influenzae,* or *S. aureus* carriers* adjunct for severe *S. aureus* **Action:** Inhibits DNA-dependent RNA polymerase activity **Dose:** *Adults. N. meningitidis and H. influenzae carrier:* 600 mg/d PO for 4 d. *TB:* 600 mg PO or IV qd or 2 ×/wk w/ combination therapy regimen. *Peds.* 10–20 mg/kg/dose PO or IV qd–bid; ↓ dose in hepatic failure **Caution:** [C, +] Amprenavir, multiple drug interactions **Contra:** Hypersensitivity, presence of active *N. meningitidis* infection **Supplied:** Caps 150, 300 mg; inj 600 mg **SE:** Orange-red discoloration of bodily fluids, ↑ LFTs, flushing, HA **Notes:** Never use as single agent for active TB; multiple drug interactions **Interactions:** ↓ Effects w/ aminosalicylic acid; ↓ effects of acetaminophen, aminophylline, amiodarone, anticoagulants, barbiturates, BBs, CCBs, chloramphenicol, clofibrate, delavirdine, digoxin, disopyramide, doxycycline, enalapril, estrogens, haloperidol, hypoglycemics, hydantoins, methadone, morphine, nifedipine, ondansetron, oral contraceptives, phenytoin, protease inhibitors, quinidine, repaglinide, sertraline, sulfapyridine, sulfones, tacrolimus, theophylline, thyroid drugs, tocainide, TCAs, theophylline, verapamil, zidovudine, zolpidem **Labs:** ↑ LFTs, uric acid; affects serum folate and vit B₁₂ levels **NIPE:** Use barrier contraception, take w/o food, reddish brown color in urine and body fluids, stains soft contact lenses

Rifapentine (Priftin)
Uses: *Pulmonary TB* **Action:** Inhibits DNA-dependent RNA polymerase. *Spectrum: M. tuberculosis* **Dose:** *Intensive phase:* 600 mg PO 2×/wk for 2 mo; separate doses by 3 or more days. *Continuation phase:* 600 mg/wk for 4 mo; should be part of 3–4 drug regimen **Caution:** [C, red/orange breast milk] ↓ efficacy of protease inhibitors, antiepileptics, BBs, CCBs **Contra:** Hypersensitivity to rifamycins **Supplied:** 150-mg tabs **SE:** Neutropenia, hyperuricemia, HTN, HA, dizziness, rash, GI upset, blood dyscrasias, ↑ LFTs, hematuria, discolored secretions **Notes:** Monitor LFTs for liver dysfunction

Rimantadine (Flumadine)
Uses: *Prophylaxis and Rx of influenza A viral infections* **Action:** Antiviral agent **Dose:** *Adults & Peds.* >9 y: 100 mg PO bid. *Peds.* 1–9 y: 5 mg/kg/d PO, 150 mg/d max; use qd in severe renal/hepatic impairment & elderly; initiate w/in 48 h of Sx onset **Caution:** [C, –] W/ cimetidine

Contra: Component and amantadine hypersensitivity **Supplied:** Tabs 100 mg; syrup 50 mg/5 mL **SE:** Orthostatic hypotension, edema, dizziness, GI upset, lowered Sz threshold **Notes:** ↑ in PRG or breast-feeding **Interactions:** ↑ Effects w/ cimetidine; ↓ effects w/ acetaminophen, ASA

Rimexolone (Vexol Ophthalmic) **Uses:** *Postop inflammation and uveitis* **Action:** Steroid **Dose:** *Adults & Peds.* >2 y: Uveitis: 1–2 gtt/h daytime and q2h at night, taper to 1 gt q4h. *Postop:* 1–2 gtt qid ≤ 2 wk **Caution:** [C, ?/–] Ocular infections **Supplied:** Susp 1%; **SE:** Blurred vision, local irritation **Notes:** Taper dose to zero **NIPE:** Shake well, ⊘ touch eye w/ dropper

Risedronate (Actonel) **Uses:** *Paget's Dz; treat/prevent glucocorticoid-induced osteoporosis or postmenopausal osteoporosis* **Action:** Bisphosphonate; inhibits osteoclast-mediated bone resorption **Dose:** *Paget's:* 30 mg/d for 2 mo. *Osteoporosis Rx/prevention:* 5 mg qd or 35 mg qwk; take 30 min before 1st food/drink of the day; maintain upright position for at least 30 min after **Caution:** [C, ?/–] Ca suppls & antacids ↓ absorption **Contra:** Hypersensitivity, hypocalcemia, esophageal abnormalities, unable to stand/sit for 30 min, ⊘ in CrCl < 30 mL/min **Supplied:** Tabs 5, 30, 35 mg **SE:** HA, diarrhea, abdominal pain, arthralgia; flu-like Sxs, rash, esophagitis, bone pain **Notes:** Monitor LFT, Ca^{2+}, PO_4^{3+}, K^+ **Interactions:** ↓ Effects w/ antacids, Ca^{2+}, food **Labs:** Interference w/ bone-imaging agents **NIPE:** EtOH intake and cigarette smoking promote osteoporosis

Risperidone (Risperdal) **Uses:** *Psychotic disorders (schizophrenia),* dementia of the elderly, bipolar disorder, mania, Tourette's disorder, autism **Action:** Benzisoxazole antipsychotic agent **Dose:** *Adults.* 0.5–6 mg PO bid. *Peds/Adolescents.* 0.25 mg PO bid, titrate up q5–7d; ↓ starting dose in elderly, renal/hepatic impairment **Caution:** [C, –]. ↑ hypotension w/ antihypertensives, clozapine **Contra:** Component hypersensitivity **Supplied:** Tabs 0.25, 0.5, 1, 2, 3, 4 mg; soln 1 mg/mL **SE:** Orthostatic hypotension, EPS w/ higher doses, tachycardia, arrhythmias, sedation, dystonias, neuroleptic malignant syndrome, sexual dysfunction, constipation, xerostomia, blood dyscrasias, cholestatic jaundice, weight gain **Notes:** Several weeks to see effect **Interactions:** ↑ Effects w/ clozapine, CNS depressants, EtOH; ↑ effects of antihypertensives; ↓ effects w/ carbamazepine; ↓ effects of levodopa **Labs:** ↑ LFTs, serum prolactin **NIPE:** ↑ Risk photosensitivity—use sunscreen, extrapyramidal effects, may alter body temp regulation

Ritonavir (Norvir) **Uses:** *HIV* **Actions:** Protease inhibitor; inhibits maturation of immature noninfectious virions to mature infectious virus **Dose:** *Adults.* Start at 300 mg PO bid and titrate over 1 wk to 600 mg PO bid (titration ↓ GI SE). *Peds.* ≥2 y: 250 mg/m^2 titrate to 400 mg bid (dose adjustments required w/ amprenavir, indinavir, nelfinavir, and saquinavir; take w/ food) **Caution:** [B, +] W/ ergotamine, amiodarone, bepridil, flecainide, propafenone, quinidine, pimozide, midazolam, triazolam **Contra:** Concurrent ergotamine, amiodarone, bepridil, flecainide, propafenone, quinidine, pimozide, midazolam, triazolam, St. John's wort **Supplied:** Caps 100 mg; soln 80 mg/mL **SE:** ↑ triglycerides, ↑ LFTs, N/V/D/C, abdominal pain, taste perversion, anemia, weakness, HA, fever, malaise, rash, paresthesias **Notes:** Store in refrigerator **Interactions:** ↑ Effects w/ erythromycin, interleukins, grapefruit juice, food; ↑ effects of amiodarone, astemizole, atorvastatin, barbiturates, bepridil, bupropion, cerivastatin, cisapride, clorazepate, clozapine, clarithromycin, despiramine, diazepam, encainide, ergot alkaloids, estazolam, flecainide, flurazepam, indinavir, ketoconazole, lovastatin, meperidine, midazolam, nelfinavir, phenytoin, pimozide, piroxicam, propafenone, propoxyphene, quinidine, rifabutin, saquinavir, sildenafil, simvastatin, SSRIs, TCAs, terfenadine, triazolam, troleandomycin, zolpidem; ↓ effects w/ barbiturates, carbamazepine, phenytoin, rifabutin, rifampin, St. John's wort, tobacco; ↓ effects of didanosine, hypnotics, methadone, oral contraceptives, sedatives, theophylline, warfarin **Labs:** ↑ Serum glucose, LFTs, triglycerides, uric acid **NIPE:** Food ↑ absorption; use barrier contraception; disulfiram-like Rxn w/ disulfiram, metronidazole

Rivastigmine (Exelon)
Uses: *Mild–moderate dementia associated w/ Alzheimer's Dz* **Action:** Enhances cholinergic activity **Dose:** 1.5 mg bid; ↑ to 6 mg bid, w/ ↑ at 2-wk intervals (take w/ food) **Caution:** [B, ?] BBs, CCBs, smoking, neuromuscular blockade, digoxin **Contra:** Hypersensitivity to rivastigmine or carbamates **Supplied:** Caps 1.5, 3, 4.5, 6 mg; soln 2 mg/mL **SE:** Dose-related GI effects, N/V/D; dizziness, insomnia, fatigue, tremor, diaphoresis, HA **Notes:** Swallow capsules whole, ⊘ break, chew, or crush; ⊘ concurrent EtOH use **Interactions:** ↑ Risk of GI bleed w/ NSAIDs; ↓ effects w/ nicotine; ↓ effects of anticholinergics **NIPE:** Take w/ food

Rizatriptan (Maxalt) (See Table 11, page 283)

Rocuronium (Zemuron)
Uses: *Skeletal muscle relaxation during rapid-sequence intubation, surgery, or mechanical ventilation* **Action:** Nondepolarizing neuromuscular blockade **Dose:** *Rapid sequence intubation:* 0.6–1.2 mg/kg IV. *Continuous inf:* 4–16 µg/kg/min IV; ↓ in hepatic impairment **Caution:** [C, ?] Aminoglycosides, vancomycin, tetracycline, polymyxins enhance blockade **Contra:** Component or pancuronium hypersensitivity **Supplied:** 10 mg/mL 5,10 mL vials **SE:** BP changes, tachycardia **Notes:** N/A **Interactions:** ↑ Effects w/ MAOIs, propranolol; ↑ vasospastic Rxn w/ ergot-containing drugs; ↑ risk of hyperreflexia, incoordination, weakness w/ SSRIs **NIPE:** Food delays drug action; ⊘ take >30 mg/24 h

Rofecoxib (Vioxx)
Uses: *Osteoarthritis, RA, acute pain, and primary dysmenorrhea* **Action:** NSAID; COX-2 inhibitor (withdrawn in 2004 by manufacturer due to indications of ↑ cardiac risk w/ long-term use)

Ropinirole (Requip)
Uses: *Rx of Parkinson's Dz* **Action:** Dopamine agonist **Dose:** Initial 0.25 mg PO tid, w/ weekly ↑ 0.25 mg per dose, to 3 mg **Caution:** [C, ?/–] Severe CV, renal, or hepatic impairment **Contra:** Component hypersensitivity **Supplied:** Tabs 0.25, 0.5, 1, 2, 5 mg **SE:** Syncope, postural hypotension, N/V, HA, somnolence, hallucinations, dyskinesias **Notes:** DC requires a 7-d taper **Interactions:** ↑ Risk of bleeding w/ ASA, NSAIDs, feverfew, garlic, gin-

ger, horse chestnut, red clover, EtOH, tobacco; ↑ effects of amitriptyline, Li, MRX, theophylline, warfarin; ↑ risk of photosensitivity w/ dong quai—use sunscreen, St. John's wort; ↓ effects w/ antacids, rifampin; ↓ effects of ACEIs, diuretics **Labs:** ↑ ALT, AST **NIPE:** Take w/ food

Rosiglitazone (Avandia) Uses: Type 2 DM Action: ↑ Insulin sensitivity **Dose:** 4–8 mg/d PO or in 2 ÷ doses (w/out regard to meals) **Caution:** [C, –] Not for DKA **Contra:** Active liver Dz, use w/ caution in ESRD (renal elimination) **Supplied:** Tabs 2, 4, 8 mg **SE:** Weight gain, hyperlipidemia, HA, edema, fluid retention, exacerbate CHF, hyper-/hypoglycemia, hepatic damage **Notes:** Take w/ or w/o meals **Interactions:** ↑ Risk of hypoglycemia w/ insulin, ketoconazole, oral hypoglycemics, fenugreek, garlic, ginseng, glucomannan; ↓ effects of oral contraceptives **Labs:** ↑ ALT, total cholesterol, LDL, HDL, ↓ Hmg, Hct **NIPE:** Use barrier contraception

Rosuvastatin (Crestor) Uses: *Rx primary hypercholesterolemia and mixed dyslipidemia* Action: HMG-CoA reductase inhibitor Dose: 5–40 mg PO daily; max 5 mg/d w/ cyclosporine, 10 mg/d w/ gemfibrozil or CrCl < 30 mL/min (⊘ Al-/Mg-based antacids for 2 h after) **Caution:** [X,?/–] **Contra:** Active liver Dz or unexplained ↑ LFT **Supplied:** Tabs 5, 10, 20, 40 mg **SE:** Myalgia, constipation, asthenia, abdominal pain, nausea, myopathy, rarely rhabdomyolysis **Notes:** May ↑ warfarin effect; monitor LFTs baseline, 12 wk, then q6mo **Interactions:** ↑ Effects of warfarin; ↑ risk of myopathy w/ cyclosporine, fibrates, niacin, statins **Labs:** ↑ ALT, AST, CK; + urine protein, Hmg; NIPE: ⊘ PRG or breast-feeding

Salmeterol (Serevent) Uses: *Asthma, exercise-induced asthma, COPD* **Action:** Sympathomimetic bronchodilator, β_2-agonist **Dose:** *Adults & Peds.* ≥12 y: 1 diskus-dose inhaled bid **Caution:** [C, ?/–] **Contra:** Acute asthma; w/in 14 d of MAOI **Supplied:** Dry powder discus **SE:** HA, pharyngitis, tachycardia, arrhythmias, nervousness, GI upset, tremors **Notes:** Not for acute attacks; should also prescribe short-acting β-agonist **Interactions:** ↑ Effects w/ MAOIs, TCAs; ↓ effects w/ BBs **Labs:** ↓ serum K^+ **NIPE:** Shake canister before use, inhale q12h, not for acute exacerbations

Saquinavir (Fortovase) Uses: *HIV infection* Action: HIV protease inhibitor **Dose:** 1200 mg PO tid w/in 2 h pc (dose adjust w/ ritonavir, delavirdine, lopinavir, and nelfinavir) **Caution:** [B, +] W/ rifampin, ketoconazole, statins, sildenafil **Contra:** Hypersensitivity, sun exposure w/o sunscreen/clothing, triazolam, midazolam, ergots **Supplied:** Caps 200 mg **SE:** Dyslipidemia, lipodystrophy, rash, hyperglycemia, GI upset, weakness, hepatic dysfunction **Notes:** Take 2h after meal. ⊘ direct sunlight **Interactions:** ↑ Effects w/ clarithromycin, delavirdine, erythromycin, indinavir, ketoconazole, nelfinavir, ritonavir, grapefruit juice, food; ↑ effects of astemizole, cisapride, clarithromycin, ergot alkaloids, erythromycin, lovastatin, midazolam, phenytoin, sildenafil, simvastatin, terfenadine, triazolam; ↓ effects w/ barbiturates, carbamazepine, dexamethasone, efavirenz, phenytoin, rifabutin, rifampin, St. John's wort; ↓ effects of oral contraceptives **Labs:** ↑ LFTs, ↓

neutrophils **NIPE:** Use barrier contraception; ↑ risk of photosensitivity—use sunscreen

Sargramostim [GM-CSF] (Prokine, Leukine) **Uses:** *Myeloid recovery following BMT or chemo* **Action:** Activates mature granulocytes and macrophages **Dose:** *Adults & Peds.* 250 μg/m²/d IV for 21 d (BMT) **Caution:** [C, ?/–] Li, corticosteroids **Contra:** >10% blasts, hypersensitivity to yeast, concurrent chemo/RT **Supplied:** Inj 250, 500 μg **SE:** Bone pain, fever, hypotension, tachycardia, flushing, GI upset, myalgia **Notes:** Rotate inj sites; use APAP PRN for pain **Interactions:** ↑ Effects w/ corticosteroids, Li **Labs:** ↑ Serum glucose, BUN, creatinine, LFTs; ↓ albumin, Ca²⁺ **NIPE:** ⊘ Exposure to infection

Scopolamine, Scopolamine Transdermal (Scopace, Transderm-Scop) **Uses:** *Prevent N/V associated w/ motion sickness, anesthesia, and opiates; mydriatic,* cycloplegic, Rx iridiocyclitis **Action:** Anticholinergic, antiemetic **Dose:** 1 patch behind ear q3d; apply > 4 h before exposure: 0.4–0.8 PO, repeat PRN q4–6h; ↓ in elderly **Caution:** [C, +] APAP, levodopa, ketoconazole, digitalis, KCl **Contra:** Narrow-angle glaucoma, GI or GU obstruction, thyrotoxicosis, paralytic ileus **Supplied:** Patch 1.5 mg, tabs 0.4 mg, ophthal 0.25% **SE:** Xerostomia, drowsiness, blurred vision, tachycardia, constipation **Notes:** ⊘ Blink excessively after admin eye drops, wait 5 min to use other eye drops; activity w/ patch requires several hours **Interactions:** ↑ Effects w/ antihistamines, amantadine, antidepressants, disopyramide, opioids, procainamide, quinidine, TCAs, EtOH; ↓ effects of acetaminophen, digoxin, ketoconazole, levodopa, K⁺, phenothiazines, riboflavin **NIPE:** ⊘ DC abruptly; wash hands after applying patch; may cause heat intolerance

Secobarbital (Seconal) [C-II] **Uses:** *Insomnia,* preanesthetic agent **Action:** Rapid-acting barbiturate **Dose:** *Adults.* 100–200 mg, 100–300 mg preop. *Peds.* 2–6 mg/kg/dose, 100 mg/max, ↓ in elderly **Caution:** [D, +] CYP2C19, 3A3/4, 3A5–7 inducer; ↑ tox w/ other CNS depressants **Contra:** Porphyria, PRG **Supplied:** Caps 100 mg **SE:** Tolerance in 1–2 wk; resp depression, CNS depression, porphyria, photosensitivity **Interactions:** ↑ Effects w/ MAOIs, valproic acid, EtOH, kava kava, valerian; ↑ effects of meperidine; ↓ effects of anticoagulants, BBs, CCBs, CNS depressants, chloramphenicol, corticosteroids, cyclosporine, digitoxin, disopyramide, doxycycline, estrogen, griseofulvin, methadone, neuroleptics, oral contraceptives, propafenone, quinidine, tacrolimus, theophylline **NIPE:** ⊘ PRG, breast-feeding; use barrier contraception

Selegiline (Eldepryl) **Uses:** Parkinson's Dz **Action:** MAOI **Dose:** 5 mg PO bid; ↓ in elderly **Caution:** [C, ?] Meperidine, SSRI, TCAs **Contra:** Concurrent meperidine **Supplied:** Tabs/ caps 5 mg **SE:** Nausea, dizziness, orthostatic hypotension, arrhythmias, tachycardia, edema, confusion, xerostomia **Notes:** ↓ carbidopa/levodopa if used in combo **Interactions:** ↑ Risk of serotonin syndrome w/ dextroamphetamine, dextromethorphan, fenfluramine, meperidine, methylphenidate, sibutramine, venlafaxine; ↑ risk of hypertension w/ dextroamphetamine.

levodopa, methylphenidate, SSRIs, tyramine containing foods, EtOH, ephedra, ginseng, ma-huang, St. John's wort **Labs:** False ↑ uric acid, urine protein; false + urine ketones, urine glucose

Selenium Sulfide (Exsel Shampoo, Selsun Blue Shampoo, Selsun Shampoo)

Uses: *Scalp seborrheic dermatitis,* itching and flaking of the scalp due to *dandruff;* tinea versicolor **Action:** Antiseborrheic **Dose:** *Dandruff, seborrhea:* Massage 5–10 mL into wet scalp, leave on 2–3 min, rinse, and repeat; use 2×/wk, then once q1–4wk PRN. *Tinea versicolor:* Apply 2.5% qd for 7 d on area and lather w/ small amounts of water; leave on skin for 10 min, then rinse **Caution:** [C, ?] **Contra:** Open wounds **Supplied:** Shampoo [OTC] 1, 2.5% **SE:** Dry or oily scalp, lethargy, hair discoloration, local irritation **Notes:** ⊘ Use more than 2×/wk **NIPE:** ⊘ Use on excoriated skin; may cause reversible hair loss; rinse thoroughly after use

Sertaconazole (Ertaczo)

Uses: *Topical Rx interdigital tinea pedis* **Action:** Imidazole antifungal. *Spectrum: Trichophyton rubrum, T. mentagrophytes, Epidermophyton floccosum* **Dose:** *Adults & Peds.* > 12: Apply between toes and immediate surrounding healthy skin bid × 4 wk **Caution:** [C, ?] **Contra:** Component allergy **Supplied:** 2% cream **SE:** Contact dermatitis, dry/burning skin, tenderness **Notes:** Use in immunocompetent Pts

Sertraline (Zoloft)

WARNING: Closely monitor Pts for worsening depression or emergence of suicidality, particularly in pediatric Pts **Uses:** *Depression, panic disorders, obsessive–compulsive disorder (OCD), posttraumatic stress disorders (PTSD),* social anxiety disorder, eating disorders, premenstrual disorders **Action:** Inhibits neuronal uptake of serotonin **Dose:** *Adults.* Depression: 50–200 mg/d PO. *PTSD:* 25 mg PO qd ×1 wk, then 50 mg PO qd, max 200 mg/d. *Peds.* 6–12 y: 25 mg PO qd. *13–17 y:* 50 mg PO qd **Caution:** [C, ?/–] W/ haloperidol (serotonin syndrome), sumatriptan, linezolid, hepatic impairment **Contra:** MAOI use w/in 14 d; concomitant pimozide **Supplied:** Tabs 25, 50, 100 mg **SE:** Can activate manic/hypomanic state; weight loss; insomnia, somnolence, fatigue, tremor, xerostomia, nausea, dyspepsia, diarrhea, ejaculatory dysfunction, ↓ libido, hepatotoxicity **Interactions:** ↑ Effects w/ cimetidine, MAOIs, tryptophan, St. John's wort; ↑ effects of clozapine, diazepam, hydantoins, sumatriptan, tolbutamide, TCAs, warfarin, EtOH; ↓ effects w/ carbamazepine, rifampin **Labs:** ↑ LFTs, triglycerides, ↓ uric acid

Sevelamer (Renagel)

Uses: Reduce serum phosphorus in ESRD **Action:** Binds intestinal phosphate **Dose:** 2–4 capsules PO tid w/ meals; adjust based on serum phosphorus **Caution:** [C, ?] **Contra:** Bowel obstruction **Supplied:** Capsules 403 mg **SE:** BP changes, N/V/D, dyspepsia, thrombosis **Notes:** ⊘ Open or chew capsules; may ↓ fat-soluble vitamin absorption; 800 mg sevelamer = 667 mg Ca acetate **Interactions:** ↓ Effects of antiarrhythmics, anticonvulsants when given w/ sevelamer **Labs:** Monitor serum bicarbonate, Ca, Cl, P **NIPE:** Must be admin with meals, take daily multivitamin, take 1 h before or 3 h after other meds

Sibutramine (Meridia) [C-IV]   **Uses:** *Obesity* **Action:** Blocks uptake of norepinephrine, serotonin, and dopamine **Dose:** 10 mg/d PO, may ↓ to 5 mg after 4 wk **Caution:** [C, –] SSRIs, Li, dextromethorphan, opioids **Contra:** MAOI w/in 14 d, uncontrolled HTN, arrhythmias **Supplied:** Caps 5, 10, 15 mg **SE:** HA, insomnia, xerostomia, constipation, rhinitis, tachycardia, HTN **Notes:** Use w/ low-calorie diet, monitor BP and HR **Interactions:** ↑ Risk of serotonin syndrome w/ dextromethorphan, ergots, fentanyl, Li, meperidine, MAOIs, naratriptan, penta-zocine, rizatriptan, sumatriptan, SSRIs, tromethorphan, tryptophan, zolmitriptan, St. John's wort; ↑ effects w/ cimetidine, erythromycin, ketoconazole; ↑ CNS depression w/ EtOH **NIPE:** ⊘ EtOH; take early in the day to avoid insomnia

Sildenafil (Viagra)   **Uses:** *Erectile dysfunction* **Action:** Smooth muscle relaxation and ↑ inflow of blood to the corpus cavernosum; inhibits phosphodi-esterase type 5 responsible for cGMP breakdown; ↑ cGMP activity **Dose:** 25–100 mg PO 1 h before sexual activity, max once daily; ↓ if >65 y; ⊘ fatty foods w/ dose **Caution:** [B, ?] Potent CYP3A4 inhibitors (eg, protease inhibitors) **Contra:** W/ nitrates; retinitis pigmentosa; hepatic/severe renal impairment **Supplied:** Tabs 25, 50, 100 mg **SE:** HA; flushing; dizziness; blue haze visual disturbance (usually reversible) **Notes:** Cardiac events in absence of nitrates debatable **Interactions:** ↑ Effects w/ amlodipine, cimetidine, erythromycin, indinavir, itraconazole, ketocona-zole, nelfinavir, protease inhibitors, ritonavir, saquinavir, grapefruit juice; ↑ risk of hypotension w/ antihypertensives, nitrates; ↓ effects w/ rifampin **NIPE:** High-fat food delays absorption; ↑ risk of cardiac arrest if used w/ nitrates

Silver Nitrate (Dey-Drop, others)   **Uses:** *Removal of granulation tis-sue and warts; prophylaxis in burns* **Action:** Caustic antiseptic and astringent **Dose:** *Adults & Peds* Apply to moist surface 2–3×/wk for several weeks or until ef-fect **Caution:** [C, ?] **Contra:** ⊘ use on broken skin **Supplied:** Topical impregnated applicator sticks, oint 10%, soln 10, 25, 50%; ophth 1% amp **SE:** May stain tissue black, usually resolves; local irritation, methemoglobinemia **Notes:** DC if redness or irritation develop; no longer used in US for newborn prevention of gonococcal conjunctivitis

Silver Sulfadiazine (Silvadene)   **Uses:** *Prevention & Rx of infection in 2nd- and 3rd-degree burns* **Action:** Bactericidal **Dose:** *Adults & Peds.* Asepti-cally cover the affected area w/ ¹⁄₁₆-in. coating bid **Caution:** [B unless near term, ?/–] **Contra:** Infants < 2 mo, PRG near term **Supplied:** Cream 1% **SE:** Itching, rash, skin discoloration, blood dyscrasias, hepatitis, allergy **Notes:** Systemic ab-sorption w/ extensive application

Simethicone (Mylicon)   **Uses:** Flatulence **Action:** Defoaming action **Dose:** *Adults & Peds.* 40–125 mg PO pc and hs PRN **Caution:** [C, ?] **Contra:** In-testinal perforation or obstruction **Supplied:** [OTC] Tabs 80, 125 mg; caps 125 mg; gtt 40 mg/0.6 mL **SE:** Diarrhea, nausea **Notes:** Available in combination prod-ucts OTC **Interactions:** ↓ Effects of topical proteolytic enzymes

Simvastatin (Zocor) Uses: ↓ Cholesterol Action: HMG-CoA reductase inhibitor Dose: 5–80 mg PO; w/ meals; ↓ in renal insufficiency Caution: [X, –] ⊘ concurrent use of gemfibrozil Contra: PRG, liver Dz Supplied: Tabs 5, 10, 20, 40 mg SE: HA, GI upset, myalgia, myopathy manifested as muscle pain, tenderness or weakness w/ creatine kinase 10× ULN, hepatitis Notes: follow LFTs Interactions: ↑ Effects w/ amprenavir, azole antifungals, cyclosporine, danazol, diltiazem, gemfibrozil, indinavir, macrolides, nefazodone, nelfinavir, ritonavir, saquinavir, verapamil, grapefruit juice; ↑ effects of digoxin, warfarin; ↓ effects w/ cholestyramine, colestipol, fluvastatin, isradipine Labs: ↑ LFTs NIPE: Take w/ food and in the evening; ⊘ PRG, breast-feeding

Sirolimus [Rapamycin] (Rapamune) WARNING: Can cause immunosuppression and infections Uses: Prophylaxis of organ rejection Action: Inhibits T-lymphocyte activation Dose: *Adults.* >40 kg: 6 mg PO on day 1, then 2 mg/d PO. *Adults.* <40 kg: *Peds.* ≥13 y: 3 mg/m² load, then 1 mg/m²/d (in water or orange juice; ⊘ drink grapefruit juice while on sirolimus); take 4 h after cyclosporine; ↓ in hepatic impairment Caution: [C, ?/–] Grapefruit juice, ketoconazole Contra: Component hypersensitivity Supplied: Soln 1 mg/mL, tab 1 mg SE: HTN, edema, CP, fever, HA, insomnia, acne, rash, ↑ cholesterol, GI upset, ↑ or ↓ K⁺, infections, blood dyscrasias, arthralgia, tachycardia, renal impairment, hepatic artery thrombosis, graft loss and death in de novo liver transplant Notes: Routine levels not needed except in liver failure (trough 9–17 ng/mL) Interactions: ↑ Effects w/ azole antifungals, cimetidine, cyclosporine, diltiazem, macrolides, nicardipine, protease inhibitors, verapamil, grapefruit juice; ↓ effects w/ carbamazepine, phenobarbital, phenytoin, rifabutin, rifapentine, rifampin; ↓ effects of live virus vaccines Labs: ↑ LFTs, BUN, creatinine, cholesterol, triglycerides NIPE: Take w/o regard to food; ⊘ PRG while taking drug and for 12 wk after drug DC

Smallpox Vaccine (Dryvax) Uses: Immunization against smallpox (variola virus) Action: Active immunization (live attenuated vaccinia virus) Dose: *Adults (routine nonemergency)* or all ages (emergency): 2–3 punctures w/ bifurcated needle dipped in vaccine into deltoid, posterior triceps muscle; check site for Rxn in 6–8 d; if major Rxn, site scabs, and heals, leaving scar; if mild/equivocal Rxn, repeat using 15 punctures Caution: [X, N/A] Contra: *Nonemergency use:* Febrile illness, immunosuppression, Hx eczema and their household contacts. *Emergency:* No absolute contraindications Supplied: Vial for reconstitution: 100 million pock-forming Units/mL SE: Malaise, fever, regional lymphadenopathy, encephalopathy, rashes, spread of inoculation to other sites administered; Stevens–Johnson syndrome, eczema vaccinatum w/severe disability

Sodium Bicarbonate [NaHCO₃] Uses: *Alkalinization of urine,* RTA, *metabolic acidosis, hyperkalemia, TCA OD* Action: Alkalinizing agent Dose: *Adults.* Cardiac arrest: Initiate ventilation, 1 mEq/kg/dose IV; can repeat 0.5 mEq/kg in 10 min once or based on acid–base status. *Metabolic acidosis:* 2–5 mEq/kg IV over 8 h and PRN based on acid–base status. *Alkalinize urine:* 4 g (48 mEq) PO, then 1–2 g q4h; adjust based on urine pH; 2 amp/1 L D_5W at 100–250 mL/h IV, monitor urine pH and serum bicarbonate. *Chronic renal failure:* 1–3 mEq/kg/d. *Distal RTA:* 1 mEq/kg/d PO. *Peds.* >1 y: Cardiac arrest: See Adult dosage. *Peds.* <1 y: ECC: Initiate ventilation; 1:1 dilution 1 mEq/mL dosed 1 mEq/kg IV; can repeat w/ 0.5 mEq/kg in 10 min ×1 or based on acid–base status. *Chronic renal failure:* See Adult dosage. *Distal RTA:* 2–3 mEq/kg/d PO. *Proximal RTA:* 5–10 mEq/kg/d; titrate based on serum bicarbonate. *Urine alkalinization:* 84–840 mg/kg/d (1–10 mEq/kg/d) in ÷ doses; adjust based on urine pH **Caution:** [C, ?] **Contra:** Alkalosis, hypernatremia, severe pulmonary edema, hypocalcemia **Supplied:** Powder, tabs; 300 mg = 3.6 mEq; 325 mg = 3.8 mEq; 520 mg = 6.3 mEq; 600 mg = 7.3 mEq; 650 mg = 7.6 mEq; inj 1 mEq/1 mL vial or amp **SE:** Belching, edema, flatulence, hypernatremia, metabolic alkalosis **Notes:** 1 g neutralizes 12 mEq of acid; 50 mEq bicarb = 50 mEq Na; can make 3 amps in 1 L D_5W to = D_5NS w/ 150 mEq bicarb **Interactions:** ↑ Effects of anorexiants, amphetamines, ephedrine, flecainide, mecamylamine, pseudoephedrine, quinidine, sympathomimetics; ↓ effects of BBs, cefpodoxime, cefuroxime, ketoconazole, Li, MRX, quinolones, salicylates, sulfonylureas, tetracyclines **Labs:** False + urinary protein **NIPE:** ⊘ Take w/in 2 h of other drugs; ↑ risk of milk-alkali syndrome w/ long-term use or when taken w/ milk

Sodium Citrate (Bicitra)

Uses: Alkalinize urine; dissolve uric acid and cysteine stones **Action:** Urinary alkalinizer **Dose:** *Adults.* 2–6 tsp (10–30 mL) diluted in 1–3 oz water pc and hs. *Peds.* 1–3 tsp (5–15 mL) diluted in 1–3 oz water pc and hs; best pc **Caution:** [C, +] **Contra:** Al-based antacids; severe renal impairment or Na-restricted diets **Supplied:** 15- or 30-mL unit dose: 16 (473 mL) or 4 (118 mL) fl oz **SE:** Tetany, metabolic alkalosis, hyperkalemia, GI upset; ⊘ use of multiple 50-mL amps; can cause hypernatremia/hyperosmolarity **Notes:** 1 mL = 1 mEq Na and 1 mEq bicarb **Interactions:** ↑ Effects of amphetamines, ephedrine, flecainide, pseudoephedrine, quinidine; ↓ effects of barbiturates, chlorpropamide, Li, salicylates **NIPE:** Dilute w/ water; take pc to ⊘ laxative effect

Sodium Oxybate (Xyrem) [C-III]

Uses: *Narcolepsy-associated cataplexy* **Action:** Inhibitory neurotransmitter **Dose:** *Adults & Peds.* ≥ 16 y: 2.25 g PO qhs, second dose 2.5–4 h later; may ↑ 9 g/d max **Caution:** [B, ?/–] **Contra:** Succinic semialdehyde dehydrogenase deficiency; potentiates EtOH **Supplied:** 500 mg/mL 180-mL PO soln **SE:** Confusion, depression, diminished level of consciousness, incontinence, significant vomiting, resp depression, psychiatric Sxs **Notes:** May lead to dependence; synonym for γ-hydroxybutyrate (GHB), abused recreationally and as a "date rape drug"; controlled distribution requires prescriber and Pt registration; must be administered when Pt in bed **Interactions:** ↑ Risk of CNS depression w/ sedatives, hypnotics, EtOH **NIPE:** Dilute w/ 2 oz water, ⊘ eat w/in 2 h of taking this drug

Sodium Phosphate (Visicol) Uses: Bowel evacuation prior to colonoscopy **Action:** Hyperosmotic laxative **Dose:** 3 tabs w/ at least 8 oz clear liquid every 15 min (20 tabs total the night before procedure; 3–5 h before colonoscopy, repeat the process) **Caution:** [C, ?] Renal impairment, electrolyte disturbances **Contra:** Megacolon, bowel obstruction, CHF, ascites, unstable angina, gastric retention, bowel perforation, colitis, hypomotility. **Supplied:** Tablets 2 g **SE:** QT prolongation, diarrhea, hypernatremia, flatulence, cramps **Interactions:** May bind with Al- & Mg-containing antacids and sucralfate; ↑ risk of hypoglycemia with bisphosphonates; ↓ absorption of other meds **Labs:** Monitor electrolytes; **NIPE:** Drink clear liq 12 h before start of this med; ⊘ take w/ drugs that prolong QT interval, ⊘ take other laxatives

Sodium Polystyrene Sulfonate (Kayexalate) Uses: *Hyperkalemia* **Action:** Na$^+$/K$^+$ ion-exchange resin **Dose:** *Adults.* 15–60 g PO or 30–60 g PR q6h based on serum K$^+$. *Peds.* 1 g/kg/dose PO or PR q6h based on serum K$^+$ (given w/agent, eg, sorbitol, to promote movement through the bowel) **Caution:** [C, M] **Contra:** Hypernatremia **Supplied:** Powder; susp 15 g/60 mL sorbitol **SE:** Can cause hypernatremia, hypokalemia, Na retention, GI upset, fecal impaction; enema acts more quickly than PO **Notes:** PO route is most effective **Interactions:** ↑ Risk of systemic alkalosis w/ Ca- or Mg-containing antacids **NIPE:** Mix w/ chilled fluid other than orange juice

Sorbitol (generic) Uses: *Constipation* **Action:** Laxative **Dose:** 30–60 mL of a 20–70% soln PRN **Caution:** [B, +] **Contra:** Anuria **Supplied:** Liq 70% **SE:** Edema, electrolyte losses, lactic acidosis, GI upset, xerostomia **Notes:** May be vehicle for many liquid formulations (eg, zinc, Kayexalate) **NIPE:** ⊘ Use unless soln clear

Sotalol (Betapace) **WARNING:** Monitor Pts for 1st 3 d of therapy to reduce risks of induced arrhythmia **Uses:** *Ventricular arrhythmias, AF* **Action:** β-Adrenergic-blocking agent **Dose:** *Adults.* 80 mg PO bid; may be ↑ to 240–320 mg/d. *Peds.* Neonates: 9 mg/m^2 tid. *1–19 mo:* 20 mg/m^2 tid. *20–23 mo:* 29.1 mg/m^2 tid. *≥ 2 y:* 30 mg/m^2 tid; ↓ in renal failure **Caution:** [B (1st tri) (D if 2nd or 3rd tri), +] **Contra:** Asthma, bradycardia, prolonged QT interval, 2nd- or 3rd-degree heart block w/o pacemaker, cardiogenic shock, uncontrolled CHF, CrCl <40 mL/min **Supplied:** Tabs 80, 120, 160, 240 mg **SE:** Bradycardia, CP, palpitations, fatigue, dizziness, weakness, dyspnea **Notes:** Betapace should not be substituted for Betapace AF because of significant differences in labeling **Interactions:** ↑ Effects w/ ASA, antihypertensives, nitrates, oral contraceptives, fluoxetine, prazosin, sulfinpyrazone, verapamil, EtOH; ↑ risk of prolonged QT interval w/ amiodarone, amitriptyline, bepridil, disopyramide, erythromycin, gatifloxacin, haloperidol, imipramine, moxifloxacin, quinidine, pimozide, procainamide, sparfloxacin, thioridazine; ↑ effects of lidocaine; ↓ effects w/ antacids, clonidine, NSAIDs, thyroid drugs; ↓ effects of hypoglycemics, terbutaline, theophylline **Labs:** ↑ BUN, serum glucose, lipoprotein, triglycerides, K⁺, uric acid **NIPE:** May ↑ sensitivity to cold; DC MAOIs 14 d before drug; take w/o food

Sotalol (Betapace AF) **WARNING:** To minimize risk of induced arrhythmia, Pts initiated/reinitiated on Betapace AF should be placed for a minimum of 3 d (on their maint dose) in a facility that can provide cardiac resuscitation, continuous ECG monitoring, and calculations of CrCl; Betapace should not be substituted for Betapace AF because of differences in labeling **Uses:** *Maintain sinus rhythm for symptomatic A fib/flutter* **Action:** β-Adrenergic-blocking agent **Dose: Adults.** Initial CrCl >60 mL/min: 80 mg PO q12h. *CrCl 40–60 mL/min:* 80 mg PO q2h; ↑ to 120 mg during hospitalization; monitor QT interval 2–4 h after each dose, w/ dose reduction or discontinuation if QT interval >500 ms. **Peds.**Neonates: 9 mg/m² tid. *1–19 mo:* 20 mg/m² tid. *20–23 mo:* 29.1 mg/m² tid. *≥ 2 y:* 30 mg/m² tid; all dosage ranges may be doubled as max daily dose; allow ≥ 36 h between dosage titrations **Caution:** [B (1st tri); D if 2nd or 3rd tri), +] **Contra:** Asthma, bradycardia, prolonged QT interval, 2nd- or 3rd-degree heart block w/o pacemaker, cardiogenic shock, uncontrolled CHF, CrCl <40 mL/min; caution if converting from previous antiarrhythmic therapy **Supplied:** Tabs 80, 120, 160 mg **SE:** Bradycardia, CP, palpitations, fatigue, dizziness, weakness, dyspnea **Notes:** Routinely evaluate renal Fxn and QT interval

Sparfloxacin (Zagam) **Uses:** *Community-acquired pneumonia, acute exacerbations of chronic bronchitis* **Action:** Quinolone antibiotic; inhibits DNA gyrase **Dose:** 400 mg PO day 1, then 200 mg q24h × 10 d; ↓ in renal impairment **Caution:** |C, ?/–] **W/** theophylline, caffeine, sucralfate, warfarin, and antacids **Contra:** QT prolongation; w/ drugs that prolong QT interval **Supplied:** Tabs 200 mg **SE:** Significant phototoxicity (even from daylight through windows); restlessness, N/V/D, rash, ruptured tendons, ↑ LFTs, sleep disorders, confusion, convulsions **Notes:** Protect from sunlight up to 5 d after last dose **Interactions:** ↑ Effects w/ cimetidine, probenecid; ↑ effects of cyclosporine, diazepam, metroprolol, theophylline, warfarin, caffeine; ↑ risk of prolonged QT interval w/ amiodarone, bepridil, disopyramide, erythromycin, pentamidine, phenothiazines, procainamide, propranolol, quinidine, sotalol, TCAs; ↓ effects w/ antacids, antineoplastics, didanosine, sucralfate **NIPE:** ↑ Risk of tendon rupture & photosensitivity—use sunscreen; take w/o regard to food; ↑ fluids to 2–3 L/d

Spironolactone (Aldactone) **Uses:** *Hyperaldosteronism, ascites from CHF or cirrhosis* **Action:** Aldosterone antagonist; K-sparing diuretic **Dose: Adults.** 25–100 mg PO qid; CHF (NYHA class III–IV) 25–50 mg/d. **Peds.** 1–3.3 mg/kg/24 h PO ÷ bid–qid. *Neonates:* 0.5–1 mg/kg/dose q8h; w/food **Caution:** [D, +] **Contra:** Hyperkalemia, renal failure, anuria **Supplied:** Tabs 25, 50, 100 mg **SE:** Hyperkalemia and gynecomastia, arrhythmia, sexual dysfunction, confusion, dizziness **Interactions:** ↑ Risk of hyperkalemia w/ ACEIs, K suppls, K-sparing diuretics, ↑ K diet; ↑ effects of Li; ↓ effects w/ salicylates; ↓ effects of anticoagulants

Labs: False $\uparrow$ of corticosteroids, digoxin **NIPE:** Take w/ food; $\uparrow$ risk of gynecomastia; maximum effects of drug may take 2–3 wk

Stavudine (Zerit)
WARNING: Lactic acidosis and severe hepatomegaly w/ steatosis and pancreatitis reported **Uses:** *Advanced HIV* **Action:** Reverse transcriptase inhibitor **Dose:** *Adults.* >60 kg: 40 mg bid. <60 kg: 30 mg bid. *Peds.* Birth–13 d: 0.5 mg/kg q12h. >14 d and <30 kg: 1 mg/kg q12h. ≥30 kg: Adult dose; ↓ in renal failure **Caution:** [C, +] **Contra:** Hypersensitivity **Supplied:** Caps 15, 20, 30, 40 mg; soln 1 mg/mL **SE:** Peripheral neuropathy, HA, chills, fever, malaise, rash, GI upset, anemias, lactic acidosis, ↑ levels on LFTs, pancreatitis **Notes:** Take w/ plenty of water **Interactions:** ↑ Risk of pancreatitis w/ didanosine; ↑ effects w/ probenecid; ↓ effects w/ zidovudine **Labs:** ↑ LFTs **NIPE:** Take w/o regard to food

Steroids, Systemic (See also Table 4, page 271)
The following relates only to the commonly used systemic glucocorticoids **Uses:** *Endocrine disorders* (adrenal insufficiency), *rheumatoid disorders, collagen–vascular Dzs, dermatologic Dzs, allergic states, cerebral edema,* nephritis, nephrotic syndrome, immunosuppression for transplantation, hypercalcemia, malignancies (breast, lymphomas), preoperatively (in any Pt who has been on steroids in the previous year, known hypoadrenalism, preop for adrenalectomy); inj into joints/tissue **Action:** Glucocorticoid **Dose:** Varies w/ use and institutional protocols. *Adrenal insufficiency, acute:* **Adults.** Hydrocortisone: 100 mg IV; then 300 mg/d ÷ q6h; convert to 50 mg PO q8h ×6 doses, taper to 30–50 mg/d ÷ bid. *Peds.* **Hydrocortisone:** 1–2 mg/kg IV, then 150–250 mg/d ÷ tid. *Adrenal insufficiency, chronic (physiologic replacement):* May need mineralocorticoid suppl such as fludrocortisone acetate. **Adults.** Hydrocortisone: 20 mg PO qAM, 10 mg PO qPM; cortisone 0.5–0.75 mg/kg/d ÷ bid; cortisone 0.25–0.35 mg/kg/d IM; dexamethasone 0.03–0.15 mg/kg/d or 0.6–0.75 mg/m²/d ÷ q6–12h PO, IM, IV. *Peds.* Hydrocortisone: 0.5–0.75 mg/kg/d PO tid; hydrocortisone succinate 0.25–0.35 mg/kg/d IM. *Asthma, acute:* **Adults.** Methylprednisolone: 60 mg PO/IV q6h or dexamethasone 12 mg IV q6h. *Peds.* Prednisolone: 1–2 mg/kg/d or prednisone 1–2 mg/kg/d ÷ qd–bid for up to 5 d; methylprednisolone 2–4 mg/kg/d IV ÷ tid; dexamethasone 0.1–0.3 mg/kg/d divided q6h. *Congenital adrenal hyperplasia:* **Peds.** Hydrocortisone: Initial dosage 30–36 mg/m²/d PO ÷ ⅓ dose qAM, ⅔ dose qPM *Maint:* 20–25 mg/m²/d ÷ bid. *Extubation/airway edema:* **Adults.** Dexamethasone: 0.5–1 mg/kg/d IM/IV ÷ q6h (start 24 h prior to extubation; continue × 4 more doses). *Peds.* Dexamethasone: 0.1–0.3 mg/kg/d ÷ q6h × 3–5 d (start 48–72h before extubation) *Immunosuppressive/antiinflammatory:* **Adults & Older Peds.** Hydrocortisone: 15–240 mg PO, IM, IV q12h *Methylprednisolone:* 4–48 mg/kg/d IV, taper to lowest effective dose *Methylprednisolone Na succinate:* 10–80 mg/d IM. **Adults.** Prednisone or prednisolone: 5–60 mg/d PO ÷ qd–qid. **Infants & Younger Children.** Hydrocortisone: 2.5–10 mg/kg/d PO ÷ q6–8h; 1–5 mg/kg/d IM/IV ÷ bid. *Nephrotic syndrome:* **Peds.** Prednisolone or prednisone: 2 mg/kg/d PO tid–qid until urine is protein-free for 5 d, use

up to 28 d; for persistent proteinuria, 4 mg/kg/dose PO qod max 120 mg/d for an additional 28 d; maint 2 mg/kg/dose qod for 28 d; taper over 4–6 wk (max 80 mg/d). *Septic shock* (controversial): *Adults.* Hydrocortisone: 500 mg–1 g IM/IV q2–6h. *Peds.* Hydrocortisone: 50 mg/kg IM/IV, repeat q4–24 h PRN. *Status asthmaticus:* *Adults & Peds* Hydrocortisone: 1–2 mg/kg/dose IV q6h; then ↓ by 0.5–1 mg/kg q6h. *Rheumatic Dz:* *Adults.* Intraarticular: Hydrocortisone acetate 25–37.5 mg large joint, 10–25 mg small joint; methylprednisolone acetate 20–80 mg large joint, 4–10 mg small joint. *Intrabursal:* Hydrocortisone acetate 25–37.5 mg. *Intraganglial:* Hydrocortisone acetate 25–37.5 mg. *Tendon sheath:* Hydrocortisone acetate 5–12.5 mg. *Perioperative steroid coverage:* Hydrocortisone 100 mg IV night before surgery, 1 h preop, intraop, and 4, 8, and 12 h postop; postop d #1 100 mg IV q6h; postop d #2 100 mg IV q8h; postop d #3 100 mg IV q12h; postop d #4 50 mg IV q12h; postop d #5 25 mg IV q12h; resume prior PO dosing if chronic use or DC if only perioperative coverage required. *Cerebral edema:* Dexamethasone 10 mg IV; then 4 mg IV q4–6h **Caution:** [C, ?/–] **Contra:** Active varicella infection, serious infection except TB, fungal infections **Supplied:** See Table 4, page 271 **SE:** All can cause ↑ appetite, hyperglycemia, hypokalemia, osteoporosis, nervousness, insomnia, "steroid psychosis," adrenal suppression **Notes:** Hydrocortisone succinate administered systemically, acetate form intraarticular; **NIPE:** Never abruptly DC steroids, especially in chronic Rx; taper dose

Streptokinase (Streptase, Kabikinase) **Uses:** *Coronary artery thrombosis, acute massive PE, DVT, and some occluded vascular grafts* **Action:** Activates plasminogen to plasmin that degrades fibrin **Dose:** *Adults.* PE: Load 250,000 Units peripheral IV over 30 min, then 100,000 Units/h IV for 24–72 h. *Coronary artery thrombosis:* 1.5 M Units IV over 60 min. *DVT or arterial embolism:* Load as w/ PE, then 100,000 Units/h for 72 h. *Peds.* 3500–4000 Units/kg over 30 min, followed by 1000–1500 Units/kg/h. *Occluded catheter* (controversial): 10,000–25,000 Units in NS to final volume of catheter (leave in place for 1h, aspirate and flush catheter w/ NS) **Caution:** [C, +] **Contra:** Streptococcal infection or streptokinase use in last 6 mo, active bleeding, CVA, TIA, spinal surgery, or trauma in last month, vascular anomalies, severe hepatic or renal Dz, endocarditis, pericarditis, severe uncontrolled HTN **Supplied:** Powder for inj 250,000, 600,000, 750,000, 1,500,000 Units **SE:** Bleeding, hypotension, fever, bruising, rash, GI upset, hemorrhage, anaphylaxis **Notes:** If maint inadequate to maintain thrombin clotting time 2–5× control, refer to the package insert for adjustments; antibodies remain 3–6 mo following dose **Interactions:** ↑ Risk of bleeding w/ anticoagulants, ASA, heparin, indomethacin, NSAIDs, dong quai, feverfew, garlic, ginger, horse chestnut, red clover; ↓ effects w/ aminocaproic acid **Labs:** ↑ PT, PTT

Streptomycin **Uses:** *TB,* streptococcal or enterococcal endocarditis **Action:** Aminoglycoside; interferes w/ protein synthesis **Dose:** *Adults.* Endocarditis: 1 g q12h 1–2 wk, then 500 mg q12h 1–4 wk; *TB:* 15 mg/kg/d (up to 1 g), directly observed therapy (DOT) 2×wk 20–30 mg/kg/dose (max 1.5gm), DOT 3×wk 25–30

mg/kg/dose (max 1g). **Peds.** 15 mg/kg/d; DOT 2×wk 20–40 mg/kg/dose (max 1 g); DOT 3×wk 25–30 mg/kg/dose (max 1 g); ↓ in renal failure, either IM or IV over 30–60 min **Caution:** [D, +] **Contra:** PRG **Supplied:** Inj 400 mg/mL (1-g vial) **SE:** ↑ incidence of vestibular and auditory toxicity, neurotoxicity, nephrotoxicity **Notes:** Monitor levels peak 20–30 μg/mL, trough < 5 μg/mL; toxic peak > 50, trough > 10 **Interactions:** ↑ Risk of nephrotoxicity w/ amphotericin B, cephalosporins, cisplatin, methoxyflurane, polymyxin B, vancomycin; ↑ risk of ototoxicity w/ carboplatin, furosemide, mannitol, urea; ↑ effects of anticoagulants **Labs:** False + urine glucose, false ↑ urine protein **NIPE:** ↑ fluid intake

Streptozocin (Zanosar) **Uses:** *Pancreatic islet cell tumors* and carcinoid tumors **Action:** DNA–DNA (interstrand) cross-linking; DNA, RNA, and protein synthesis inhibitor **Dose:** Refer to specific protocol; ↓ in renal failure **Caution:** [D, ?/–] **Contra:** Caution in renal failure, PRG **Supplied:** Inj 1 g **SE:** N/V, duodenal ulcers; myelosuppression rare (20%) and mild; nephrotoxicity (proteinuria and azotemia often heralded by hypophosphatemia) dose-limiting; hypo-/hyperglycemia may occur; phlebitis and pain at inj site of inj **Notes:** Monitor renal Fxn **Interactions:** ↑ Risk of nephrotoxicity w/ aminoglycosides, amphotericin B, cisplatin, vancomycin; ↑ effects of doxorubicin; ↓ effects w/ phenytoin **NIPE:** ⊘ PRG, breast-feeding; ↑ fluid intake to 2–3 L/d

Succimer (Chemet) **Uses:** *Lead poisoning (lead levels > 45 μg/mL)* **Action:** Heavy-metal chelating agent **Dose:** *Adults & Peds.* 10 mg/kg/dose q8h × 5 d, then 10 mg/kg/dose q12h for 14 d; ↓ in renal impairment **Caution:** [C, ?] **Contra:** Hypersensitivity **Supplied:** Caps 100 mg **SE:** Rash, fever, GI upset, hemorrhoids, metallic taste, drowsiness, ↑ LFTs **Notes:** Monitor lead levels, maintain adequate hydration, may open capsules **Labs:** False ↑ urinary ketones, false ↑ serum CPK, false ↓ uric acid **NIPE:** ⊘ Take w/ other chelating agents; ↑ fluid intake to 2–3 L/d

Succinylcholine (Anectine, Quelicin, Sucostrin) **Uses:** *Adjunct to general anesthesia to facilitate ET intubation and to induce skeletal muscle relaxation during surgery or mechanically supported ventilation* **Action:** Depolarizing neuromuscular blocking agent **Dose:** *Adults.* 1–1.5 mg/kg IV over 10–30 s, followed by 0.04–0.07 mg/kg PRN or Inf—10–100mcg/kg/min inf. *Peds.* 1–2 mg/kg/dose IV, followed by 0.3–0.6 mg/kg/dose q5min or use of CI ⊘; ↓ in severe liver Dz **Caution:** [C, M] **Contra:** At risk for malignant hyperthermia; myopathy; recent major burn, multiple trauma, extensive skeletal muscle denervation **Supplied:** Inj 20, 50, 100 mg/mL; powder for inj 500 mg, 1 g/vial **SE:** May precipitate malignant hyperthermia, resp depression, or prolonged apnea; multiple drugs potentiate succinylcholine; observe for CV effects (arrhythmias, hypotension, brady/tachycardia); ↑ intraocular pressure, postoperative stiffness, salivation, myoglobinuria **Notes:** May be given IVP or inf or IM in the deltoid **Interactions:** ↑ Effects w/ amphotericin B, aprotinin, BBs, clindamycin, lidocaine, Li, metoclopramide, oral contraceptives, oxytocin, phenothiazines, procainamide, procaine, quinidine, quinine, trimethaphan; ↓ effect w/ diazepam **Labs:** ↑ Serum K⁺

Sucralfate (Carafate) **Uses:** *Duodenal ulcers,* gastric ulcers, stomatitis, GERD, preventing stress ulcers, esophagitis **Action:** Forms ulcer-adherent complex that protects against acid, pepsin, and bile acid **Dose:** *Adults.* 1 g PO qid, 1 h ac and hs. *Peds.* 40–80 mg/kg/d ÷ q6h; continue 4–8 wk unless healing demonstrated by x-ray or endoscopy; separate from other drugs by 2 h; take on empty stomach ac **Caution:** [B, +] **Contra:** Component hypersensitivity **Supplied:** Tabs 1 g; susp 1 g/10 mL **SE:** Constipation frequent; diarrhea, dizziness, xerostomia **Notes:** Al may accumulate in renal failure **Interactions:** ↓ Effects of cimetidine, digoxin, levothyroxine, phenytoin, quinolones, quinidine, ranitidine, tetracyclines, theophylline, warfarin **NIPE:** Take w/o food

Sulfacetamide (Bleph-10, Cetamide, Sodium Sulamyd) **Uses:** *Conjunctival infections* **Action:** Sulfonamide antibiotic **Dose:** 10% oint apply qid and hs; soln for keratitis apply q2–3h based on severity **Caution:** [C, M] **Contra:** Sulfonamide sensitivity; age <2 mo **Supplied:** Oint 10%; soln 10, 15, 30% **SE:** Irritation, burning; blurred vision, brow ache, Stevens–Johnson syndrome, photosensitivity **Interactions:** ↓ Effects w/ tetracyclines **NIPE:** Not compatible w/ Ag-containing preps; purulent exudate inactivates drug; ↑ risk of photosensitivity—use sunscreen

Sulfacetamide & Prednisolone (Blephamide, others) **Uses:** *Steroid-responsive inflammatory ocular conditions w/ infection or a risk of infection* **Action:** Antibiotic and antiinflammatory **Dose:** *Adults and Peds.* >2 y: Apply oint to lower conjunctival sac qd–qid; soln 1–3 gtt 2–3 h while awake **Caution:** [C, ?/–] Sulfonamide sensitivity; age <2 mo **Supplied:** Oint sulfacetamide 10%/prednisolone 0.5%, sulfacetamide 10%/prednisolone 0.2%, sulfacetamide 10%/prednisolone 0.25%; susp sulfacetamide 10%/prednisolone 0.25%, sulfacetamide 10%/prednisolone 0.5%, sulfacetamide 10%/prednisolone 0.2% **SE:** Irritation, burning; blurred vision, brow ache, Stevens–Johnson syndrome, photosensitivity **Notes:** Ophth susp can be used as an otic agent **Interactions:** ↓ Effects w/ tetracyclines **NIPE:** Not compatible w/ Ag-containing preps; purulent exudate inactivates drug; ↑ risk of sensitivity to light; ⊘ DC abruptly

Sulfasalazine (Azulfidine, Azulfidine EN) **Uses:** *Ulcerative colitis, RA, juvenile RA,* active Crohn's, ankylosing spondylitis, psoriasis **Action:** Sulfonamide; actions unclear **Dose:** *Adults.* Initially, 1 g PO tid–qid; ↑ to a max of 8 g/d in 3–4 ÷ doses; maint 500 mg PO qid. *Peds.* Initially, 40–60 mg/kg/24 h PO ÷ q4–6h; maint. 20–30 mg/kg/24 h PO ÷ q6h. *RA* >6 y: 30–50 mg/kg/d in 2 doses, start w/ ¼–⅓ described maint dose, ↑ weekly until dose reached at 1 mo. 2 g/d max; ↓ in renal failure **Caution:** [B (D if near term), M] **Contra:** Sulfonamide or salicylate sensitivity, porphyria, GI or GU obstruction; ⊘ in hepatic impairment **Supplied:** Tabs 500 mg; EC tabs 500 mg; PO susp 250 mg/5 mL **SE:** Can cause severe GI upset; discolors urine; dizziness, HA, photosensitivity, oligospermia, anemias, Stevens–Johnson syndrome **Notes:** May cause yellow-orange skin discoloration or stain contact lenses; ⊘ long sunlight exposure **Interactions:** ↑ Effects of anticoagulants, hypoglycemics, MRX, phenytoin, zidovudine; ↓ effects w/ antibiotics; ↓ effects of digoxin, folic acid, Fe, procaine, proparacaine, sulfonylureas, tetracaine **Labs:** False + urinary glucose; false ↑ serum conjugated bilirubin, creatinine; false ↓ serum unconjugated bilirubin, K+ **NIPE:** Take pc; ↑ fluids to 2–3 L/d; ↑ risk of photosensitivity—use sunscreen; skin & urine may become yellow-orange

Sulfinpyrazone (Anturane) **Uses:** *Acute and chronic gout* **Action:** Inhibits renal tubular absorption of uric acid **Dose:** 100–200 mg PO bid for 1 wk, ↑ PRN to maint of 200–400 mg bid; max 800 mg/d; take w/ food or antacids, and plenty of fluids; ⊘ salicylates **Caution:** [C (D if near term), ?/–] **Contra:** ⊘ in renal impairment, ⊘ salicylates; peptic ulcer; blood dyscrasias, near term PRG, hypersensitivity **Supplied:** Tabs 100 mg; caps 200 mg **SE:** N/V, stomach pain, urolithiasis, leukopenia **Notes:** Take w/ plenty of water **Interactions:** ↑ Effects of anticoagulants, hypoglycemics, MRX; ↓ effects w/ ASA, cholestyramine, niacin, salicylates, EtOH; ↓ effects of acetaminophen, BBs, nitrofurantoin, theophylline, verapamil **Labs:** ↓ Serum uric acid **NIPE:** Take w/ food, ↑ fluids to 2–3 L/d

Sulindac (Clinoril) **Uses:** *Arthritis and pain* **Action:** NSAID; inhibits prostaglandins **Dose:** 150–200 mg bid w/ food **Caution:** [B (D if 3rd tri or near term), ?] **Contra:** NSAID or ASA sensitivity, ulcer, GI bleeding **Supplied:** Tabs 150, 200 mg **SE:** Dizziness, rash, GI upset, pruritus, edema, ↓ renal blood flow, renal failure (? fewer renal effects than other NSAIDs), peptic ulcer, GI bleeding **Interactions:** ↑ Effects w/ NSAIDs, probenecid; ↑ effects of aminoglycosides, anticoagulants, cyclosporine, digoxin, Li, MRX, K-sparing diuretics; ↑ risk of bleeding w/ ASA, NSAIDs, EtOH, dong quai, feverfew, garlic, ginger, horse chestnut, red clover; ↓ effects w/ antacids, ASA; ↓ effects of BBs, captopril, diuretics, hydralazine **Labs:** ↑ Serum Cl, Na, glucose, LFTs, PT **NIPE:** Take w/ food; ↑ risk of photosensitivity—use sunscreen; may take several weeks for full drug effect

Sumatriptan (Imitrex) **Uses:** Acute Rx of migraine attacks **Action:** Vascular serotonin receptor agonist **Dose:** *Adults.* SQ: 6 mg SQ as a single dose PRN; repeat PRN in 1 h to a max of 12 mg/24 h. *PO:* 25 mg, repeat in 2 h, PRN, 100 mg/d max PO dose; max 300 mg/d. *Nasal spray:* 1 spray into 1 nostril, may repeat in 2 h to a max of 40 mg/24 h. *Peds. Nasal spray: 6–9 y:* 5–20 mg/d. *12–17 y:* 5–20 mg, up to 40 mg/d **Caution:** [C, M] **Contra:** Angina, ischemic heart Dz, uncontrolled HTN, ergot use, MAOI use w/in 14 d **Supplied:** Inj 6 mg/mL; orally disintegrating tabs 25, 50, 100 mg; nasal spray 5, 20 mg **SE:** Pain and bruising at the inj site; dizziness, hot flashes, paresthesias, CP, weakness, numbness, coronary vasospasm, HTN **Interactions:** ↑ Effects of weakness, incoordination and hyperreflexia w/ ergots, MAOIs, and SSRIs, horehound, St. John's wort **NIPE:** Admin drug as soon as possible after onset of migraine

Tacrine (Cognex) **Uses:** *Mild/moderate Alzheimer's dementia* **Action:** Cholinesterase inhibitor **Dose:** 10–40 mg PO qid to 160 mg/d; separate doses from food **Caution:** [C, ?] **Contra:** Previous tacrine-induced jaundice **Supplied:** Caps 10, 20, 30, 40 mg **SE:** ↑ LFT, HA, dizziness, GI upset, flushing, confusion, ataxia, myalgia, bradycardia **Notes:** Serum conc > 20 ng/mL assoc w/ more SE **Interactions:** ↑ Effects w/ cimetidine, quinolones, SSRIs, ↑ effects of BBs, cholinergics, cholinesterase inhibitors, succinylcholine, theophylline; ↓ effects w/ tobacco, food; ↓ effects of anticholinergics, levodopa **Labs:** ↑ ALT **NIPE:** If taken w/ food ↓ drug plasma levels by 30%; may take up to 6 wk for ALT elevations

Tacrolimus [FK 506] (Prograf, Protopic) **Uses:** Prophylaxis against organ rejection, eczema **Action:** Macrolide immunosuppressant **Dose:** *Adults.* IV: 0.05–0.1 mg/kg/d cont inf. PO: 0.15–0.3 mg/kg/d ÷ 2 doses. *Peds.* IV: 0.03–0.05 mg/kg/d as cont inf. PO: 0.15–0.2 mg/kg/d PO ÷ q 12 h. *Adults & Peds. Eczema:* Apply bid, continue 1 wk after clearing; ↓ in hepatic/renal impairment **Caution:** [C, –] ⊘ use w/ cyclosporine **Contra:** Component hypersensitivity **Supplied:** Caps 1, 5 mg; inj 5 mg/mL; oint 0.03, 0.1% **SE:** Neurotoxicity and nephrotoxicity, HTN, edema, HA, insomnia, fever, pruritus, hypo-/hyperkalemia, hyperglycemia, GI upset, anemia, leukocytosis, tremors, paresthesias, pleural effusion, Szs, lymphoma **Notes:** Monitor drug levels

Tadalafil (Cialis) **Uses:** Erectile dysfunction **Action:** Phosphodiesterase inhibitor **Dose:** *Adults.* 10 mg PO before sexual activity w/o regard to meals (20 mg max); ↓ 5 mg (10 mg max) in renal and mild hepatic insufficiency **Caution:** [B, –] **Contra:** Nitrates, α-blockers (except tamsulosin), severe hepatic insufficiency **Supplied:** 5-, 10-, 20-mg tabs **SE:** HA, flushing, dyspepsia, rhinitis, back pain, myalgia **Notes:** Longest acting of class (36 h) **Interactions:** ↑ Effects w/ ketoconazole, ritonavir, and other cytochrome P450 CYP3A4 inhibitors; ↑ hypotension w/ antihypertensives, EtOH; ↓ effects w/ P450 CYP3A4 inducers such as rifampin, antacids **NIPE:** ↑ Risk of priapism; use barrier contraception to prevent STDs

Talc (Sterile Talc Powder) **Uses:** ↓ recurrence of malignant pleural effusions (pleurodesis) **Action:** Sclerosing agent **Dose:** Mix slurry: 50 mL NS w/5-g vial, mix, distribute 25 mL into two 60-mL syringes, volume to 50 mL/syringe w/ NS. Infuse each into chest tube, flush w/ 25 mL NS. Keep tube clamped and have Pt change positions q15min for 2 h, unclamp tube **Caution:** [X, –] **Contra:** Further surgery on site planned **Supplied:** 5 g powder **SE:** Pain, infection **Notes:** May add 10–20 mL 1% lidocaine/syringe; must have chest tube in place, monitor closely while tube clamped (tension pneumothorax), not antineoplastic

Tamoxifen (Nolvadex) **Uses:** *Breast CA (postmenopausal, estrogen receptor-+), reduction of breast CA in women at high-risk, metastatic male breast CA,* mastalgia, pancreatic CA, gynecomastia, ovulation induction **Action:** Nonsteroidal antiestrogen; mixed agonist–antagonist effect **Dose:** 20–40 mg/d (typically 10 mg bid or 20 mg/d) **Caution:** [D, –]**Contra:** Caution in leukopenia, thrombocytopenia, hyperlipidemia **Supplied:** Tabs 10, 20 mg **SE:** Uterine malignancy and thrombotic events noted in breast CA prevention trials; menopausal Sxs (hot flashes, N/V) in premenopausal Pts; vaginal bleeding and menstrual irregularities; skin rash, pruritus vulvae, dizziness, HA, peripheral edema; acute flare of bone metastasis pain and hypercalcemia; retinopathy reported (high dose) Notes: ↑ Risk of PRG in premenopausal women by inducing ovulation Interactions: ↑ Effects w/ bromocriptine, grapefruit juice; ↑ effects of warfarin, cyclosporine, warfarin; ↓ effects w/ antacids, aminoglutethimide, letrozole, medroxyprogesterone, rifamycins Labs: ↑ Ca²⁺, T₄, BUN, creatinine, LFTs NIPE: ⊘ PRG or breast-feeding; use barrier contraception; ↑ risk of photosensitivity—use sunscreen

Tamsulosin (Flomax)
Uses: *BPH* Action: Antagonist of prostatic α-receptors Dose: 0.4 mg/d PO; ⊘ crush, chew, or open caps Caution: [B, ?] Contra: Female gender Supplied: Caps 0.4, 0.8 mg SE: HA, dizziness, syncope, somnolence, ↓ libido, GI upset, retrograde ejaculation, rhinitis, rash, angioedema Notes: Not for use as antihypertensive Interactions: ↑ Effects w/ cimetidine; ↑ hypotension w/ doxazosin, prazosin, terazosin NIPE: Ensure − test results for prostate CA before drug admin

Tazarotene (Tazorac)
Uses: *Facial acne vulgaris; stable plaque psoriasis up to 20% body surface area* Action: Keratolytic Dose: Adults & Peds. >12 y: Acne: Cleanse face, dry, and apply thin film qd hs on acne lesions. Psoriasis: Apply hs Caution: [X, ?/–] Contra: Retinoid sensitivity Supplied: Gel 0.05, 0.1% SE: Burning, erythema, irritation, rash, photosensitivity, desquamation, bleeding, skin discoloration Notes: DC if excessive pruritus, burning, skin redness or peeling occur until Sxs resolve Interactions: ↑ Risk of photosensitivity w/ quinolones, phenothiazines, sulfonamides, tetracyclines, thiazide diuretics NIPE: ⊘ PRG or breast-feeding; use contraception; use sunscreen for ↑ photosensitivity risk

Tegaserod Maleate (Zelnorm)
Uses: *Short-term Rx of constipation-predominant IBS in women* Action: 5HT4 serotonin agonist Dose: 6 mg PO bid pc for 4–6 wk; may continue for 2nd course Caution: [B, ?/–] Contra: Severe renal, moderate–severe hepatic impairment, Hx of bowel obstruction, gallbladder Dz, sphincter of Oddi dysfunction, abdominal adhesions Supplied: Tabs 2, 6 mg SE: ⊘ Administer if diarrhea present, as GI motility ↑; DC if abdominal pain worsens Notes: Maintain adequate hydration NIPE: Take ac

Telithromycin (Ketek)
Uses: *Exacerbation of chronic bacterial bronchitis, sinusitis, community-acquired pneumonia* Action: Ketolide antibiotic, related to macrolides, blocks protein synthesis. Spectrum: Gram(+), gram(–) cocci (esp. H. influenzae, S. pneumoniae, M. catarrhalis, Toxoplasma, and anaerobic bacteria) Dose: Bronchitis, sinusitis: 800 mg PO daily ×5d. Pneumonia: 800 mg PO daily × 10 d Caution: [C, ?] CYP inducers (eg, rifampin, phenytoin, carbamazepine, phenobarbital) may ↓ telithromycin levels, use w/hepatically metabolized drugs Contra: W/ cisapride or pimozide, macrolide sensitivity Supplied: Tabs 400 mg SE: N/V/D, dizziness, prolonged QTc interval, ↑ LFTs Notes: Monitor for pseudomembranous colitis Interactions: ↑ QT interval & arrhythmias w/ antiarrhythmics, mesoridazine, quinolone antibiotics, thioridazine; ↑ effects of alprazolam, atorvastatin, benzodiazepines, CCBs, carbamazepine—cisapride, colchicine, cyclosporine, digoxin, ergot alkaloids, felodipine, lovastatin, mirtazapine, midazo-

lam, nateglinide, nefazodone, pimozide, sildenafil, simvastatin, sirolimus, tacrolimus, tadalafil, triazolam, vardenafil, venlafaxine, verapamil; ↑ effects with azole antifungals, ciprofloxin, clarithromycin, diclofenac, doxycycline, erythromycin, imatinib, INH, nefazodone, nicardipine, propofol, protease inhibitors, quinidine, verapamil; ↓ effect with aminoglutethimide, carbamazepine, nafcillin, nevirapine, phenobarbital, phenytoin, rifampin, rifamycins **NIPE:** Take w/o regard to food; ⊘ chew or crush tablets.

Telmisartan (Micardis) Uses: *HTN, CHF,* DN Action: Angiotensin II receptor antagonist **Dose:** 40–80 mg/d **Caution:** [C (1st tri; D 2nd and 3rd tri), ?/–] **Contra:** Angiotensin II receptor antagonist sensitivity **Supplied:** Tabs 40, 80 mg **SE:** Edema, GI upset, HA, angioedema, renal impairment, orthostatic hypotension **Interactions:** ↑ Effects w/ EtOH; ↑ effects of digoxin; ↓ effects of warfarin **Labs:** ↑ Creatinine, ↓ Hmg **NIPE:** Take w/o regard to food; ⊘ PRG; use barrier contraception

Temazepam (Restoril) [C-IV] Uses: *Insomnia,* anxiety, depression, panic attacks **Action:** Benzodiazepine **Dose:** 15–30 mg PO hs PRN; ↓ dose in elderly **Caution:** [X, ?/–] Potentiates CNS depressive effects of opioids, barbs, EtOH, antihistamines, MAOIs, TCAs **Contra:** Narrow-angle glaucoma **Supplied:** Caps 7.5, 15, 30 mg **SE:** Confusion, dizziness, drowsiness, hangover **Notes:** Abrupt DC after >10 d use may cause withdrawal **Interactions:** ↑ Effects w/ cimetidine, disulfiram, kava kava, valerian; ↑ CNS depression w/ anticonvulsants, CNS depressants, EtOH; ↑ effects of haloperidol, phenytoin; ↓ effects w/ aminophylline, dyphylline, oral contraceptives, oxtriphylline, rifampin, theophylline, tobacco; ↓ effects of levodopa **NIPE:** ⊘ DC abruptly after prolonged use, use in PRG or breast-feeding

Tenecteplase (TNKase) Uses: *Restore perfusion and reduce mortality w/ AMI* **Action:** Thrombolytic; tPA **Dose:** 30–50 mg (see following table)

Tenecteplase Dosing

Weight (kg)	TNKase (mg)	TNKase[a] Volume (mL)
<60	30	6
≥60–70	35	7
≥70–80	40	8
≥80–90	45	9
≥90	50	10

[a]From one vial of reconstituted TNKase.

Caution: [C, ?], ↑ bleeding w/ concurrent NSAIDs, ticlodipine, clopidogrel, GPIIb/IIIa antagonists **Contra:** Bleeding, CVA, major surgery (intracranial, intraspinal) or trauma w/in 2 mo **Supplied:** Inj 50 mg, reconstitute w/ 10 mL sterile water **SE:** Bleeding, hypersensitivity **Notes:** ⊘ shake when reconstituting; do not use D_5W either in the IV line or to reconstitute **Interactions:** ↑ Risk of bleeding w/ anticoagulants, ASA, clopidogrel, dipyridamole, ticlopidine, vitamin K antagonists; ↓ effects w/ aminocaproic acid **NIPE:** Eval for S/Sxs bleeding

Tenofovir (Viread) Uses: *HIV infection* **Action:** Nucleotide RT inhibitor **Dose**: 300 mg PO qd w/ a meal **Caution:** [B, ?/–] Dianosine (separate admin times), lopinavir, ritonavir **Contra:** CrCl <60 mL/min; caution w/ known risk factors for liver Dz **Supplied:** Tabs 300 mg **SE:** GI upset, metabolic syndrome, hepatotoxicity; separate didanosine doses by 2 h **Notes:** Take w/ fatty meal **Interactions:** ↑ Effects w/ acyclovir, cidofovir, ganciclovir, indinavir, lopinavir, ritonavir, valacyclovir, food; ↓ effects of didanosine, lamivudine, ritonavir **Labs:** ↑ LFTs, triglycerides, serum and urine glucose **NIPE:** Take w/ food, take 2 h before or 1 h after didanosine, lopinavir/ritonavir

Terazosin (Hytrin) Uses: *BPH and HTN* **Action:** α_1-Blocker (blood vessel and bladder neck/prostate) **Dose:** Initially, 1 mg PO hs; ↑ 20 mg/d max **Caution:** [C, ?] ↑ hypotension w/BB, CCB, ACEI **Contra:** α-Antagonist sensitivity **Supplied:** Tabs 1, 2, 5, 10 mg; caps 1, 2, 5, 10 mg **SE:** Hypotension and syncope following 1st dose; dizziness, weakness, nasal congestion, peripheral edema common; palpitations, GI upset **Notes:** Caution w/1st dose syncope; if for HTN, combine w/ thiazide diuretic **Interactions:** ↑ Effects w/ antihypertensives, diuretics; ↑ effects of finasteride; ↓ effects w/ NSAIDs, α-blockers, ephedra, garlic, ginseng, saw palmetto, yohimbe; ↓ effects of clonidine **Labs:** ↓ Albumin, Hmg, Hct, WBCs **NIPE:** Take w/o regard to food, ⊘ DC abruptly

Terbinafine (Lamisil) Uses: *Onychomycosis, athlete's foot, jock itch, ringworm,* cutaneous candidiasis, pityriasis versicolor **Action:** Inhibits squalene epoxidase resulting in fungal death **Dose:** *PO:* 250 mg/d PO for 6–12 wk. *Topical:* Apply to area; ↓ in renal/hepatic impairment **Caution:** [B, –] May ↑ effects of drug metab by CYP2D6 **Contra:** Liver Dz or kidney failure **Supplied:** Tabs 250 mg; cream 1% **SE:** HA, dizziness, rash, pruritus, alopecia, GI upset, taste perversion, neutropenia, retinal damage, Stevens–Johnson syndrome **Notes:** Effect may take months due to need for new nail growth; ⊘ use occlusive dressings **Interactions:** ↑ Effects w/ cimetidine; ↓ effects of dextromethorphan, theophylline, caffeine; ↓ effects w/ rifampin; ↓ effects of cyclosporine **Labs:** LFT abnormalities

Terbutaline (Brethine, Bricanyl) Uses: *Reversible bronchospasm (asthma, COPD); inhibition of labor (tocolytic)* **Action:** Sympathomimetic **Dose:** *Adults.* Bronchodilator: 2.5–5 mg PO qid or 0.25 mg SQ; may repeat in 15 min (max 0.5 mg in 4 h). *Met-dose inhaler:* 2 inhal q4–6h. *Premature labor:* Acutely 2.5–10 mg/min/IV, gradually ↑ as tolerated q10–20min; maint 2.5–5 mg PO q4–6h until term **Peds.** PO: 0.05–0.15 mg/kg/dose PO tid; max 5 mg/24h; ↓ in renal failure **Caution:** [B, +] ↑ toxicity w/MAOIs, TCAs; diabetes, HTN, hyperthyroidism **Contra:** Tachycardia, component hypersensitivity **Supplied:** Tabs 2.5, 5 mg; inj 1 mg/mL; met-dose inhaler **SE:** HTN, hyperthyroidism; high doses may precipitate β₁-adrenergic effects; nervousness, trembling, tachycardia, HTN, dizziness **Notes:** Caution w/ DM **Interactions:** ↑ Effects w/ MAOIs, TCAs; ↓ effects w/ BBs **Labs:** ↑ LFTs, serum glucose **NIPE:** Take oral dose w/ food

Terconazole (Terazol 7) **Uses:** *Vaginal fungal infections* **Action:** Topical antifungal **Dose:** 1 applicatorful or 1 supp intravaginally hs for 3–7 d **Caution:** [C, ?] **Contra:** Component hypersensitivity **Supplied:** Vaginal cream 0.4%, vaginal supp 80 mg **SE:** Vulvar or vaginal burning **Notes:** Insert high into vagina **NIPE:** Insert cream or supp high into vagina, complete full course of Rx, ⊘ intercourse during drug Rx. ↑ risk of breakdown of latex condoms & diaphragms w/ drug

Teriparatide (Forteo) **Uses:** *Severe/refractory osteoporosis* **Action:** PTH (recombinant) **Dose:** 20 μg SQ qd in thigh or abdomen **Caution:** [C, ?/–] **Contra:** Osteosarcoma in animals; ⊘ administer if Paget's Dz, prior radiation, bone mets, hypercalcemia; caution in urolithiasis **Supplied:** 3-mL prefilled device (discard after 28 d) **SE:** Symptomatic orthostatic hypotension on administration, N/D, ↑ Ca, leg cramps **Notes:** ⊘ for use > 2 y **Labs:** ↑ Serum Ca²⁺, uric acid, urine Ca²⁺ **NIPE:** ⊘ Take if Hx Paget's Dz, bone mets or malignancy, or Hx radiation therapy; take w/o regard to food; not used to prevent osteoporosis

Testosterone (AndroGel, Androderm, Striant, Testim, Testoderm) [CIII] **Uses:** *Male hypogonadism* **Action:** Testosterone replacement; ↑ lean body mass and libido **Dose:** All daily dosing: *AndroGel:* 5g gel. *Androderm:* two 2.5-mg or one 5-mg patch qd. *Striant:* 30-mg buccal tabs bid. *Testim:* one 5-g gel tube. *Testoderm:* one 4- or 6-mg scrotal patch **Caution:** [N/A, N/A] **Supplied:** *AndroGel, Testim:* 5-g gel (50-mg test); *Androderm:* 2.5-, 5-mg patches; *Striant:* 30-mg buccal tabs; *Testoderm:* 4- or 6-mg scrotal patch **SE:** Site Rxns, acne, edema, weight gain, gynecomastia, hypertension, ↑ in sleep apnea, prostate enlargement **Notes:** Injectable testosterone enanthate (Delatestryl; Testro-LA) and cypionate (Depo-Testosterone) require inj every 14-28 d w/ highly variable serum levels; PO agents methyltestosterone and oxandrolone associated w/ hepatitis and hepatic tumors; transdermal/mucosal forms preferred **Interactions:** ↑ Effects of anticoagulants, cyclosporine, insulin, hypoglycemics, oxyphenbutazone; ↑ effects with grapefruit juice; ↓ effects with St. John's wort **Labs:** ↑ AST, creatinine, Hgb, Hct, LDL, serum alkaline phosphatase, bilirubin, Ca, K & Na; ↓ HDL, thyroid hormones **NIPE:** Wear gloves if handling transdermal patches; topical drug may cause virilization in female partners. Apply Testoderm to dry shaved scrotal skin (⊘ use chemical depilatories), Androderm to nonscrotal skin, AndroGel to shoulder and upper arms, buccal system, on gum above incisors

Tetanus Immune Globulin **Uses:** *Passive immunization against tetanus* (suspected contaminated wound and unknown immunization status) **Ac-**

tion: Passive immunization **Dose:** *Adults & Peds* 250–500 Units IM (higher doses if delayed therapy) **Caution:** [C, ?] **Contra:** Thimerosal sensitivity **Supplied:** Inj 250-unit vial or syringe **SE:** Pain, tenderness, erythema at inj site; fever, angioedema, muscle stiffness, anaphylaxis **Notes:** May begin active immunization series at different inj site if required **Interactions:** ↓ Immune response when admin w/ Td **NIPE:** Drug does not cause AIDs or hepatitis

Tetanus Toxoid **Uses:** *Tetanus prophylaxis* **Action:** Active immunization **Dose:** Based on previous immunization status **Caution:** [C, ?] **Contra:** Chloramphenicol use, neurologic Sxs w/ previous use, active infection (for routine primary immunization) **Supplied:** Inj tetanus toxoid, fluid, 4–5 Lf Units/0.5 mL; tetanus toxoid, adsorbed, 5, 10 Lf Units/0.5 mL **SE:** Local erythema, induration, sterile abscess; chills, fever, neurologic disturbances **Interactions:** Delay of active immunity if given w/ tetanus immune globulin; ↓ immune response if given to Pts taking corticosteroids or immunosuppressive drugs **NIPE:** Stress the need of timely completion of immunization series

Tetracycline (Achromycin V, Sumycin) **Uses:** *Broad-spectrum antibiotic* **Action:** Bacteriostatic; inhibits protein synthesis. *Spectrum:* Gram(+): *Staphylococcus, Streptococcus.* Gram(–): *H. pylori.* Atypicals: *Chlamydia, Rickettsia,* and *Mycoplasma* **Dose:** *Adults.* 250–500 mg PO bid–qid. *Peds.* >8 y: 25–50 mg/kg/24 h PO q6–12h; ↓ in renal/hepatic impairment **Caution:** [D, +] **Contra:** PRG, antacids, dairy products; children ≤8 y **Supplied:** Caps 100, 250, 500 mg; tabs 250, 500 mg; PO susp 250 mg/5 mL **SE:** Photosensitivity, GI upset, renal failure, pseudotumor cerebri, hepatic impairment **Notes:** Can stain tooth enamel and depress bone formation in children **Interactions:** ↑ Effects of anticoagulants, digoxin; ↓ effects w/ antacids, cimetidine, laxatives, penicillin, Fe suppl, dairy products; ↓ effects of oral contraceptives **Labs:** False − of urinary glucose, serum folate; false ↑ serum glucose; **NIPE:** ⊘ Take w/ dairy products, take w/o food; use barrier contraception

Thalidomide (Thalomid) **Uses:** *Erythema nodosum leprosum (ENL).* graft-versus-host Dz, aphthous ulceration in HIV-+ Pts **Action:** Inhibits neutrophil chemotaxis, ↓ monocyte phagocytosis **Dose:** *GVHD:* 100–1600 mg PO qd. *Stomatitis:* 200 mg bid for 5 d, then 200 mg qd for up to 8 wk. *ENL:* 100–300 mg PO qhs **Cautions:** [X, –] May ↑ HIV viral load; Hx Szs **Contra:** PRG; sexually active males not using latex condoms, or females not using 2 forms of contraception **SE:** Dizziness, drowsiness, rash, fever, orthostasis, Stevens–Johnson syndrome, peripheral neuropathy, Szs **Supplied:** 50-mg cap **Notes:** MD must register w/ STEPS risk management program; informed consent necessary; immediately DC if skin rash develops **Interactions:** ↑ Effects of barbiturates, CNS depressants, chlorpromazine, reserpine, ETOH; ↑ peripheral neuropathy with INH, Li, metronidazole, phenytoin **Labs:** Monitor LFTs, WBC, differential, PRG test before start of therapy & monthly during therapy **NIPE:** If also taking drugs that ↓ hormonal contraceptives (carbamazepine, griseofulvin, phenytoin, rifabutin, rifampin) use two other contraceptive methods; take 1 h pc—food will effect absorption; photosensitivity—use sunscreen; ⊘ PRG & breast-feeding

Theophylline (Theolair, Somophyllin, others) Uses: *Asthma, bronchospasm* Action: Relaxes smooth muscle of the bronchi and pulmonary blood vessels Dose: *Adults.* 900 mg PO ÷ q6h; SR products may be ÷ q8–12h (maint). *Peds.* 16–22 mg/kg/24 h PO ÷ q6h; SR products may be ÷ q8–12h (maint); ↓ dose in hepatic failure Interactions: [C, +] Multiple interactions (eg, caffeine, smoking, carbamazepine, barbiturates, BBs, ciprofloxacin, E-mycin, INH, loop diuretics) Contra: Arrhythmia, hyperthyroidism, uncontrolled Szs Supplied: Elixir 80, 150 mg/15 mL; liq 80, 160 mg/15 mL; caps 100, 200, 250 mg; tabs 100, 125, 200, 225, 250, 300 mg; SR caps 50, 75, 100, 125, 200, 250, 260, 300 mg; SR tabs 100, 200, 250, 300, 400, 450, 500 mg SE: N/V, tachycardia, and Szs; nervousness, arrhythmias Notes: See drug levels in Table 2, page 265 Interactions: ↑ effects w/ allopurinol, BBs, CCBs, cimetidine, corticosteroids, macrolide antibiotics, oral contraceptives, quinolones, rifampin, tacrine, tetracyclines, verapamil, zileuton; ↑ effects of digitalis; ↓ effects w/ barbiturates, loop diuretics, thyroid hormones, tobacco, St John's wort; ↓ effects of benzodiazepines, Li, phenytoin Labs: False + ↑ uric acid, ↑ bilirubin, ESR NIPE: Use barrier contraception; take w/ food if GI upset; caffeine foods ↑ drug effects; smoking ↓ drug effects

Thiamine [Vitamin B₁] Uses: *Thiamine deficiency (beriberi), alcoholic neuritis, Wernicke's encephalopathy* Action: Dietary suppl Dose: *Adults.* Deficiency: 100 mg/d IM for 2 wk, then 5–10 mg/d PO for 1 mo. *Wernicke's encephalopathy:* 100 mg IV single dose, then 100 mg/d IM for 2 wk. *Peds.* 10–25 mg/d IM for 2 wk, then 5–10 mg/24 h PO for 1 mo Caution: [A (C if doses exceed RDA), +] Contra: Component hypersensitivity Supplied: Tabs 5, 10, 25, 50, 100, 500 mg; inj 100, 200 mg/mL SE: Angioedema, paresthesias, rash, anaphylaxis w/ rapid IV administration Notes: IV thiamine use associated w/ anaphylactic Rxn; must give IV slowly Interactions: ↑ Effects of neuromuscular blocking drugs; Labs: False + uric acid; interference w/ theophylline levels

Thiethylperazine (Torecan) Uses: *N/V* Action: Antidopaminergic antiemetic Dose: 10 mg PO, PR, or IM qd–tid; ↓ in hepatic failure Caution: [X, ?] Contra: Phenothiazine and sulfite sensitivity, PRG Supplied: Tabs 10 mg; supp 10 mg; inj 5 mg/mL SE: EPS, xerostomia, drowsiness, orthostatic hypotension, tachycardia, confusion Interactions: ↑ Effects w/ atropine, CNS depressants, epinephrine, Li, MAOIs, TCAs, EtOH; ↑ effects of antihypertensives, phenytoin; ↓ effects of bromocriptine, cabergoline, levodopa Labs: ↑ Serum prolactin level, interferes w/ PRG test NIPE: May cause tardive dyskinesia; ↑ risk of photosensitivity—use sunscreen

6-Thioguanine [6-TG] (Tabloid) Uses: *AML, ALL, CML* Action: Purine-based antimetabolite (substitutes for natural purines interfering w/ nucleotide synthesis) Dose: 2–3 mg/kg/d; ↓ in severe renal/hepatic impairment Caution: [D, −] Contra: Resistance to mercaptopurine Supplied: Tabs 40 mg SE:

Myelosuppression (especially leukopenia and thrombocytopenia), N/V/D, anorexia, stomatitis, rash, hyperuricemia, rare hepatotoxicity **Interactions:** ↑ Bleeding w/ anticoagulants, NSAIDs, salicylates, thrombolytics **Labs:** ↑ Serum and urine uric acid **NIPE:** Take w/o food; ↑ fluids to 2–3 L/d; ⊘ exposure to infection

Thioridazine (Mellaril)
WARNING: Dose-related QT prolongation **Uses:** *Schizophrenia,* psychosis **Action:** Phenothiazine antipsychotic **Dose:** *Adults.* Initially, 50–100 mg PO tid; maint 200–800 mg/24 h PO in 2–4 ÷ doses. *Peds. >2 y:* 0.5–3 mg/kg/24 h PO in 2–3 ÷ doses **Caution:** [C, ?] Phenothiazines, QT$_c$-prolonging agents, AI **Contra:** Phenothiazine sensitivity **Supplied:** Tabs 10, 15, 25, 50, 100, 150, 200 mg; PO conc 30, 100 mg/mL; PO susp 25, 100 mg/5 mL **SE:** Low incidence of EPS; ventricular arrhythmias; hypotension, dizziness, drowsiness, neuroleptic malignant syndrome, Szs, skin discoloration, photosensitivity, constipation, sexual dysfunction, blood dyscrasias, pigmentary retinopathy, hepatic impairment **Notes:** ⊘ EtOH, dilute PO conc in 2–4 oz liquid **Interactions:** ↑ Effects w/ BBs; ↑ effects of anticholinergics, antihypertensives, antihistamines, CNS depressants, nitrates, EtOH; ↓ effects w/ barbiturates, Li, tobacco; ↓ effects of levodopa **Labs:** False + and − urinary PRG test; false + urine bilirubin and amylase; ↑ serum LFTs; **NIPE:** ↑ Risk of photosensitivity—use sunscreen, take w/ food; ⊘ DC abruptly; ↓ temp regulation; urine color change to reddish brown

Thiothixene (Navane)
Uses: *Psychotic disorders* **Action:** Antipsychotic **Dose:** *Adults & Peds.* >12 y: Mild–moderate psychosis: 2 mg PO tid, up to 20–30 mg/d. *Severe psychosis:* 5 mg PO bid; ↑ to a max of 60 mg/24 h PRN. *IM use:* 16–20 mg/24 h ÷ bid–qid; max 30 mg/d. *Peds. <12 y:* 0.25 mg/kg/24 h PO ÷ q6–12h **Caution:** [C, ?] **Contra:** Phenothiazine sensitivity **Supplied:** Caps 1, 2, 5, 10, 20 mg; PO conc 5 mg/mL; inj 2, 5 mg/mL **SE:** Drowsiness, EPS most common; hypotension, dizziness, drowsiness, neuroleptic malignant syndrome, Szs, skin discoloration, photosensitivity, constipation, sexual dysfunction, blood dyscrasias, pigmentary retinopathy, hepatic impairment **Notes:** Dilute PO conc immediately before administration **Interactions:** ↑ Effects w/ BBs; ↑ effects of anticholinergics, antihistamines, BBs, CNS depressants, nitrates, EtOH; ↓ effects w/ barbiturates, Li, tobacco, caffeine; ↓ effects of levodopa **Labs:** ↑ Serum glucose, cholesterol; ↓ serum uric acid; false + urinary PRG test **NIPE:** ↑ risk of photosensitivity—use sunscreen; take w/ food; ⊘ DC abruptly; ↓ temp regulation; darkens urine color

Tiagabine (Gabitril)
Uses: *Adjunctive therapy in Rx of partial Szs,* bipolar disorder **Action:** Inhibition of GABA **Dose:** *Adults and Peds.* ≥ 12 y: Initially 4 mg/d PO, ↑ by 4 mg during 2nd wk; ↑ PRN by 4–8 mg/d based on response, 56 mg/d max **Caution:** [C, M] **Contra:** Component hypersensitivity **Supplied:** Tabs 4, 12, 16, 20 mg **SE:** Dizziness, HA, somnolence, memory impairment, tremors **Notes:** Use gradual withdrawal; used in combination w/ other anticonvulsants **Interactions:** ↑ Effects w/ valproate; ↑ effects of CNS depressants,

EtOH; ↓ effects w/ barbiturates, carbamazepine, phenobarbital, phenytoin, primidone, rifampin, ginkgo biloba **NIPE:** Take w/ food; ○ DC abruptly

Ticarcillin (Ticar)   **Uses:** Infections due to gram(–) bacteria (*Klebsiella, Proteus, E. coli, Enterobacter, P. aeruginosa,* and *Serratia*) involving the skin, bone, resp tract, urinary tract, and abdomen, and septicemia **Action:** 4th-gen PCN, bactericidal; inhibits cell wall synthesis. *Spectrum:* Some gram(+), includes strep, fair enterococcus, not MRSA, gram(–), enhanced w/aminoglycoside use, good anaerobes (*Bactericides*) **Dose:** *Adults.* 3 g IV q4–6h. *Peds.* 200–300 mg/kg/d IV ÷ q4–6h; ↓ dose in renal failure **Caution:** [B, +] Penicillin sensitivity **Supplied:** Inj **SE:** Often used in combination w/ aminoglycosides; interstitial nephritis, anaphylaxis, bleeding, rash, hemolytic anemia **Notes:** Used w/ aminoglycosides **Interactions:** ↑ Effects w/ probenecid; ↑ effects of anticoagulants, MRX; ↓ effects w/ tetracyclines, ↓ effects of aminoglycosides **Labs:** False ↑ urine glucose; ↑ serum AST, ALT, alkaline phosphatase **NIPE:** Monitor for S/Sxs superinfection; frequent loose stools may be due to pseudomembranous colitis

Ticarcillin/Potassium Clavulanate (Timentin)   **Uses:** *Infections involving the skin, bone, resp tract, urinary tract, and abdomen, and septicemia* **Action:** 4th-gen PCN bactericidal; inhibits cell wall synthesis; clavulanic acid blocks β-lactamase. *Spectrum:* Good gram(+) but not MRSA; good gram(–) and anaerobes **Dose:** *Adults.* 3.1 g IV q4–6h. *Peds.* 200–300 mg/kg/d IV ÷ q4–6h; ↓ dose in renal failure **Caution:** [B, +/–] Penicillin sensitivity **Supplied:** Inj **SE:** Hemolytic anemia **Notes:** Often used in combination w/ aminoglycosides; penetrates CNS w/ meningeal irritation; may cause false + proteinuria **Interactions:** ↑ Effects w/ probenecid; ↑ effects of anticoagulants, MRX; ↓ effects w/ tetracyclines, ↓ effects of aminoglycosides, oral contraceptives **Labs:** False ↑ urine glucose, false + urine proteins **NIPE:** Monitor for S/Sxs superinfection; frequent loose stools may be due to pseudomembranous colitis; use barrier contraception

Ticlopidine (Ticlid)   **WARNING:** Neutropenia/agranulocytosis, TTP, and aplastic anemia reported **Uses:** *↓ Risk of thrombotic stroke.* protect grafts status post CABG, diabetic microangiopathy, ischemic heart Dz, DVT prophylaxis, graft prophylaxis after renal transplant **Action:** Plt aggregation inhibitor **Dose:** 250 mg PO bid w/ food **Caution:** [B, ?/–], ↑ toxicity of ASA, anticoagulation, NSAIDs, theophylline **Contra:** Bleeding, hepatic impairment, neutropenia, thrombocytopenia **Supplied:** Tabs 250 mg **SE:** Bleeding, GI upset, rash, ↑ on LFTs **Notes:** Follow CBC 1st 3 mo **Interactions:** ↑ Effects w/ anticoagulants, cimetidine, dong quai, evening primrose oil, feverfew, garlic, ginkgo biloba, ginseng, grapeseed extract, red clover; ↑ effects of ASA, carbamazepine, phenytoin, theophylline; ↓ effects w/ antacids; ↓ effects of cyclosporine, digoxin **Labs:** ↑ ALT, AST, serum alkaline phosphatase, cholesterol, triglycerides **NIPE:** Take w/ food

Timolol (Blocadren)   **WARNING:** Exacerbation of ischemic heart Dz following abrupt withdrawal **Uses:** *HTN and MI* **Action:** β-adrenergic receptor blocker, β_1, β_2 **Dose:** *HTN:* 10–20 mg bid, up to 60 mg/d. *MI:* 10 mg bid **Caution:**

[C (1st tri); D if 2nd or 3rd tri), +] **Contra:** Uncomplicated CHF, cardiogenic shock, bradycardia, heart block, COPD, asthma **Supplied:** Tabs 5, 10, 20 mg **SE:** Sexual dysfunction, arrhythmia, dizziness, fatigue, CHF **Interactions:** ↑ Effects w/ anti-hypertensives, ciprofloxacin, fentanyl, quinindine, ↑ bradycardia and myocardial depression w/ cardiac glycosides, diltiazem, tarcine, verapamil; ↑ effects of epinephrine, ergots, flecainide, lidocaine, nifedipine, phenothiazines, prazosin, verapamil; ↓ effects w/ barbiturates, cholestyramine, colestipol, NSAIDs, penicillin, rifampin, salicylates, sulfinpyrazone; ↓ effect of hypoglycemics, sulfonylureas, theophylline **Labs:** ↑ Serum glucose, BUN, K⁺, lipoprotein, triglycerides, uric acid **NIPE:** ⊘ DC abruptly; ↑ cold sensitivity.

Timolol, Ophthalmic (Timoptic)
Uses: *Glaucoma* **Action:** BB **Dose:** 0.25% 1 gt bid; ↓ to qd when controlled; use 0.5% if needed; 1 gt/d gel **Caution:** [C (1st tri); D 2nd or 3rd), ?/+] **Supplied:** Soln 0.25/0.5%; Timoptic XE (0.25, 0.5%) gel-forming soln **SE:** Local irritation. See Timolol **Additional NIPE:** Depress lacrimal sac 1 min after admin to lessen systemic absorption, admin other drops 10 min before gel

Tinzaparin (Innohep)
Uses: *Rx of DVT w/ or w/out PE* **Action:** LMW heparin **Dose:** 175 Units/kg SQ qd at least 6 d until warfarin dose stabilized **Caution:** [B, ?] Pork hypersensitivity, active bleeding, mild–moderate renal dysfunction **Contra:** Hypersensitivity to sulfites, heparin, benzyl EtOH, HIT **Supplied:** 20,000 Units/mL **SE:** Bleeding, bruising, thrombocytopenia, pain at inj site, ↑ LFTs **Notes:** Anti-Xa levels monitoring tool; no effect on bleeding time, plt Fxn, PT, or aPTT **Interactions:** ↑ Bleeding w/ anticoagulants, cephalosporins, dextran, NSAIDs, penicillins, salicylates, thrombolytics **Labs:** ↑ ALT, AST **NIPE:** ⊘ Rub inj site, admin deep SQ inj, rotate abdominal inj sites

Tioconazole (Vagistat)
Uses: *Vaginal fungal infections* **Action:** Topical antifungal **Dose:** 1 applicatorful intravaginally hs (single dose) **Caution:** [C, ?] **Contra:** Component hypersensitivity **Supplied:** Vaginal oint 6.5% **SE:** Local burning, itching, soreness, polyuria **Notes:** Insert high into vagina **Interactions:** Risk of inactivation of nonoxynol-9 spermacidal **NIPE:** Insert high into vaginal canal; may cause staining of clothing; refrain from intercourse during drug therapy; risk of latex breakdown of condoms and diaphragm

Tiotropium (Spiriva)
Uses: Bronchospasm w/ COPD, bronchitis, and emphysema **Action:** Synthetic anticholinergic similar to atropine **Dose:** 1 cap/d inhaled using HandiHaler device, ⊘ use w/spacer **Caution:** [C, ?/–] BPH, narrow-angle glaucoma, MyG, renal impairment **Contra:** Acute bronchospasm **Supplied:** Caps 18 μg **SE:** URI, xerostomia **Notes:** Monitor FEV₁ or peak flow **Interactions:** ↑ Effects with other anticholinergic drugs **Labs:** Monitor peak flow & PFT **NIPE:** ⊘ For acute resp episode; take daily at same time each day

Tirofiban (Aggrastat)
Uses: *ACS* **Action:** Glycoprotein IIB/IIIa inhibitor **Dose:** Initial 0.4 μg/kg/min for 30 min, followed by 0.1 μg/kg/min; use in combination w/ heparin; ↓ in renal insufficiency **Caution:** [B, ?/–] **Contra:** Bleed-

ing, intracranial neoplasm, vascular malformation, stroke/surgery/trauma w/in last 30 d, severe HTN **Supplied:** Inj 50, 250 µg/mL **SE:** Bleeding, bradycardia, coronary dissection, pelvic pain, rash **Interactions:** ↑ Bleeding risks w/ anticoagulants, antiplatlets, NSAIDs, salicylates, dong quai, feverfew, garlic, ginger, ginkgo, horse chestnut; ↓ effects w/ levothyroxine, omeprazole **Labs:** ↓ Hmg, Hct, plts; **NIPE:** ⊘ Breast-feeding

Tobramycin (Nebcin) Uses: *Serious gram(−) infections* **Action:** Aminoglycoside; inhibits protein synthesis. *Spectrum:* Gram(−) bacteria (including *Pseudomonas*) **Dose:** **Adults.** 1–2.5 mg/kg/dose IV q8–24h. **Peds.** 2.5 mg/kg/dose IV q8h; ↓ w/ renal insufficiency **Caution:** [C, M] **Contra:** Aminoglycoside sensitivity **Supplied:** Inj 10, 40 mg/mL **SE:** Nephrotoxic and ototoxic **Notes:** Monitor CrCl and serum concs for dosage adjustments (see Table 2, page 265) **Interactions:** ↑ Effects w/ carbenicillin, NSAIDs, ticarcillin; ↑ nephrotoxic, neurotoxic, and/or ototoxic effects w/ aminoglycosides, amphotericin B, cephalosporins, cisplatin, furosemide, mannitol, methoxyflurane, polymyxin B, urea, vancomycin **Labs:** ↑ LFTs, BUN, creatinine, serum protein; ↓ serum K+, Na+, Ca2+, Mg2+ **NIPE:** ↑ Fluids to 2–3 L/d; monitor for superinfection

Tobramycin Ophthalmic (AKTob, Tobrex) Uses: *Ocular bacterial infections* **Action:** Aminoglycoside **Dose:** 1–2 gtt q4h; oint bid–tid; if severe, use oint q3–4h, or 2 gtt q30–60min, then less frequently **Caution:** [C, M] **Contra:** Aminoglycoside sensitivity **Supplied:** Oint and soln tobramycin 0.3% **SE:** Ocular irritation. See Tobramycin. **Additional NIPE:** Depress lacrimal sac for 1 min to prevent systemic absorption; ↑ risk of blurred vision & burning

Tobramycin & Dexamethasone Ophthalmic (TobraDex) Uses: *Ocular bacterial infections associated w/ significant inflammation* **Action:** Antibiotic w/ antiinflammatory **Dose:** 0.3% oint apply q3–8h or soln 0.3% apply 1–2 gtt q1–4h **Caution:** [C, M] **Contra:** Aminoglycoside sensitivity **Supplied:** Oint and soln tobramycin 0.3% and dexamethasone 0.1% **SE:** Local irritation or edema **Notes:** Use under ophthalmologist's direction. See Tobramycin. **Additional NIPE:** Eval intraocular pressure and lens if prolonged use

Tolazamide (Tolinase) Uses: *Type 2 DM* **Action:** Sulfonylurea; stimulates pancreatic insulin release; ↑ peripheral insulin sensitivity at peripheral sites; ↓ hepatic glucose output **Dose:** 100–500 mg/d (no benefit >1 g/d) **Caution:** [C, +/−] Elderly, hepatic or renal impairment **Supplied:** Tabs 100, 250, 500 mg **Notes/SE:** HA, dizziness, GI upset, rash, hyperglycemia, photosensitivity, blood dyscrasias **Interactions:** ↑ Effects w/ chloramphenicol, cimetidine, clofibrate, insulin, MAOIs, phenylbutazone, probenecid, salicylates, sulfonamides, garlic, ginseng; ↓ effects w/ diuretics **NIPE:** Risk of disulfiram-type Rxn w/ EtOH; take w/ food; use sunscreen

Tolazoline (Priscoline) Uses: *Peripheral vasospastic disorders* **Action:** Competitively blocks α-adrenergic receptors **Dose:** **Adults.** 10–50 mg IM/IV/SQ qid. **Neonates.** 1–2 mg/kg IV over 10–15 min, then 1–2 mg/kg/h (adjust w/ ↓ renal

Fxn) Caution: [C, ?] Contra: CAD Supplied: Inj 25 mg/mL SE: Hypotension, peripheral vasodilation, tachycardia, arrhythmias, GI upset, blood dyscrasias, renal failure, GI bleeding Interactions: ↓ BP w/ epinephrine, norepinephrine, phenylephrine NIPE: Risk of disulfiram-type Rxn w/ EtOH

Tolbutamide (Orinase) Uses: *Type 2 DM* Action: Sulfonylurea; ↑ pancreatic insulin release; ↑ peripheral insulin sensitivity; ↓ hepatic glucose output Dose: 500–1000 mg bid; ↓ dose in hepatic failure Caution: [C, +] Contra: Sulfonylurea sensitivity Supplied: Tabs 500 mg SE: HA, dizziness, GI upset, rash, photosensitivity, blood dyscrasias, hypoglycemia Interactions: ↑ Effects w/ anticoagulants, antidepressants, chloramphenicol, insulin, H_2 antagonists, MAOIs, metformin, NSAIDs, phenylbutazone, probenecid, salicylates; ↓ effects w/ BBs, CCBs, cholestyramine, corticosteroids, hydantoins, INH, oral contraceptives, phenothiazines, phenytoin, rifampin, sympathomimetics, thiazides, thyroid drugs NIPE: Risk of disulfiram-type Rxn w/ EtOH; take w/ food; use barrier contraception; ↑ risk of photosensitivity—use sunscreen

Tolcapone (Tasmar) Uses: *Adjunct to carbidopa/levodopa in Parkinson's D2* Action: Catechol-O-methyltransferase inhibitor slows metabolism of levodopa Dose: 100 mg PO w/ first daily levodopa/carbidopa dose, followed by doses 6 and 12 h later; ↓ in renal impairment Caution: [C, ?] Contra: Hepatic impairment; nonselective MAOI Supplied: Tablets 100 mg, 200 mg SE: Constipation, xerostomia, vivid dreams, hallucinations, anorexia, N/D, orthostasis, liver failure Notes: ⊘ Abruptly DC or ↓ dose; monitor LFTs Interactions: ↑ Effects of apomorphine, dobutalmine, CNS depressants, desipramine, isoproterenol, levodopa, methyldopa, SSRIs, TCAs, warfarin, EtOH, gout kola, kava kava, St. John's wort, valerian; ↑ risk of hypertensive crisis with nonselective MAO inhibitors (phenelzine, tranylcypromine) Labs: Monitor AST,ALT NIPE: May give w/o regard to food but food ↓ bioavailability of drug; may experience hallucinations

Tolmetin (Tolectin) Uses: *Arthritis and pain* Action: NSAID; inhibits prostaglandins Dose: 200–600 mg tid; 2000 mg/d max Caution: [C (D in 3rd tri or near term), +] Contra: NSAID or ASA sensitivity Supplied: Tabs 200, 600 mg; caps 400 mg SE: Dizziness, rash, GI upset, edema, GI bleeding, renal failure Interactions: ↑ Effect of aminoglycosides, anticoagulants, cyclosporine, digoxin, insulin, Li, MRX, K-sparing diuretics, sulfonylureas; ↓ effect w/ ASA, food; ↓ effect of furosemide, thiazides Labs: ↑ ALT, AST, serum K^+, BUN, ↓ Hmg, Hct NIPE: Take w/ food if GI upset; ↑ risk of photosensitivity—use sunscreen

Tolnaftate (Tinactin) Uses: *Tinea pedis, tinea cruris, tinea corporis, tinea manus, tinea versicolor* Action: Topical antifungal Dose: Apply to area bid for 2–4 wk Caution: [C, ?] Contra: Nail and scalp infections Supplied: OTC 1% liq; gel; powder; cream; soln SE: Local irritation Notes: ⊘ Ocular contact, infection should improve in 7–10 d

Tolterodine (Detrol, Detrol LA) Uses: *Overactive bladder (frequency, urgency, incontinence)* Action: Anticholinergic Dose: Detrol 1–2 mg PO bid; Detrol LA 2–4 mg/d **Caution:** [C, ?/–] CYP2D6 & 3A3/4 inhibitor **Contra:** Urinary retention, gastric retention, or uncontrolled narrow-angle glaucoma **Supplied:** Tabs 1, 2 mg; Detrol LA tabs 2, 4 mg **SE:** Xerostomia, blurred vision **Interactions:** ↑ Effects w/ azole antifungals, macrolides, grapefruit juice, food; ↑ anticholinergic effects w/ amantadine, amoxapine, bupropion, clozapine, cyclobenzaprine, disopyramide, olanzapine, phenothiazines, TCAs **NIPE:** May cause blurred vision

Topiramate (Topamax) **Uses:** *Adjunctive Rx for complex partial Szs & tonic–clonic Szs,* bipolar disorder, neuropathic pain **Action:** Anticonvulsant **Dose:** *Adults.* Total dose 400 mg/d; see product information for 8-wk titration schedule. *Peds.* 2–16 y: Initially, 1–3 mg/kg/d PO qhs; titrate per product info to 5–9 mg/kg/d; ↓ in renal failure **Caution:** [C, ?/–] **Contra:** Component hypersensitivity **Supplied:** Tabs 25, 100, 200 mg; caps sprinkles 15, 25, 50 mg **SE:** May cause metabolic acidosis, kidney stones; fatigue, dizziness, psychomotor slowing, memory impairment, GI upset, tremor, nystagmus; acute secondary angle closure glaucoma requiring drug DC **Notes:** May be associated w/ weight loss; metabolic acidosis generally responsive to dose reduction or DC; DC requires taper **Interactions:** ↑ CNS effects w/ CNS depressants, EtOH; ↑ effects of phenytoin; ↓ effects w/ carbamazepine, phenytoin, valproate, ginkgo biloba; ↓ effects of digoxin, oral contraceptives **Labs:** ↑ LFTs **NIPE:** Take w/o regard to food; ⊘ DC abruptly; use barrier contraception; ↑ fluids to 2–3 L/d

Topotecan (Hycamtin) **WARNING:** Chemo precautions, bone marrow suppression possible **Uses:** *Ovarian CA (cisplatin-refractory), small-cell lung CA,* sarcoma, pediatric non-small-cell lung CA **Action:** Topoisomerase I inhibitor; interferes w/ DNA synthesis **Dose:** 1.5 mg/m²/d as a 1-h IV inf for 5 consecutive days, repeated q3wk; ↓ in renal failure **Caution:** [D, –] **Contra:** PRG, breast-feeding **Supplied:** 4-mg vials **SE:** Myelosuppression, N/V/D, drug fever, skin rash **Interactions:** ↑ Myelosuppression w/ cisplatin, other neoplastic drugs, radiation therapy; ↑ in duration of neutropenia w/ filgrastim **Labs:** ↑ AST, ALT, bilirubin **NIPE:** Monitor CBC; ⊘ PRG, breast-feeding, immunizations; ⊘ exposure to infection; use barrier contraception

Torsemide (Demadex) **Uses:** *Edema, HTN, CHF, and hepatic cirrhosis* **Action:** Loop diuretic; inhibits reabsorption of Na⁺ and Cl⁻ in ascending loop of Henle and distal tubule **Dose:** 5–20 mg/d PO or IV **Caution:** [B, ?] **Contra:** Sulfonylurea sensitivity **Supplied:** Tabs 5, 10, 20, 100 mg; inj 10 mg/mL **SE:** Orthostatic hypotension, HA, dizziness, photosensitivity, electrolyte imbalance, blurred vision, renal impairment **Notes:** 20 mg torsemide = 40 mg furosemide **Interactions:** ↑ Risk of ototoxicity w/ aminoglycosides, cisplatin; ↑ effects w/ thiazides; ↑ effects of anticoagulants, antihypertensives, Li, salicylates; ↓ effects w/ barbiturates, carbamazepine, cholestyramine, NSAIDs, phenytoin, phenobarbital, probenicid, dandelion **NIPE:** Monitor electrolytes, BUN, creatinine, glucose, uric acid; take w/o regard to food; monitor for S/Sxs tinnitus

Tramadol (Ultram)   Uses: *Moderate–severe pain* **Action:** Centrally acting analgesic **Dose:** *Adults.* 50–100 mg PO q4–6h PRN, not to exceed 400 mg/d. *Peds.* 0.5–1 mg/kg PO q 4–6h PRN **Caution:** [C, ?/–] **Contra:** Opioid dependency; MAOIs **Supplied:** Tabs 50 mg **SE:** Dizziness, HA, somnolence, GI upset, resp depression, anaphylaxis (sensitivity to codeine) **Notes:** ↓ Sz threshold, tolerance or dependence may develop **Interactions:** ↑ Effects w/ cimetidine, CNS depressants, MAOIs, phenothiazines, quinidine, TCAs, EtOH, St. John's wort; ↑ effects of digoxin, warfarin; ↓ effects w/ carbamazepine **Labs:** ↑ Creatinine, LFTs, ↓ Hmg **NIPE:** Take w/o regard to food

Tramadol/Acetaminophen (Ultracet)   Uses: *Short-term Rx acute pain (<5 d)* **Action:** Centrally acting analgesic; nonnarcotic analgesic **Dose:** 2 tabs PO q4–6h PRN; 8 tabs/d max. *Elderly/renal impairment:* Lowest possible dose; 2 tabs q12h max if CrCl <30 **Caution:** [C, –] Szs, hepatic/renal impairment, or Hx addictive tendencies **Contra:** Acute intoxication **Supplied:** Tab 37.5 mg tramadol/325 mg APAP **SE:** SSRIs, TCAs, opioids, MAOIs ↑ risk of Szs; dizziness, somnolence, tremor, headache, N/V/D, constipation, xerostomia, liver toxicity, rash, pruritus, ↑ sweating, physical dependence **Notes:** ⊘ EtOH **Interactions:** ↑ Effects w/ cimetidine, CNS depressants, MAOIs, phenothiazines, quinidine, TCAs, EtOH, St. John's wort; ↑ effects of digoxin, warfarin; ↓ effects w/ carbamazepine **Labs:** ↑ Creatinine, LFTs, ↓ Hmg **NIPE:** Take w/o regard to food; ⊘ take other acetaminophen-containing drugs

Trandolapril (Mavik)   **WARNING:** Use in PRG in 2nd/3rd tri can result in fetal death **Uses:** *HTN,* CHF, LVD, post-AMI **Action:** ACEI **Dose:** *HTN:* 2–4 mg/d. *CHF/LVD:* 4 mg/d; ↓ in severe renal/hepatic impairment **Caution:** [D, +] ACEI sensitivity, angioedema w/ ACEIs **Supplied:** Tabs 1, 2, 4 mg **SE:** Hypotension, bradycardia, dizziness, hyperkalemia, GI upset, renal impairment, cough, angioedema **Notes:** Afro-Americans, minimal effective dose is 2 mg vs 1 mg in Caucasians **Interactions:** ↑ Effects w/ diuretics; ↑ effects of insulin, Li; ↓ effects w/ ASA, NSAIDs; **NIPE:** ⊘ Take if PRG or breast-feeding; ⊘ K-containing salt substitutes

Trastuzumab (Herceptin)   Uses: *Metastatic breast cancer overexpress the HER2/neu protein* **Action:** Monoclonal antibody; binds human epidermal growth factor receptor 2 protein (HER2); mediates cellular cytotoxicity **Dose:** Refer to specific protocol **Caution:** [B, ?] CV dysfunction, hypersensitivity/inf Rxns **Contra:** None known **Supplied:** Injectable **SE:** Anemia, cardiomyopathy, nephritic syndrome, pneumonitis **Notes:** Inf-related Rxns minimized w/ acetaminophen, diphenhydramine, and meperidine **Interactions:** ↑ Risk of cardiac dysfunction with anthracyclines, cyclophosphamide, doxorubicin, epirubicin; **Labs:** Monitor cardiac function; **NIPE:** ⊘ Use dextrose inf soln; ⊘ breast-feed for 6 mo following drug therapy

Trazodone (Desyrel)   Uses: *Depression,* hypnotic, augment other antidepressants **Action:** Antidepressant; inhibits reuptake of serotonin and norepinephrine **Dose:** *Adults & Adolescents.* 50–150 mg PO qd–qid; max 600 mg/d. *Sleep:* 50

mg PO, qhs, PRN **Caution:** [C, ?/–] **Contra:** Component hypersensitivity **Supplied:** Tabs 50, 100, 150, 300 mg **SE:** Dizziness, HA, sedation, nausea, xerostomia, syncope, confusion, tremor, hepatitis, EPS **Notes:** May take 1–2 wk for symptomatic improvement **Interactions:** ↑ Effects w/ fluoxetine, phenothiazines; ↑ risk of serotonin syndrome w/ MAOIs, SSRIs, venlafaxine, St. John's wort; ↑ CNS depression w/ barbiturates, CNS depressants, opioids, sedatives, EtOH; ↑ hypotension w/ antihypertensive, neuroleptics; nitrates, EtOH; ↑ effects of clonidine, digoxin, phenytoin; ↓ effects w/ carbamazepine **NIPE:** Take w/ food; ↑ fluids to 2–3 L/d; ⊘ DC abruptly; ↑ risk of priapism

Treprostinil Sodium (Remodulin) **Uses:** *NYHA class II–IV pulmonary arterial hypertension* **Action:** Vasodilation, inhibition of plt aggregation **Dose:** 0.625–1.25 ng/kg/min cont inf **Caution:** [B, ?/–] **Contra:** Component hypersensitivity **Supplied:** 1, 2.5, 5, 10 mg/mL inj **SE:** Additive effects w/ anticoagulants, antihypertensives; inf site Rxns **Notes:** Initiate in monitored setting; ⊘ DC or reduce dose abruptly **Interactions:** ↑ Effects w/ antihypertensives; ↑ effects of anticoagulants **NIPE:** Teach care of inf site and pump; use barrier contraception; once med vial used discard after 14 d

Tretinoin, Topical [Retinoic Acid] (Retin-A, Avita, Renova) **Uses:** *Acne vulgaris, sun-damaged skin, wrinkles* (photoaging), some skin CAs **Action:** Exfoliant retinoic acid derivative **Dose:** *Adults & Peds.* >12 y: Apply qd hs (if irritation develops, ↓ frequency). *Photoaging:* Start w/ 0.025%, ↑ to 0.1% over several months (apply only q3d if on neck area; dark skin may require bid application) **Caution:** [C, ?] **Contra:** Retinoid sensitivity **Supplied:** Cream 0.025, 0.05, 0.1%; gel 0.01, 0.025, 0.1%; microformulation gel 0.1%; liq 0.05% **SE:** ⊘ sunlight; edema; skin dryness, erythema, scaling, changes in pigmentation, stinging, photosensitivity **Interactions:** ↑ photosensitivity w/ quinolones, phenothiazines, sulfonamides, tetracyclines, thiazides, dong quai, St. John's wort; ↑ skin irritation w/ topical sulfur, resorcinol, benzoyl peroxide, salicylic acid; ↓ effects w/ vitamin A suppl and foods w/ excess vitamin A such as fish oils **NIPE:** ⊘ Apply to mucous membranes, wash skin and apply med after 30 min, wash hands after application; ⊘ breast-feeding, PRG use contraception; use sunscreen

Triamcinolone (Azmacort) **Uses:** *Chronic asthma* **Actions:** Topical steroid **Dose:** Two inhalations tid–qid or 4 inhal bid **Caution:** [C, ?] **SE:** Cough, oral candidiasis **Contra:** Component hypersensitivity **Supplied:** Inhaler 100 μg/met spray **Notes:** Instruct Pts to rinse their mouth after use; not for acute asthma **Interactions:** ↑ Effects w/ salmeterol, troleandomycin; ↓ effects with barbiturates, hydantoins, phenytoin, rifampin; ↓ effects of diuretics, insulin, oral hypoglycemics, K suppl, salicylates, somatrem, live virus vaccines **Labs:** ↑ serum glucose, lipids, amylase, sodium; ↓ skin test reaction, serum Ca, K+, thyroxine **NIPE:** Use bronchodilator several minutes before triamcinolone; allow 1 min between repeat inhalations

Triamcinolone & Nystatin (Mycolog-II) Uses: *Cutaneous candidiasis* **Action:** Antifungal and antiinflammatory **Dose:** Apply lightly to area bid; max 25 mg/d **Caution:** [C, ?] **Contra:** Varicella; systemic fungal infections **Supplied:** Cream and oint 15, 30, 60, 120 mg **SE:** Local irritation, hypertrichosis, changes in pigmentation **Notes:** For short-term use (<7 d) **Interactions:** ↓ Effects w/ barbiturates, phenytoin, rifampin; ↓ effects of salicylates, vaccines **NIPE:** ∅ Eyes; ∅ apply to open skin/wounds, eyes, mucous membranes

Triamterene (Dyrenium) Uses: *Edema associated w/ CHF, cirrhosis* **Action:** K-sparing diuretic **Dose:** *Adults.* 100–300 mg/24 h PO ÷ qd–bid. *Peds.* 2–4 mg/kg/d in 1–2 ÷ doses; ↓ dose in renal/hepatic impairment **Caution:** [B (manufacturer; D expert opinion), ?/–] **Contra:** Hyperkalemia, renal impairment, DM; caution w/ other K-sparing diuretics **Supplied:** Caps 50, 100 mg **SE:** Hyperkalemia, blood dyscrasias, liver damage, and other Rxns **Interactions:** ↑ Risk of hyperkalemia w/ ACEIs, K suppls, K-sparing drugs, K-containing drugs, K salt substitutes; ↑ effects w/ cimetidine, indomethacin; ↑ effects of amantadine, antihypertensives, Li; ↓ effects of digitalis **Labs:** False ↑ serum digoxin **NIPE:** Take w/ food, blue discoloration of urine, ↑ risk of photosensitivity—use sunscreen

Triazolam (Halcion) [C-IV] Uses: *Short-term management of insomnia* **Action:** Benzodiazepine **Dose:** 0.125–0.25 mg/d PO hs PRN; ↓ dose in elderly **Caution:** [X, ?/–] **Contra:** Narrow-angle glaucoma; cirrhosis; concurrent amprenavir, ritonavir, or nelfinavir **Supplied:** Tabs 0.125, 0.25 mg **SE:** Tachycardia, CP, drowsiness, fatigue, memory impairment, GI upset **Notes:** Additive CNS depression w/ EtOH and other CNS depressants **Interactions:** ↑ Effects w/ azole antifungals, cimetidine, clarithromycin, ciprofloxin, CNS depressants, disulfiram, digoxin, erythromycin, fluvoxamine, INH, protease inhibitors, troleandomycin, verapamil, EtOH, grapefruit juice, kava kava, valerian; ↓ effects of levodopa; ↓ effects w/ carbamazepine, phenytoin, rifampin, theophylline **NIPE:** ∅ PRG or breast-feeding; ∅ DC abruptly after long-term use

Triethanolamine (Cerumenex) [OTC] Uses: *Cerumen (ear wax) removal* **Action:** Ceruminolytic agent **Dose:** Fill the ear canal and insert the cotton plug; irrigate w/ water after 15 min; repeat PRN **Caution:** [C, ?] **Contra:** Perforated tympanic membrane, otitis media **Supplied:** Soln 6, 12 mL **SE:** Local dermatitis, pain, erythema, pruritus **NIPE:** Warm soln to body temp before use for better effect

Triethylenetriphosphamide (Thio-Tepa, Tespa, TSPA) Uses: *Hodgkin's and NHLs; leukemia; breast, ovarian, and bladder CAs* (IV and intravesical therapy), preparative regimens for allogeneic and ABMT in high doses **Action:** Polyfunctional alkylating agent **Dose:** 0.5 mg/kg q1–4wk, 6 mg/m² IM or IV ×4 d q2–4wk, 15–35 mg/m² by cont IV inf over 48 h; 60 mg into the bladder and retained 2 h q1–4wk; 900–125 mg/m² in ABMT regimens (highest dose w/o ABMT is 180 mg/m²); 1–10 mg/m² (typically 15 mg) IT 1 or 2 ×/wk; 0.8 mg/kg in

1–2 L of soln may be instilled intraperitoneally; ↓ in renal failure **Caution:** [D, –]
Contra: Component hypersensitivity **Supplied:** Inj 15 mg **SE:** Myelosuppression,
N/V, dizziness, HA, allergy, paresthesias, alopecia

Trifluoperazine (Stelazine) **Uses:** *Psychotic disorders* **Action:** Phenothiazine; blocks postsynaptic CNS dopaminergic receptors in the brain **Dose:**
Adults. 2–10 mg PO bid. *Peds.* 6–12 y: 1 mg PO qd–bid initially, gradually ↑ to 15
mg/d; ↓ dose in elderly/debilitated Pts **Caution:** [C, ?/–] **Contra:** Hx blood
dyscrasias; phenothiazine sensitivity **Supplied:** Tabs 1, 2, 5, 10 mg; PO conc 10
mg/mL; inj 2 mg/mL **SE:** Orthostatic hypotension, EPS, dizziness, neuroleptic malignant syndrome, skin discoloration, lowered Sz threshold, photosensitivity, blood
dyscrasias **Notes:** PO conc must be diluted to 60 mL or more prior to administration; requires several weeks for onset of effects

Trifluridine (Viroptic) **Uses:** *Herpes simplex keratitis and conjunctivitis*
Action: Antiviral **Dose:** 1 gt q2h (max 9 gtt/d); ↓ to 1 gt q4h after healing begins;
treat up to 14 d **Caution:** [C, M] **Contra:** Component hypersensitivity **Supplied:**
Soln 1% **SE:** Local burning, stinging **Interactions:** ↑ Hypotensive effects w/ antihypertensives, nitrates, sulfadoxine-pyrimethamine, EtOH; ↑ effects of anticholinergics; ↑ CNS depression w/ antihistamines, CNS depressants, narcotics, EtOH; ↓
effects w/ barbiturates, Li, caffeine, tobacco; ↓ effects of guanadrel, guanethidine,
levodopa **Labs:** ↑ LFTs, serum prolactin levels, ↑ Hmg, Hct, plts, false PRG test results + or – **NIPE:** Use sunscreen due to photosensitivity; affects body temperature
regulation; reddish brown urine color change; ⊘ DC abruptly after long-term use

Trihexyphenidyl (Artane) **Uses:** *Parkinson's Dz* **Action:** Blocks excess acetylcholine at cerebral synapses **Dose:** 2–5 mg PO qd–qid **Caution:** [C, +]
Contra: Narrow-angle glaucoma, GI obstruction, MyG, bladder obstructions **Supplied:** Tabs 2, 5 mg; SR caps 5 mg; elixir 2 mg/5 mL **SE:** Dry skin, constipation,
xerostomia, photosensitivity, tachycardia, arrhythmias **Interactions:** ↑ Effects w/
MAOIs, phenothiazines, quinidine, TCAs; ↑ effects of amantadine, anticholinergics, digoxin; ↓ effects w/ antacids, tacrine; ↓ effects of chlorpromazine, haloperidol, tacrine **Labs:** False ↑ T3, T4 **NIPE:** Take w/ food; monitor for urinary
hesitancy or retention; ⊘ DC abruptly; ↑ risk of heat stroke

Trimethobenzamide (Tigan) **Uses:** *N/V* **Action:** Inhibits medullary
chemoreceptor trigger zone **Dose:** *Adults.* 250 mg PO or 200 mg PR or IM tid–qid
PRN. *Peds.* 20 mg/kg/24 h PO or 15 mg/kg/24 h PR or IM in 3–4 ÷ doses **Caution:**
[C, ?] **Contra:** Benzocaine sensitivity **Supplied:** Caps 100, 250 mg; supp 100, 200
mg; inj 100 mg/mL **SE:** Drowsiness, hypotension, dizziness; hepatic impairment,
blood dyscrasias, Szs, parkinsonian-like syndrome **Notes:** In the presence of viral
infections, may mask emesis or mimic CNS effects of Reye's syndrome **Interactions:** ↑ CNS depression w/ antidepressants, antihistamines, opioids, sedatives,
EtOH; ↑ risk of extrapyramidal effects

Trimethoprim (Trimpex, Proloprim) **Uses:** *UTI due to susceptible
gram(+) and gram(–) organisms;* suppression of UTI **Action:** Inhibits dihydrofo-

late reductase. *Spectrum:* Many gram(+) and (–) except *Bacteroides, Branhamella, Brucella, Chlamydia, Clostridium, Mycobacterium, Mycoplasma, Nocardia, Neisseria, Pseudomonas,* and *Treponema* **Dose: Adults.** 100 mg/d PO bid or 200 mg/d PO. **Peds.** 4 mg/kg/d in 2 ÷ doses; ↓ in renal failure **Caution:** [C, +] **Contra:** Megaloblastic anemia due to folate deficiency **Supplied:** Tabs 100, 200 mg; PO soln 50 mg/5 mL **SE:** Rash, pruritus, megaloblastic anemia, hepatic impairment, blood dyscrasias **Notes:** Take w/ plenty of water **Interactions:** ↑ Effects w/ dapsone; ↑ effects of dapsone, phenytoin, procainamide; ↓ efficacy w/ rifampin **Labs:** ↑ LFTs, BUN, creatinine **NIPE:** ↑ Fluids to 2–3 L/d; ↑ risk of folic acid deficiency

Trimethoprim (TMP)–Sulfamethoxazole (SMX) [Co-Trimoxazole] (Bactrim, Septra)

Uses: *UTI Rx and prophylaxis, otitis media, sinusitis, bronchitis* **Action:** SMX-inhibiting synthesis of dihydrofolic acid; TMP-inhibiting dihydrofolate reductase to impair protein synthesis. *Spectrum:* Includes *Shigella, P. jiroveci* (formerly *carinii*), and *Nocardia* infections, *Mycoplasma, Enterobacter* sp, *Staphylococcus, Streptococcus,* and more **Dose: Adults.** 1 DS tab PO bid or 5–20 mg/kg/24 h (based on TMP) IV in 3–4 ÷ doses. *P. jiroveci:* 15–20 mg/kg/d IV or PO (TMP) in 4 ÷ doses. *Nocardia:* 10–15 mg/kg/d IV or PO (TMP) in 4 ÷ doses. *UTI prophylaxis:* 1 PO qd. **Peds.** 8–10 mg/kg/24 h (TMP) PO ÷ into 2 doses or 3–4 doses IV; ⊘ use in newborns; ↓ in renal failure; maintain hydration **Caution:** [B (D if near term), +] **Contra:** Sulfonamide sensitivity, porphyria, megaloblastic anemia w/ folate deficiency, significant hepatic impairment **Supplied:** Regular tabs 80 mg TMP/400 mg SMX; DS tabs 160 mg TMP/800 mg SMX; PO susp 40 mg TMP/200 mg SMX/5 mL; inj 80 mg TMP/400 mg SMX/5 mL **SE:** Allergic skin Rxns, photosensitivity, GI upset, Stevens–Johnson syndrome, blood dyscrasias, hepatitis **Notes:** Synergistic combination, interacts w/ warfarin **Interactions:** ↑ Effect of dapsone, MRX, phenytoin, sulfonylureas, warfarin, zidovudine; ↓ effects w/ rifampin; ↓ effect of cyclosporine **Labs:** ↑ Serum bilirubin, alkaline phosphatase, creatinine **NIPE:** ↑ Risk of photosensitivity—use sunscreen; ↑ fluids to 2–3 L/d

Trimetrexate (Neutrexin)

WARNING: Must be used w/ leucovorin to ⊘ toxicity **Uses:** *Moderate to severe PCP* **Action:** Inhibits dihydrofolate reductase **Dose:** 45 mg/m² IV q24h for 21 d; administer w/ leucovorin 20 mg/m² IV q6h for 24 d; ↓ in hepatic impairment **Caution:** [D, ?/–] **Contra:** MTX sensitivity **Supplied:** Inj **SE:** Sz, fever, rash, GI upset, anemias, ↑ LFTs, peripheral neuropathy, renal impairment **Notes:** Use cytotoxic cautions; inf over 60 min **Interactions:** ↑ Effects w/ azole antifungals, cimetidine, erythromycin; ↓ effects w/ rifabutin, rifampin; ↓ effects of pneumococcal immunization **Labs:** ↑ LFTs, SCr **NIPE:** ⊘ PRG, breast-feeding use contraception; ⊘ exposure to infection

Triptorelin (Trelstar Depot, Trelstar LA)

Uses: *Palliation of advanced CAP* **Action:** LHRH analogue; ↓ gonadotropin secretion when given continuously; transient surge in LH, FSH, testosterone, and estradiol after first dose; w/ chronic/continuous use (usually 2–4 wk), sustained ↓ LH and FSH w/ ↓ testicular and ovarian steroidogenesis similar to surgical castration **Dose:** 3.75 mg IM monthly or 11.25 mg IM q3mo **Caution:** [X, N/A] **Contra:** Not indicated in females **Supplied:** Inj depot 3.75 mg; LA 11.25 mg **SE:** Dizziness, emotional lability, fatigue, headache, insomnia HTN, diarrhea, vomiting, impotence, urinary retention, UTI, pruritus, anemia, inj site pain, musculoskeletal pain, allergic Rxns **Interactions:** ↑ Risk of severe hyperprolactinemia w/ antipsychotics, metoclopramide **Labs:** Suppression of pituitary-gonadal Fxn **NIPE:** ⊘ PRG or breastfeeding; may cause hot flashes; initial ↑ bone pain

Trospium Chloride (Sanctura) **Uses:** Overactive bladder **Action:** Anticholinergic **Dose:** 20 mg PO bid; CrCl <30 mL/min, 20 mg qhs; >75 y ↓ dose; take 1 h ac or on empty stomach **Caution:** [C, ?] Hepatic impairment **Contra:** Urinary/gastric retention, narrow-angle glaucoma **Supplied:** 20-mg tabs **SE:** Xerostomia, constipation, HA **Notes:** Food impairs absorption **Interactions:** ↑ Effects may be seen when used with amiloride, digoxin, morphine, metformin, procainamide, quinidine, quinine, ranitidine, tenofovir, triamterene, trimethoprim, vancomycin; ↑ effects of these drugs may be seen amiloride, digoxin, morphine, metformin, procainamide, quinidine, quinine, ranitidine, tenofovir, triamterene, trimethoprim, vancomycin **NIPE:** Take w/o food 1 h ac

Trovafloxacin (Trovan) **WARNING:** Trovan has been associated w/ serious liver injury leading to need for liver transplantation and/or death. **Uses:** *Life-threatening infections* including pneumonia, complicated intraabdominal, gynecologic/pelvic, or skin infections **Action:** Fluoroquinolone antibiotic; inhibits DNA gyrase. *Spectrum:* Broad-spectrum gram(+) and gram(−), including anaerobes; TB typically resistant **Dose:** 200 mg/d; ↓ in hepatic impairment **Caution:** [C, –] Use w/ caution in children **Contra:** Hepatic impairment **Supplied:** Inj 5 mg/mL in 40 and 60 mL; tabs 100, 200 mg **SE:** Liver failure, dizziness, HA, nausea, rash **Notes:** Use restricted to hospitals; hepatotoxicity led to restricted availability **Interactions:** ↑ Risk of photosensitivity with dong quai, St John's wort; ↑ risk of tendon rupture if used with corticosteroids ↓ effects with antacids containing Al or Mg, Fe salts, Mg, sucralfate, vitamins/minerals containing Fe, zinc; IV morphine; dairy products **Labs:** Monitor LFTs **NIPE:** Admin antacids or IV morphine 2 h after trovafloxacin on empty stomach, take w/o regard to food and w/ 8 oz water, risk of photosensitivity–use sunscreen

Urokinase (Abbokinase) **Uses:** *PE, DVT, restore patency to IV catheters* **Action:** Converts plasminogen to plasmin that causes clot lysis **Dose:** *Adults & Peds* Systemic effect: 4400 Units/kg IV over 10 min, followed by 4400–6000 Units/kg/h for 12 h. *Restore catheter patency:* Inject 5000 Units into catheter and aspirate **Caution:** [B, +] **Contra:** ⊘ use w/in 10 d of surgery, delivery, or organ biopsy; bleeding, CVA, vascular malformation **Supplied:** Powder for inj 5000 Units/mL, 250,000-unit vial **SE:** Bleeding, hypotension, dyspnea, bronchospasm, anaphylaxis, cholesterol embolism **Interactions:** ↑ Risk of bleeding w/ anticoagulants, ASA, heparin, indomethacin, NSAIDs, phenylbutazone, feverfew, garlic, ginger, ginkgo biloba; ↓ effects w/ aminocaproic acid **Labs:** ↑ PT, PTT; ↓ fibrinogen, plasminogen

Valacyclovir (Valtrex) Uses: *Herpes zoster; genital herpes* **Action:** Prodrug of acyclovir; inhibits viral DNA replication. *Spectrum:* Herpes simplex I and II **Dose:** 1 g PO tid. *Genital herpes:* 500 mg bid × 7 d. *Herpes prophylaxis:* 500–1000 mg/d; ↓ in renal failure **Caution:** [B, +] **Supplied:** Caplets 500 mg **SE:** HA, GI upset, dizziness, pruritus, photophobia **Interactions:** ↑ Effects w/ cimetidine, probenecid **Labs:** ↑ LFTs, creatinine **NIPE:** Take w/o regard to food; ↑ fluids to 2–3 L/d; begin drug at first sign of S/Sxs

Valdecoxib (Bextra) (withdrawn in 2005 by manufacturer) Uses: *RA, osteoarthritis, primary dysmenorrhea* **Action:** COX-2 inhibition **Dose:** *Arthritis:* 10 mg PO qd. *Dysmenorrhea:* 20 mg PO bid, PRN **Caution:** [C, ?] Asthma, urticaria, allergic-type Rxns after ASA or NSAIDs, sulfonamide hypersensitivity **Supplied:** Tabs 10, 20 mg **SE:** ↑ LFT, GI ulceration or bleeding; dizziness, edema, HTN, HA, peptic ulcer, renal failure; serious hypersensitivity Rxns have occurred, including Stevens–Johnson syndrome **Interactions:** ↑ Effects w/ azole antifungals; ↑ effects of dextromethorphan, Li, warfarin; ↓ effects of ACEIs, diuretics **Labs:** ↑ LFTs, BUN, creatinine **NIPE:** Take w/ food if GI upset; ↑ fluids to 2–3 L/d

Valganciclovir (Valcyte) Uses: *CMV* **Action:** Ganciclovir prodrug; inhibits viral DNA synthesis **Dose:** Induction, 900 mg PO bid w/ food × 21 d, then 900 mg PO qd; ↓ in renal dysfunction **Caution:** [C, ?/–] Use w/ imipenem/cilastatin, nephrotoxic drugs **Contra:** Hypersensitivity to acyclovir, ganciclovir, valganciclovir; ANC < 500/mm²; plt < 25 K; Hgb < 8 g/dL **Supplied:** Tabs 450 mg **SE:** Bone marrow suppression **Notes:** Monitor CBC and Cr **Interactions:** ↑ Effects w/ cytotoxic drugs, immunosuppressive drugs, probenecid; ↑ risks of nephrotoxicity w/ amphotericin B, cyclosporine; ↑ effects w/ didanosine **Labs:** ↑ SCr **NIPE:** Take w/ food; ⊘ PRG, breast-feeding, EtOH, NSAIDs; use contraception for at least 3 mo after drug Rx

Valproic Acid (Depakene, Depakote) Uses: *Rx epilepsy, mania; prophylaxis of migraines,* Alzheimer's behavior disorder **Action:** Anticonvulsant; ↑ availability of GABA **Dose:** *Adults & Peds.* Szs: 30–60 mg/kg/24 h PO ÷ tid (after initiation of 10–15 mg/kg/24 h). *Mania:* 750 mg in 3 ÷ doses, ↑ 60 mg/kg/d max. *Migraines:* 250 mg bid, ↑ 1000 mg/d max; ↓ dose in hepatic impairment **Caution:** [D, +] **Contra:** Severe hepatic impairment **Supplied:** Caps 250 mg; syrup 250 mg/5 mL **SE:** somnolence, dizziness, GI upset, diplopia, ataxia, rash, thrombocytopenia, hepatitis, pancreatitis, prolonged bleeding times, alopecia, weight gain, hyperammonemic encephalopathy reported in Pts w/ urea cycle disorders **Notes:** Monitor LFTs and serum levels (see Table 2, page 265); phenobarbital and phenytoin may alter levels **Interactions:** ↑ Effects w/ clarithromycin, erythromycin, felbamate, INH, salicylates, troleandomycin; ↑ effects of anticoagulants, lamotrigine, nimodipine, phenobarbital, primidone, zidovudine; ↑ CNS depression w/ CNS depressants, haloperidol, loxapine, maprotiline, MAOIs, phenothiazines, thioxanthenes, TCAs, EtOH; ↓ effects w/ cholestyramine, colestipol; ↓ effects of clozapine, rifampin **Labs:** ↑ LFTs; altered TFTs, false + urinary ketones **NIPE:** Take w/ food for GI upset; ⊘ PRG, breast-feeding; DC abruptly

Valsartan (Diovan) **WARNING:** Use during 2nd/3rd tri of PRG can cause fetal harm **Uses:** *HTN, CHF, DN* **Action:** Angiotensin II receptor antagonist **Dose:** 80–160 mg/d **Caution:** [C (1st tri; D 2nd and 3rd tri), ?/–] W/ K-sparing diuretics or K suppls **Contra:** Severe hepatic impairment, biliary cirrhosis, biliary obstruction, primary hyperaldosteronism, bilateral renal artery stenosis **Supplied:** Caps 80, 160 mg **SE:** Hypotension, dizziness **Interactions:** ↑ Effects w/ diuretics, Li; ↑ risk of hyperkalemia w/ K-sparing diuretics, K suppls, trimethoprim **Labs:** ↑ LFTs, K⁺, ↓ Hmg, Hct **NIPE:** Take w/o regard to food; ⊘ PRG, breast-feeding; use contraception

Vancomycin (Vancocin, Vancoled) **Uses:** *Serious MRSA infections; enterococcal infections; PO Rx of C. difficile pseudomembranous colitis* **Action:** Inhibits cell wall synthesis. **Spectrum:** Gram(+) bacteria & some anaerobes (includes MRSA, Staphylococcus sp, Enterococcus sp, Streptococcus sp, C. difficile) **Dose:** *Adults.* 1 g IV q12h; for colitis 125–500 mg PO q6h. *Peds.* 40–60 mg/kg/24 h IV in ÷ doses q6–12 h. *Neonates.* 10–15 mg/kg/dose q12h; (↓ in renal insufficiency **Caution:** [C, M] **Contra:** Component hypersensitivity; ⊘ in Hx hearing loss **Supplied:** Caps 125, 250 mg; powder for PO soln; powder for inj 500 mg, 1000 mg, 10 g/vial **SE:** Ototoxic and nephrotoxic; GI upset (PO), neutropenia **Notes:** See drug levels (see Table 2, page 265); not absorbed PO, local effect in gut only; give IV dose slowly (over 1–3 h) to prevent "red-man syndrome" (a red flushing of the head, neck, and upper torso); IV product may be given PO for colitis **Interactions:** ↑ Ototoxicity and nephrotoxicity w/ ASA, aminoglycosides, cyclosporine, cisplatin, loop diuretics; ↓ effects of MRX **Labs:** ↑ BUN; **NIPE:** Take w/ food, ↑ fluid to 2–3 L/d

Vardenafil (Levitra) **WARNING:** May prolong QT$_c$ interval **Uses:** *Erectile dysfunction* **Action:** Phosphodiesterase 5 inhibitor **Dose:** 10 mg PO 60 min before sexual activity; 2.5 mg if administered w/ CYP3A4 inhibitor; administer no more than once daily or in doses greater than 20 mg **Caution:** [B, –] W/ CV, hepatic, or renal Dz **Contra:** Nitrates **Supplied:** 2.5-mg, 5-mg, 10-mg, 20-mg tabs **SE:** Hypotension, headache, dyspepsia, priapism **Notes:** Concomitant α-blockers may cause hypotension **Interactions:** ↑ Effects w/ erythromycin, keotconazole, indinavir, ritonavir; ↑ effects of α-blockers, nitrates; ↓ effects of indinavir, ritonavir **NIPE:** Take w/o regard to food; ↑ risk of priapism

Varicella Virus Vaccine (Varivax) **Uses:** *Prevention of varicella (chickenpox) infection* **Action:** Active immunization; live attenuated virus **Dose:** *Adults & Peds.* 0.5 mL SQ, repeat 4–8 wk **Caution:** [C, M] **Contra:** Immunocompromise; neomycin-anaphylactoid Rxn, blood dyscrasias; immunosuppressive drugs; ⊘ PRG for 3 mo after **Supplied:** Powder for inj **SE:** May cause mild varicella infection; fever, local Rxns, irritability, GI upset **Notes:** Recommended for all children and adults who have not had chickenpox **Interactions:** ↓ Effects w/ acyclovir, immunosuppressant drugs **NIPE:** ⊘ Aalicylates for 6 wk after immunization; ⊘ PRG for 3 mo after immunization

Vasopressin [Antidiuretic Hormone, ADH] (Pitressin) Uses:
DI; Rx postop abdominal distension; adjunct Rx of GI bleeding & esophageal varices; pulseless VT & VF, adjunct systemic vasopressor (IV drip) **Action:** Posterior pituitary hormone, potent GI vasoconstrictor, potent peripheral vasoconstrictor **Dose: *Adults & Peds*** DI: 2.5–10 Units SQ or IM tid–qid or 1.5–5.0 Units IM q1–3d of the tannate. *GI hemorrhage:* 0.2–0.4 Units/min; ↓ dose in cirrhosis; caution in vascular Dz. *VT/VF:* 40 Units IVP × 1. *Vasopressor:* 0.01–0.1 Units/kg/min **Caution:** [B, +] **Contra:** Hypersensitivity **Supplied:** Inj 20 Units/mL **SE:** HTN, arrhythmias, fever, vertigo, GI upset, tremor **Notes:** Addition of vasopressor to concurrent norepinephrine or epinephrine infs **Interactions:** ↑ Vasopressor effects w/ guanethidine, neostigmine; ↑ antidiuretic effects w/ carbamazepine, chlorpropamide, clofibrate, phenformin urea, TCAs; ↓ antidiuretic effects w/ demeclocycline, epinephrine, heparin, Li, phenytoin, EtOH **Labs:** ↑ cortisol level **NIPE:** Take 1–2 glasses H₂O w/ drug

Vecuronium (Norcuron) Uses:
Skeletal muscle relaxation during surgery or mechanical ventilation **Action:** Nondepolarizing neuromuscular blocker **Dose: *Adults & Peds*** 0.08–0.1 mg/kg IV bolus; maint 0.010–0.015 mg/kg after 25–40 min; additional doses q12–15min PRN; ↓ dose in severe renal/hepatic impairment **Caution:** [C, ?] Drug interactions causing ↑ effect of vecuronium (eg, aminoglycosides, tetracycline, succinylcholine) **Supplied:** Powder for inj 10 mg **SE:** Bradycardia, hypotension, itching, rash, tachycardia, CV collapse **Notes:** Fewer cardiac effects than w/ pancuronium **Interactions:** ↑ Neuromuscular blockade w/ aminoglycosides, BBs, CCBs, clindamycin, furosemide, lincomycin, quinidine, tetracyclines, thiazide diuretics, verapamil; ↑ resp depression w/ opioids; ↓ effects w/ phenytoin **NIPE:** Will not provide pain relief or sedation

Venlafaxine (Effexor) WARNING:
Closely monitor for worsening depression or emergence of suicidality, particularly in pediatric Pts **Uses:** *Depression, generalized anxiety,* social anxiety disorder; obsessive–compulsive disorder, chronic fatigue syndrome, ADHD, autism **Action:** Potentiation of CNS neurotransmitter activity **Dose:** 75–375 mg/d ÷ into 2–3 equal doses; ↓ dose in renal/hepatic impairment **Caution:** [C, ?/–] **Contra:** MAOIs **Supplied:** Tabs 25, 37.5, 50, 75, 100 mg; ER caps 37.5, 75, 150 mg **SE:** HTN, ↑ mean HR, HA, somnolence, GI upset, sexual dysfunction; actuates mania or Szs **Notes:** ⊘ EtOH **Interactions:** ↑ Effects w/ cimetidine, desipramine, haloperidol, MAOIs; ↑ risk of serotonin syndrome w/ buspirone, Li, meperidine, sibutramine, sumatriptan, SSRIs, TCAs, trazodone, St. John's wort **Labs:** ↑ LFTs, creatinine **NIPE:** Take w/ food; ⊘ DC abruptly; DC MAOI 14 days before start of this drug; ↑ fluids to 2–3 L/d; may take 2–3 wk for full effects

Verapamil (Calan, Isoptin)   Uses: *Angina, HTN, PSVT, AF, atrial flutter,* migraine prophylaxis, hypertrophic cardiomyopathy, bipolar Dz **Action:** CCB **Dose: Adults.** Arrhythmias: 2nd line for PSVT w/ narrow QRS complex and adequate BP 2.5–5 mg IV over 1–2 min; repeat 5–10 mg in 15–30 min PRN (30 mg max). *Angina:* 80–120 mg PO tid, ↑ 480 mg/24 h max. *HTN:* 80–180 mg PO tid or SR tabs 120–240 mg PO qd to 240 mg bid. **Peds** <1 y: 0.1–0.2 mg/kg IV over 2 min (may repeat in 30 min). *1–16y:* 0.1–0.3 mg/kg IV over 2 min (may repeat in 30 min); 5 mg max. *PO: 1–5 y:* 4–8 mg/kg/d in 3 ÷ doses. >5 y: 80 mg q6–8h; ↓ in renal/hepatic impairment **Caution:** [C, +] Amiodarone/BBs/flecainide can cause bradycardia; statins, midazolam, tacrolimus theophylline levels may be ↑ **Contra:** Conduction disorders, cardiogenic shock; caution w/ elderly Pts **Supplied:** Tabs 40, 80, 120 mg; SR tabs 120, 180, 240 mg; SR caps 120, 180, 240, 360 mg; inj 5 mg/2 mL **SE:** Gingival hyperplasia, constipation, hypotension, bronchospasm, heart rate or conduction disturbances **Interactions:** ↑ Effects w/ antihypertensives, nitrates, quinidine, EtOH, grapefruit juice; ↑ effects of buspirone, carbamazepine, cyclosporine, digoxin, prazosin, quinidine, theophylline, warfarin; ↓ effects w/ antineoplastics, barbiturates, NSAIDs, ↓ effects of Li, rifampin **Labs:** ↑ ALT, AST, alkaline phosphatase **NIPE:** Take w/ food; ↑ fluids and bulk foods to prevent constipation

Vinblastine (Velban, Velbe)   WARNING: Chemotherapeutic agent; handle w/ caution Uses: *Hodgkin's and NHLs, mycosis fungoides, CAs (testis, renal cell, breast, non-small-cell lung, AIDS-related Kaposi's sarcoma,* choriocarcinoma), histiocytosis **Action:** Inhibits microtubule assembly **Dose:** 0.1–0.5 mg/kg/wk (4–20 mg/m²); ↓ in hepatic failure **Caution:** [D, ?] **Contra:** Intrathecal use **Supplied:** Inj 1 mg/mL **SE:** Myelosuppression (especially leukopenia), N/V (rare), constipation, neurotoxicity (like vincristine but less frequent), alopecia, rash; myalgia tumor pain **Interactions:** ↑ Effects w/ erythromycin, itraconazole; ↓ effects w/ glutamic acid, tryptophan; ↓ effects of phenytoin **Labs:** ↑ Uric acid **NIPE:** ↑ Fluids to 2–3 L/d; ⊘ PRG or breast-feeding; use contraception for at least 2 mo after drug; photosensitivity—use sunscreen; ⊘ admin immunizations

Vincristine (Oncovin, Vincasar PFS)   WARNING: Chemotherapeutic agent; handle w/ caution***Fatal if administered intrathecally*** Uses: *ALL, breast and small-cell lung carcinoma, sarcoma (eg, Ewing's, rhabdomyosarcoma), Wilms' tumor, Hodgkin's and NHLs, neuroblastoma, multiple myeloma* **Action:** Promotes disassembly of mitotic spindle, causing metaphase arrest **Dose:** 0.4–1.4 mg/m² (single doses 2 mg/max); ↓ dose in hepatic failure **Caution:** [D, ?] **Contra:** Intrathecal use **Supplied:** Inj 1 mg/mL **SE:** Neurotoxicity commonly dose limiting, jaw pain (trigeminal neuralgia), fever, fatigue, anorexia, constipation and paralytic ileus, bladder atony; no significant myelosuppression w/ standard doses; soft tissue necrosis possible w/ extravasation **Interactions:** ↑ Effects w/ CCBs; ↑ effects of MRX; ↑ risk of bronchospasm w/ mitomycin; ↓ effects of digoxin, phenytoin **NIPE:** ↑ Fluids to 2–3 L/d; reversible hair loss; ⊘ exposure to infection; ⊘ admin immunizations

Vinorelbine (Navelbine) **WARNING:** Chemotherapeutic agent; handle w/ caution **Uses:** *Breast and non-small-cell lung CA* (alone or w/ cisplatin) **Action:** Inhibits polymerization of microtubules, impairing mitotic spindle formation; semisynthetic vinca alkaloid **Dose:** 30 mg/m²/wk; ↓ dose in hepatic failure **Caution:** [D, ?] **Contra:** Intrathecal use **Supplied:** Inj 10 mg **SE:** Myelosuppression (especially leukopenia), mild GI effects, and infrequent neurotoxicity (6–29%); constipation and paresthesias (rare); tissue damage can result from extravasation **Interactions:** ↑ Risk of granulocytopenia w/ cisplatin, ↑ pulmonary effects w/ mitomycin, paclitaxel **Labs:** ↑ LFTs **NIPE:** ⊘ PRG or breast-feeding; use contraception; ⊘ infectious environment; ↑ fluids to 2–3 L/d

Vitamin B₁ See Thiamine

Vitamin B₆ See Pyridoxine

Vitamin B₁₂ See Cyanocobalamin

Vitamin K See Phytonadione

Voriconazole (VFEND) **Uses:** *Invasive aspergillosis, serious fungal infections* **Action:** Inhibits ergosterol synthesis. *Spectrum:* Several types of fungus including *Aspergillus, Scedosporium* sp, *Fusarium* sp **Dose: *Adults and Peds.*** ≥ 12 y: IV: 6 mg/kg q12h × 2, then 4 mg/kg bid; may ↓ to 3 mg/kg per dose. *PO: <40 kg:* 100 mg q12h, up to 150 mg; *>40 kg:* 200 mg q 12 h, up to 300 mg; ↓ dose in mild–moderate hepatic impairment; IV only one dose in renal impairment/ESRD **Caution:** [D, ?/–] **Contra:** Severe hepatic impairment **Supplied:** Tabs 50, 200 mg; 200-mg inj **SE:** Visual changes, fever, rash, GI upset, ↑ LFTs **Notes:** Must screen for multiple drug interactions (eg, ↑ dose when given w/ phenytoin); administer PO doses on empty stomach **Interactions:** ↑ Effects w/ delaviridine, efavirenz; ↑ effects of benzodiazepines, buspirone, CCBs, cisapride, cyclosporine, ergots, pimozide, quinidine, sirolimus, sulfonylureas, tacrolimus; ↓ effects w/ carbamazepine, mephobarbital, phenobarbital, rifampin, rifabutin **NIPE:** Take w/o food; ↑ risk of photosensitivity—use sunscreen; ⊘ PRG or breast-feeding

Warfarin (Coumadin) **Uses:** *Prophylaxis and Rx of PE and DVT, AF w/ embolization,* other postop indications **Action:** Inhibits vitamin K-dependent production of clotting factors in the order VII-IX-X-II **Dose: *Adults.*** Adjust to keep INR 2.0–3.0 for most; mechanical valves INR is 2.5–3.5. *ACCP guidelines:* 5 mg initially (unless rapid therapeutic INR needed), use 7.5–10 mg or if Pt elderly or has other bleeding risk factors ↓. *Alternative:* 10–15 mg PO, IM, or IV qd for 1–3 d; maint 2–10 mg/d PO, IV, or IM; follow daily INR initially to adjust dosage. ***Peds.*** 0.05–0.34 mg/kg/24 h PO, IM, or IV; follow PT/INR to adjust dosage; monitor vitamin K intake; ↓ in hepatic impairment or elderly **Caution:** [X, +] **Contra:** Severe hepatic or renal Dz, bleeding, peptic ulcer, PRG **Supplied:** Tabs 1, 2, 2.5, 3, 4, 5, 6, 7.5, 10 mg; inj **SE:** Bleeding caused by overanticoagulation (PT >3× control or INR >5.0–6.0) or injury and INR w/in therapeutic range; bleeding, alopecia, skin necrosis, purple toe syndrome **Notes:** INR preferred test; to rapidly correct overanticoagulation, use vitamin K, FFP or both; highly teratogenic; do *not* use in PRG. Caution Pt on taking warfarin w/ other meds, especially ASA. *Common warfarin interactions:* Potentiated by APAP, EtOH (w/ liver Dz), amiodarone, cimetidine, ciprofloxacin, co-trimoxazole, erythromycin, fluconazole, flu vaccine, INH, itraconazole, metronidazole, omeprazole, phenytoin, propranolol, quinidine, tetracycline. Inhibited by barbiturates, carbamazepine, chlordiazepoxide, cholestyramine, dicloxacillin, nafcillin, rifampin, sucralfate, high-vitamin K foods **Labs:** ↑ PTT; false ↓ serum theophylline levels **NIPE:** Reddish discoloration of urine; ⊘ PRG or breast-feeding; use barrier contraception; monitor for bleeding

Zafirlukast (Accolate) **Uses:** *Adjunctive Rx of asthma* **Action:** Selective and competitive inhibitor of leukotrienes **Dose:** *Adults and Peds.* ≥ 12 y:. 20 mg bid. *Peds.* 5–11 y: 10 mg PO bid (empty stomach) **Caution:** [B, –] Interacts w/ warfarin to ↑ INR **Contra:** Component hypersensitivity **Supplied:** Tabs 20 mg **SE:** Hepatic dysfunction, usually reversible on discontinuation; HA, dizziness, GI upset; Churg–Strauss syndrome **Notes:** Not for acute asthma, take on empty stomach **Interactions:** ↑ Effects w/ ASA; ↑ effects of CCBs, cyclosporine; ↑ risk of bleeding w/ warfarin; ↓ effects w/ erythromycin, theophylline, food **Labs:** ↑ ALT **NIPE:** Take w/o food; ⊘ use for acute asthma attack

Zalcitabine (Hivid) **WARNING:** Use w/ caution in Pts w/ neuropathy, pancreatitis, lactic acidosis, hepatitis **Uses:** *HIV* **Action:** Antiretroviral agent **Dose:** *Adults.* 0.75 mg PO tid. *Peds.* 0.015–0.04 mg/kg PO q 6h; ↓ dose in renal failure **Caution:** [C, +] **Contra:** Component hypersensitivity **Supplied:** Tabs 0.375, 0.75 mg **SE:** Peripheral neuropathy, pancreatitis, fever, malaise, anemia, hypo-/ hyperglycemia, hepatic impairment **Notes:** May be used in combination w/ zidovudine **Interactions:** ↑ Risk of peripheral neuropathy w/ amphotericin B, aminoglycosides, cisplatin, didanosine, disulfiram, foscarnet, INH, phenytoin, ribavirin, vincristine; ↑ effects w/ cimetidine, metoclopramide; probenecid; ↓ effects w/ antacids **Labs:** ↑ LFTs, lipase, triglycerides **NIPE:** Use barrier contraception; take w/o regard to food

Zaleplon (Sonata) **Uses:** *Insomnia* **Action:** A nonbenzodiazepine sedative–hypnotic, a pyrazolopyrimidine **Dose:** 5–20 mg hs PRN; ↓ dose in renal/hepatic insufficiency, elderly **Caution:** [C, ?/–] Caution in mental/psychological conditions **Contra:** Component hypersensitivity **Supplied:** Caps 5, 10 mg **SE:** HA, edema, amnesia, somnolence, photosensitivity **Notes:** Take immediately before desired onset **Interactions:** ↑ CNS depression w/ cimetidine, CNS depressants, imipramine, thoridazine, EtOH; ↓ effects w/ carbamazepine, phenobarbital, phenytoin, rifampin **NIPE:** Rapid effects of drug; take w/o food ⊘ DC abruptly

Zanamivir (Relenza) **Uses:** *Influenza A and B* **Action:** Inhibits viral neuraminidase **Dose:** *Adults & Peds.* >7 y: 2 inhal (10 mg) bid for 5 d; initiate w/in 48 h of Sxs **Caution:** [C, M] **Contra:** Pulmonary Dz **Supplied:** Powder for inhal 5

mg **SE:** Bronchospasm, HA, GI upset **Notes:** Uses a Diskhaler for administration **Labs:** ↑?LFTs, CPK **NIPE:** Does not reduce risk of transmitting virus

Zidovudine (Retrovir)
WARNING: Neutropenia, anemia, lactic acidosis, and hepatomegaly w/ steatosis **Uses:** *HIV infection, prevention of maternal transmission of HIV* **Action:** Inhibits RT **Dose:** *Adults.* 200 mg PO tid or 300 mg PO bid or 1–2 mg/kg/dose IV q4h. *PRG:* 100 mg PO 5×/d until the start of labor, then during labor 2 mg/kg over 1 h followed by 1 mg/kg/h until clamping of the umbilical cord. *Peds.* 160 mg/m²/dose q8h; ↓ dose in renal failure **Caution:** [C, ?/–] **Contra:** Life-threatening hypersensitivity **Supplied:** Caps 100 mg; tabs 300 mg; syrup 50 mg/5 mL; inj 10 mg/mL **SE:** Hematologic toxicity, HA, fever, rash, GI upset, malaise **Interactions:** ↑ Effects w/ fluconazole, phenytoin, probenecid, trimethoprim, valproic acid, vinblastine, vincristine; ↑ hematologic toxicity w/ adriamycin, dapsone, ganciclovir, interferon-α; ↓ effects w/ rifampin, ribavirin, stavudine **NIPE:** Take w/o food monitor for S/Sxs opportunistic infection; monitor for anemia

Zidovudine and Lamivudine (Combivir)
WARNING: Neutropenia, anemia, lactic acidosis, and hepatomegaly w/ steatosis **Uses:** *HIV infection* **Action:** Combination of RT inhibitors **Dose:** *Adults & Peds.* >12 y: 1 tab bid; ↓ in renal failure **Caution:** [C, ?/–] **Contra:** Component hypersensitivity **Supplied:** Caps zidovudine 300 mg/lamivudine 150 mg **SE:** Hematologic toxicity, HA, fever, rash, GI upset, malaise, pancreatitis **Notes:** Combination product ↓ daily pill burden **Interactions:** ↑ Effects w/ fluconazole, phenytoin, probenecid, trimethoprim, valproic acid, vinblastine, vincristine; ↑ hematologic toxicity w/ adriamycin, dapsone, ganciclovir, interferon-α; ↓ effects w/ rifampin, ribavirin, stavudine **NIPE:** Take w/o food; monitor for S/Sxs opportunistic infection; monitor for anemia

Zileuton (Zyflo)
Uses: *Chronic Rx of asthma* **Action:** Inhibitor of 5-lipoxygenase **Dose:** *Adults and Peds.* ≥ 1? y: 600 mg PO qid **Caution:** [C, ?/–] **Contra:** Hepatic impairment **Supplied:** Tabs 600 mg **SE:** Hepatic damage, HA, GI upset, leukopenia **Notes:** Monitor LFTs every month × 3, then q2–3 mo; must take on a regular basis; not for acute asthma **Interactions:** ↑ Effects of propranolol, terfenadine, theophylline, warfarin **Labs:** ↑ LFTs, ↑ WBCs; **NIPE:** Take w/o regard to food

Ziprasidone (Geodon)
Uses: *Schizophrenia, acute agitation* **Action:** Atypical antipsychotic **Dose:** 20 mg PO bid w/ food, may ↑ in 2-d intervals up to 80 mg bid; agitation 10–20 mg IM PRN up to 40 mg/d; separate 10 mg doses by 2 h and 20 mg doses by 4h **Caution:** [C, –] W/ hypokalemia/hypomagnesemia **Contra:** QT prolongation, recent MI, uncompensated HF, meds that prolong QT interval **Supplied:** Caps 20, 40, 60, 80 mg; Inj 20 mg/mL **SE:** Bradycardia; rash, somnolence, resp disorder, EPS, weight gain, orthostatic hypotension **Notes:** Monitor electrolytes **Interactions:** ↑ Effects w/ ketoconazole; ↑ effects of antihypertensives; ↑ CNS depression w/ anxiolytics, sedatives, opioids, EtOH; TCAs; thioridazine, risk of prolonged QT w/ cisapride, chlorpromazine, clarithromycin,

diltiazem, erythromycin, levofloxacin, mefloquine, pentamidine, TCAs, thiori-dazine; ↓ effects w/ amphetamines, carbamazepine; ↓ effects of levodopa **Labs:** ↑ Prolactin, cholesterol, triglycerides **NIPE:** May take weeks before full effects, take w/ food, ↑ risk of tardive dyskinesia

Zoledronic Acid (Zometa) Uses: *Hypercalcemia of malignancy (HCM).* ↓ skeletal-related events in CAP, multiple myeloma, and metastatic bone lesions **Action:** Bisphosphonate; inhibits osteoclastic bone resorption **Dose:** *HCM:* 4 mg IV over at least 15 min; may re-treat in 7 d if adequate renal Fxn. *Bone lesions/myeloma:* 4 mg IV over at least 15 min, repeat q3–4wk PRN; prolonged w/ Cr ↑ **Caution:** [C, ?/–] Loop diuretics, aminoglycosides; ASA-sensitive asthmatics **Contra:** Bisphosphonate hypersensitivity **Supplied:** Vial 4 mg **SE:** Adverse effects ↑ w/ renal dysfunction; fever, flu-like syndrome, GI upset, insomnia, anemia; electrolyte abnormalities **Notes:** Requires vigorous prehydration; ⊘ exceed recommended doses/inf duration to minimize dose-related renal dysfunction; follow Cr **Interactions:** ↑ Risk of hypocalcemia w/ diuretics; ↑ risk of nephrotoxicity w/ aminoglycosides, thalidomide **NIPE:** ↑ Fluids to 2–3 L/d

Zolmitriptan (Zomig) Uses: *Acute Rx migraine* **Action:** Selective serotonin agonist; causes vasoconstriction **Dose:** Initial 2.5 mg PO, may repeat after 2 h to 10 mg max in 24 h **Caution:** [C, ?/–] **Contra:** Ischemic heart Dz, Prinzmetal's angina, uncontrolled HTN, accessory conduction pathway disorders, ergots, MAOIs **Supplied:** Tabs 2.5, 5 mg **SE:** Dizziness, hot flashes, paresthesias, chest tightness, myalgia, diaphoresis **Interactions:** ↑ Effects w/ cimetidine, MAOIs, oral contraceptives, propranolol; ↑ risk of prolonged vasospasms w/ ergots; ↑ risk of serotonin syndrome w/ sibutramine, SSRIs **NIPE:** Admin to relieve migraines; not for prophylaxis

Zolpidem (Ambien) [C-IV] Uses: *Short-term Rx of insomnia* **Action:** Hypnotic agent **Dose:** 5–10 mg PO hs PRN; ↓ in elderly, hepatic insufficiency **Caution:** [B, –] **Contra:** Breast-feeding **Supplied:** Tabs 5, 10 mg **SE:** HA, dizziness, drowsiness, nausea, myalgia **Notes:** May be habit-forming **Interactions:** ↑ CNS depression w/ CNS depressants, sertraline, EtOH ↑ effects of ketoconazole; ↓ effects of rifampin; **NIPE:** Take w/o food; ⊘ DC abruptly if long-term use; may develop tolerance to drug

Zonisamide (Zonegran) Uses: *Adjunct Rx complex partial Szs* **Action:** Anticonvulsant **Dose:** Initial 100 mg/d PO; may ↑ to 400 mg/d **Caution:** [C, –] ↑ toxicity w/ CYP3A4 inhibitor; ↓ levels w/ concurrent carbamazepine, phenytoin, phenobarbital, valproic acid **Contra:** Hypersensitivity to sulfonamides; oligohydrosis and hypothermia in peds **Supplied:** Caps 100 mg **SE:** Dizziness, drowsiness, confusion, ataxia, memory impairment, paresthesias, psychosis, nystagmus, diplopia, tremor; anemia, leukopenia; GI upset, nephrolithiasis, Stevens–Johnson syndrome; monitor for ↓ sweating and ↑ body temperature **Notes:** Swallow capsules whole **Interactions:** ↓ Effects w/ carbamazepine, phenobarbital, phenytoin, valproic acid **Labs:** ↑ serum alkaline phosphatase, ALT, AST, creatinine, BUN, ↓ glucose, Na **NIPE:** ⊘ DC

COMMONLY USED MEDICINAL HERBS

Arnica (*Arnica montana*) **Uses:** ↓ Swelling & inflammation from acne, blunt injury, bruises, rashes, sprains **Action:** Sesquiterpenoids have shown antibacterial, antiinflammatory, & analgesic properties; **Available forms:** Topical cream, spray, oint, tinc; for poultice dilute tinc 3–10 × w/ water & apply PRN **Contra:** Poisonous, ⊘ take internally; ⊘ if Pt allergic to arnica, chrysanthemums, marigold, sunflowers **Notes/SE:** Arrhythmias, abdominal pain, cardiac arrest, contact dermatitis, coma, death, hepatic failure, HTN, nervousness, restlessness **Interactions:** ↑ Risk of bleeding w/ ASA, heparin, warfarin, angelica, anise, asafetida, bogbean, boldo, capsicum, celery, chamomile, clove, danshen, fenugreek, feverfew, garlic, ginger, ginkgo, ginseng, horse chestnut, horseradish, licorice, meadowsweet, onion, papain, passion flower, poplar bark, prickly ash, quassia wood, red clover, turmeric, wild carrot, wild lettuce, willow; ↓ effects of antihypertensives **Labs:** None **NIPE:** ⊘ Apply to broken skin. ⊘ use in PRG & lactation, serious liver & kidney damage w/ internal use, ingestion of flowers & root can cause death, prolonged topical use ↑ risk of allergic reaction

Astragalus (*Astragalus membranaceus*) **Uses:** Rx of resp infections, enhancement of immune system, & heart failure **Action:** Root saponins ↑ diuresis, ↓ BP; antiinflammatory action related to the stimulation of macrophages, ↑ antibody formation & ↑ T-lymphocyte proliferation **Available forms:** Caps/tabs 1–4 g tid, PO; liq ext 4–8 mL/d (1:2 ratio) ÷ doses; dry ext 250 mg (1:8 ratio) tid, PO **Notes/SE:** Immunosuppression w/ doses > 28 g **Interactions:** ↑ Effect of acyclovir, anticoagulants, antihypertensives, antithrombotics, antiplts, interleukin-2, interferon; ↓ effect of cyclophosphamide **Labs:** ↑ PT, INR **NIPE:** Use cautiously in immunosuppressed Pts or those w/ autoimmune Dz

Butcher's Broom (*Ruscus aculeatus*) **Uses:** Rx of circulatory disorders such as PVD, varicose veins, & leg edema; hemorrhoids; diuretic; laxative; inflammation; arthritis **Action:** Vasoconstriction due to direct activation of the α-receptors of the smooth-muscle cells in vascular walls **Available forms:** Raw ext 7–11 mg once/d, PO; tea 1 tsp in 1 cup water; topical oint apply PRN **Notes/SE:** GI upset, N/V **Interactions:** ↑ Effects of anticoagulants, MAOIs; ↓ effects of antihypertensives **Labs:** None **NIPE:** Hypertensive crisis may occur if admin w/ MAOIs; ⊘ use in PRG & lactation

Black Cohosh (*Cimicifuga racemosa*) **Uses:** Antitussive; smooth muscle relaxant; management of menopausal symptoms esp hot flashes, sleep disturbance & anxiety, premenstrual syndrome, & dysmenorrhea. Antiinflammatory, peripheral vasodilation, & sedative effects **Action:** Estrogenic activity w/ some studies showing ↓ in LH; vasodilation activity causing ↑ blood flow & hypotensive effects; antimicrobial activity **Available forms:** Dried root/rhizome caps 40–200 mg ONCE/D; fluid ext (1:1) 2–4 mL or 1 tsp once/d; tinc (1:5) 3–6 mL or 1–2 tsp once/d; powdered ext (4:1) 250–500 mg once/d; Remifemin Menopause (standardized ext brand name) 20 mg bid **Notes/SE:** Hypotension, bradycardia, N/V, anorexia, HA, miscarriage, nervous system & visual disturbances **Interactions:** ↑ Effects of antihypertensives, estrogen HRT, oral contraceptives, hypnotics, sedatives; tinc may cause a reaction w/ disulfiram & metronidazole; ↑ antiproliferative effect w/ tamoxifen; ↓ effects of ferrous fumarate, ferrous gluconate, ferrous sulfate **Labs:** May ↓ LH levels & plt counts **NIPE:** Tinc contains large % of EtOH, ⊘ use in PRG or lactation or give to children

Chamomile (*Matricaria recutita*) **Uses:** Antiinflammatory, antipyretic, antimicrobial, antispasmodic, astringent, sedative **Action:** Ingredients include α-bisabolol oil, which ↓ inflammation, antispasmodic activity, ↑ healing times for burns & ulcers, & inhibits ulcer formation; apigenin contributes to the anti-inflammatory effect, antispasmodic & sedative effect; azulene inhibits histamine release; chamazulene reduces inflammation & has antioxidant & antimicrobial effects **Available forms:** Teas 3–5 g (1 tbsp) flower heads steeped in water tid–qid, also use as a gargle or compress; fluid ext 1:1 -45% EtOH 1–3 mL tid **Notes/SE:** Allergic reactions if Pt allergic to Compositae family (ragweed, sunflowers, asters), eg, angioedema, eczema, contact dermatitis & anaphylaxis **Interactions:** ↑ Effects of CNS depressants, EtOH, anticoagulants, antiplts; ↑ risk of miscarriage; ↓ effects of drugs metabolized by CY 450 3A4, eg, alprazolam, atorvastatin, diazepam, ketoconazole, verapamil **Labs:** Monitor anticoagulant levels **NIPE:** ⊘ in PRG, lactation, children < age 2 y, patients w/ asthma or hay fever

Chondroitin Sulfate **Uses:** Combine w/ glucosamine to Rx arthritis; use as an anticoagulant **Action:** Attracts fluid & nutrients into the joints; inhibits thrombi **Available forms:** 1200 mg once/d, PO, & usually given w/ glucosamine 1500 mg once/d, PO for normal weight adults; **Notes/SE:** Diarrhea, dyspepsia, HA, N/V, restlessness **Interactions:** ↑ Effects of anticoagulants, aspirin, NSAIDs **Labs:** None **NIPE:** ⊘ in PRG & lactation

Dong Quai (*Angelica polymorpha, sinensis*) **Uses:** Dysmenorrhea, PMS, menorrhagia, chronic pelvic infection, irregular menstruation. Other reported uses include anemia, HTN, HA, rhinitis, neuralgia, & hepatitis **Action:** Root exts contain at least six coumarin derivatives that have anticoagulant, vasodilating, antispasmodic, & CNS-stimulating activity. Studies demonstrate weak estrogen-agonist actions of the ext **Available forms:** Caps 500 mg, 1–2 caps PO, tid; liq ext 1–2 gtt, tid; tea 1–2 g, tid **Notes/SE:** Diarrhea, bleeding, photosensitivity, fever **Interactions:** ↑ Effects of anticoagulants, antiplts, estrogens, warfarin; ↑ anticoagulant activity w/ chamomile, dandelion, horse chestnut, red clover; ↑ risk of disulfiram-like reaction w/ disulfiram, metronidazole; **Labs:** ↑ PT, PTT, INR

NIPE: Photosensitivity—use sunscreen, ⊘ if breast-feeding or PRG; tincs & exts contain EtOH up to 60%; stop herb 14 d prior to dental or surgical procedures

Echinacea (*Echinacea purpurea*)
Uses: Immune system stimulant; prevention/Rx of colds, flu; as supportive therapy for colds & chronic infections of the resp tract & lower urinary tract **Action:** Stimulates phagocytosis & cytokine production & ↑ resp cellular activity; topically exerts anesthetic, antimicrobial, & antiinflammatory effects **Available forms:** Caps w/ powdered herb equivalent to 300–500 mg, PO, tid; pressed juice 6–9 mL, PO, once/d; tinc 2–4 mL, PO, tid (1:5 dilution); tea 2 tsp (4 g) of powdered herb in 1 cup of boiling water **Notes/SE:** Fever, taste perversion, urticaria, angioedema; **Contra:** ⊘ in Pts w/ autoimmune Dz, collagen Dz, HIV, leukemia, MS, TB **Interactions:** ↑ Risk of disulfiram-like reaction w/ disulfiram, metronidazole; ↑risk of exacerbation of HIV or AIDS w/ echinacea & amprenavir, other protease inhibitors; ↓effects of azathioprine, basiliximab, corticosteroids, cyclosporine, daclizumab, econazole vaginal cream, muromonab-CD3, mycophenolate, prednisone, tacrolimus **Labs:** ↑ ALT, AST, lymphocytes, ESR **NIPE:** Large doses of herb interferes w/ sperm activity; ⊘ w/ breast-feeding or PRG; ⊘ continuously for longer than 8 wk w/o a 3-wk break in Rx

Ephedra/Ma Huang
Uses: CNS stimulant, appetite suppressant, weight-loss herb, asthma, headaches, nasal congestion, arthralgia **Action:** Active ingredient of ext is ephedrine that stimulates CNS, ↑ HR, BP, & peripheral vasoconstriction; acts on β-receptors & α-receptors **Available forms:** Ext 1–3 mL, PO, tid; tea 1–5 g herb in 1 pt boiling water; caps max daily dose of 300 mg **Notes/SE:** Anxiety, confusion, dizziness, HA, insomnia, irritability, restlessness, nervousness, arrhythmias, HTN, palpitations, constipation, urinary retention, uterine contractions, dermatitis **Contra:** ⊘ Narrow-angle glaucoma, seizures, CAD, PRG, lactation **Interactions:** ↑Sympathomimetic effects w/ BBs, guanethidine, yohimbe; ↑ cardiac rhythm disturbance w/ anesthetics, cardiac glycosides, halothane; ↑ psychotic episodes w/ caffeine, EtOH; ↑ effects of CNS stimulants, pseudoephedrine, theophylline ; ↑ risk of HTN crisis w/ MAOIs, oxytocics, phenelzine, TCAs; ↓effects of oral hypoglycemics **Labs:** ↑ ALT, AST, total bilirubin, urine bilirubin, serum glucose **NIPE:** Tincs & exts contain EtOH; linked to several deaths; monitor for behavioral mood changes

Feverfew (*Tanacetum parthenium*)
Uses: Antiinflammatory for arthritis, asthma, digestion problems, fever, migraines, menstrual complaints, threatened abortion **Action:** Active ingredient, parthenolide, inhibits serotonin release, prostaglandin synthesis, plt aggregation, & histamine release from mast cells; several ingredients inhibit activation of polymorphonuclear leukocytes & leukotriene synthesis **Available forms:** Freeze-dried leaf ext 25 mg once/d; caps 300 mg–400 mg tid PO; tinc 15-ñ30 gtt once/d to 0.2–0.7 mg of parthenolide **Notes/SE:** Mouth ulcers, muscle stiffness, joint pain, GI upset, rash **Contra:** ⊘ in PRG & lactation or w/ ragweed allergy **Interactions:** ↑ Effects of anticoagulants,

antiplts, ↓ effects of Fe absorption **Labs:** ↑ PT, INR, PTT **NIPE:** ⊘ DC herb abruptly or may experience joint stiffness & pain, headaches, insomnia

Garlic (*Allium sativum*)
Uses: Antithrombotic, antilipidemic, antitumor, antimicrobial, antiasthmatic, antiinflammatory **Action:** Inhibits gram(+) & gram(−) organisms, exerts cholesterol-lowering by preventing gastric lipase fat digestion & fecal excretion of sterols & bile acids & it inhibits free radicals **Available forms:** Teas, tabs, caps, ext, oil, dried powder, syrup, fresh bulb **Notes/SE:** Dizziness, diaphoresis, HA, N/V, hypothyroidism, contact dermatitis, allergic reactions, oral mucosa irritation, systemic garlic odor, ↓ Hgb production, lysis of RBCs **Interactions:** ↑ Effects of anticoagulants, antiplts, insulin, oral hypoglycemics; ↓ effects w/ acidophilus **Labs:** ↓ Total cholesterol, LDL, triglycerides, plt aggregation, iodine uptake; ↑ PT, serum IgE **NIPE:** ⊘ in PRG, lactation, prior to surgery, GI disorders; report bleeding, bruising, petechiae, tarry stools, monitor CBC, PT

Ginger (*Zingiber officinale*)
Uses: Antiemetic ↑ N/V; antiinflammatory relieves pain & swelling of muscle injury, osteoarthritis & rheumatoid arthritis; antispasmodic action relieves colic, flatulence & indigestion; antiplt; antipyretic; antioxidant; antiinfective against gram(+) & gram(−) bacteria **Action:** Antiinflammatory effect inhibits prostaglandin, thromboxane, & leukotriene biosynthesis; antiemetic effects due to action on the GI tract; antiplt effect due to the inhibition of thromboxane formation; + inotropic effect on CV system **Available forms:** Dosage form & strength depends on Dz process *General use:* Dried ginger caps 1 g once/d, PO; fluid ext 0.7–2 mL once/d, PO, (2:1 ratio); tabs 500 mg bid–qid, PO; tinc 1.7–5 mL once/d, PO, (1:5 ratio) **Interactions:** ↑ Risk of bleeding w/ anticoagulants, antiplts; ↑ risk of disulfiram-like reaction w/ disulfiram, metronidazole **Labs:** ↑ PT **NIPE:** Store herb in cool, dry area; ⊘ in PRG, lactation; lack of standardization for herb dosing

Ginkgo Biloba
Uses: Effective w/ circulatory disorders, cerebrovascular Dz, & dementia; used to improve alertness & attention span **Action:** Ext flavonoids release neurotransmitters & inhibit monoamine oxidase, which enhances cognitive function; vascular protective action results from relaxation of blood vessels, ↑ tissue perfusion, inhibition of plt aggregation; eradicates free radicals & ↓ polymorphonuclear neutrophils **Available forms:** Dosage depends on diagnosis *General uses:* Tabs & caps 40–ñ80 mg tid, PO; tinc 0.5 mL tid, PO; ext 40–80 mg tid, PO **Notes/SE:** Anxiety, diarrhea, flatulence, HA, heart palpitations, N/V, restlessness **Interactions:** ↑ Effect of MAOIs; ↑ risk of bleeding w/ anisindione, dalteparin, dicumerol, garlic, heparin, salicylates, warfarin; ↑ risk of coma w/ trazodone; ↓ effect of carbamazepine, gabapentin, insulin, oral hypoglycemics, phenobarbital, phenytoin; ↑ seizure threshold w/ bupropion, TCAs **Labs:** ↑ PT **NIPE:** ⊘ in PRG & lactation; tincs contain up to 60% EtOH; ⊘ 2 wk prior to surgery

Ginseng (*Panax quinquefolius*)
Uses: ↑ Physical endurance, concentration, appetite, sleep & stress resistance; ↓ fatigue; antioxidant; aids in glucose control **Action:** Dried root contains ginsenosides, which ↑ natural killer cell activ-

ity, & nuclear RNA synthesis, & motor activity **Available forms:** No standard dosage *General use:* Caps 200 mg–500 mg once/d, PO: tea 3 g steeped in boiling water tid PO, tinc 1–2 mg once/d, PO (1:1 dilution) **Notes/SE:** Anxiety, anorexia, chest pain, diarrhea, HTN, N/V, palpitations **Interactions:** ↑ Effects of estrogen, hypoglycemics, CNS stimulants, caffeine, ephedra; ↑ risk of bleeding w/ ibuprofen; ↑ risk of HA, irritability & visual hallucinations w/ MAOIs; ↓ effects of anisindione, dicumarol, furosemide, heparin, warfarin **Labs:** ↑ Digoxin level falsely; ↓ glucose, PT, INR **NIPE:** ⊘ Use continuously for > 3 mo; ⊘ during PRG or lactation; eval for ginseng abuse syndrome w/ symptoms of diarrhea, depression, edema, HTN, insomnia, rash & restlessness

Glucosamine Sulfate (chitosamine) Uses: Used w/ chondroitin for the Rx of arthritis **Action:** Stimulate the production of cartilage components **Available forms:** Caps/tabs 1500 mg once/d, PO & chondroitin sulfate 1200 mg once/d, PO for adults of normal weight **Notes/SE:** Abdominal pain, anorexia, constipation or diarrhea, drowsiness, HA, heartburn, N/V, rash **Interactions:** ↑ Effects of hypoglycemics; **Labs:** Monitor serum glucose levels in diabetics **NIPE:** Take w/ food to reduce GI effects; no uniform standardization of herb

Hawthorn (*Crataegus laevigata*) Uses: Rx of HTN, arrhythmias, heart failure, stable angina pectoris, insomnia **Action:** ↑ myocardial contraction by ↓ oxygen consumption, ↓ peripheral resistance, dilating coronary blood vessels, ACE inhibition **Available forms:** Tinc 1–2 mL (1:5 ratio) tid, PO; liq ext 0.5–1 mL, (1:1 ration) tid, PO **Notes/SE:** Arrhythmias, fatigue, hypotension, N/V, sedation **Interactions:** ↑ Effects of antihypertensives, cardiac glycosides, CNS depressants,& herbs such as adonis, lily of the valley, squill ↓; effects of Fe **Labs:** False ↑ of digoxin **NIPE:** ⊘ in PRG & lactation; many tincs contain EtOH

Kava Kava (*Piper methysticum*) Uses: ↓ Anxiety, stress, & restlessness; sedative effect **Action:** Appears to act directly on the limbic system **Available forms:** Standardized ext (70% kavalactones) 100 mg bid–tid, PO **Notes/SE:** ↑ Reflexes, HA, dizziness, visual changes, hematuria, SOB **Interactions:** ↑ Effects of antiplts, benzodiazepines, CNS depressants, MAOIs, phenobarbital; ↑ absorption when taken w/ food; ↑ in parkinsonism symptoms w/ kava & antiparkinsonian drugs **Labs:** ↑ ALT, AST, urinary RBCs; ↓ albumin, total protein, bilirubin, urea, plts, lymphocytes **NIPE:** ⊘ Take for > 3 mo; ⊘ during PRG & lactation

Licorice (*Glycyrrhiza glabra*) Uses: Expectorant, shampoo, GI complaints **Action:** ↑ Mucous secretions, ↓ peptic activity, ↓ scalp sebum secretion **Available forms:** Liq ext, bulk dried root, tea; 15 g once/d PO of licorice root; intake > 50 g once/d may cause toxicity **Notes/SE:** HTN, arrhythmias, edema, hypokalemia, HA, lethargy, rhabdomyolysis **Interactions:** ↑ Drug effects of diuretics, corticosteroids, may prolong QT interval w/ loratadine, procainamide, quinidine, terfenadine; **Labs:** None **NIPE:** Monitor for electrolyte & ECG changes, HTN, mineralocorticord-like effects; toxicity more likely w/ prolonged intake of small doses than one large dose

Melatonin (MEL) **Uses:** Insomnia, jet lag, antioxidant, immunostimulant **Action:** Hormone produce by the pineal gland in response to darkness; declines w/ age **Available forms:** ER caps 1–3 mg once/d 2 h before hs, PO **Notes/SE:** HA, confusion, sedation, HTN, tachycardia, hyperglycemia **Interactions:** ↑ anxiolytic effects of benzodiazepines; ↑ risk of insomnia w/ cerebral stimulants, methamphetamine, succinylcholine **Labs:** None **NIPE:** ⊘ during PRG & lactation

Milk thistle (*Silybum marianum*) **Uses:** Rx of hepatotoxicity, dyspepsia, liver protectorant **Action:** stimulates protein synthesis, which leads to liver cell regeneration **Available forms:** Tinc 70–120 mg (70% silymarin) tid, PO **Notes/SE:** Diarrhea, menstrual stimulation, N/V **Interactions:** ↑ Effects of drugs metabolized by the cytochrome P-450, CYP3A4, CYP2C9 enzymes **Labs:** ↑ PT; ↓ LFTs, serum glucose **NIPE:** ⊘ in PRG & lactation; ⊘ in Pts allergic to ragweed, chrysanthemums, marigolds, daisies

Saw Palmetto (*Serenoa repens*) **Uses:** Rx of benign prostatic hypertrophy (BPH) stages 1 & 2 (inhibits testosterone-5-α-reductase), ↑ sperm production, ↑ breast size (estrogenic), ↑ sexual vigor, mild diuretic, treat chronic cystitis **Action:** Theorized that sitosterols inhibit conversion of testosterone to dihydrotestosterone (DHT), which reduces the prostate gland, also competes w/ DHT on receptor sites resulting in antiestrogenic effects **Available forms:** Caps/tabs 160 mg bid, PO; tinc 20–30 gtt qid (1:2 ration); fluid ext, standardized 160 mg bid PO or 320 mg once/d PO **Notes/SE:** Abdominal pain, back pain, diarrhea, dysuria, HA, HTN, N/V, impotence **Contra:** ⊘ PRG, lactation **Interactions:** ↑ Effects of adrenergics, anticoagulants, antiplts, hormones, Fe **Labs:** May affect semen analysis, may cause false – PSA **NIPE:** Take w/ meals to ↓ GI upset, do baseline PSA prior to taking herb, no standardization of herb content

Spirulina (*Spirulina spp*) **Uses:** Rx of obesity & as a nutritional supplement **Action:** Contains 65% protein, all amino acids, carotenoids, B-complex vitamins, essential fatty acids & Fe; has been shown to inhibit replicating viral cells **Available forms:** Caps/tabs or powder admin 3–5 g ac, PO **Notes/SE:** Anorexia, N/V **Interactions:** ↑ Effects of anticoagulants; ↓ effects of thyroid hormones due to high iodine content; ↓ absorption of vitamin B_{12} **Labs:** ↑ Serum Ca, serum alkaline phosphatase; monitor PT, INR **NIPE:** May contain ↑ levels of Hg & radioactive ion content

St. John's Wort (*Hypericum perforatum*) **Uses:** Depression, anxiety, antiinflammatory, antiviral **Action:** MAOI in vitro, not in vivo; bacteriostatic & bacteristatic, ↑ capillary blood flow, uterotonic activity in animals **Available forms:** Teas, tabs, caps, tinc, oil ext for topical use **Notes/SE:** Photosensitivity (use sunscreen)rash, dizziness, dry mouth, GI distress **Interactions:** Enhance MAOI activity, EtOH, narcotics, MAOIs, sympathomimetics **Labs:** ↑ GH; ↓ digoxin, serum iron, serum prolactin, theophylline; **NIPE:** ⊘ in PRG, breast-feeding, or in children, ⊘ w/ SSRIs, MAOIs, EtOH, ⊘ sun exposure

Tea Tree (*Melaleuca alternifolia*) **Uses:** Rx of superficial wounds (bacterial, viral,& fungal, insect bites, minor burns, cold sores, acne **Action:** Broad-spectrum antibiotic activity against *E. coli, S. aureus, C. albicans* **Available forms:** Topical creams, lotions, oint, oil apply topically PRN **Notes/SE:** Ataxia, contact dermatitis, diarrhea, drowsiness, GI mucosal irritation **Interactions:** ↓ Effects of drugs that affect histamine release **Labs:** ↑ Neutrophil count **NIPE:** Caution Pt to use externally only; ⊘ apply to broken skin

Valerian (*Valeriana officinalis*) **Uses:** Antianxiety, antispasmodic, dysmenorrheal, restlessness, sedative **Action:** Inhibits uptake & stimulates release of GABA, which ↑ GABA concentration extracellularly & causes sedation **Available forms:** Ext 400–900 mg PO 30 min < HS, tea 2–3 g (1 tsp of crude herb) qid, PRN, tinc 3–5 mL (½–1 tsp) (1:5 ratio) PO qid, PRN **Notes/SE:** GI upset, HA, insomnia, N/V, palpitations, restlessness, vision changes **Interactions:** ↑ Effects of barbiturates, benzodiazepines, opiates, EtOH, catnip, hops, kava, passion flower, skullcap; ↓ effects of MAOIs, phenytoin, warfarin **Labs:** ↑ ALT, AST, total bilirubin, urine bilirubin **NIPE:** Periodic check of LFTs, unknown effects in PRG & lactation, full effect may take 2–4 wk, taper herb to avoid withdrawal symptoms after long-term use

Yohimbine (*Pausinystalia yohimbe*) **Uses:** Rx for impotence, aphrodisiac **Action:** Peripherally affects autonomic nervous system by ↓ adrenergic activity & ↑ cholinergic activity; ↑ blood flow **Available forms:** Tabs 5.4 mg tid, PO; doses at 20–30 mg/d may ↑ BP & heart rate **Notes/SE:** Anxiety, dizziness, dysuria, genital pain, HTN, tachycardia, tremors **Interactions:** ↑ Effects of CNS stimulants, MAOIs, SSRIs, caffeine, ETOH; ↑ risk of toxicity w/ α-adrenergic blockers, phenothiazines; ↑ yohimbe toxicity w/ sympathomimetics; ↑ BP w/ foods containing tyramine **Labs:** ↑ BUN, creatinine **NIPE:** ⊘ w/ caffeine-containing foods w/ herb, may exacerbate mania in patients w/ psychiatric disorders

TABLES

TABLE 1
Quick Guide to Dosing of Acetaminophen Based on the Tylenol Product Line

	Suspension[a] Drops and Original Drops 80 mg/0.8 mL Dropperful	Chewable[a] Tablets 80-mg tabs	Suspension[a] Liquid and Original Elixir 160 mg/5 mL	Junior[a] Strength 160-mg Caplets/Chewables	Regular[b] Strength 325-mg Caplets/Tablets	Extra Strength[b] 500-mg Caplets/Gelcaps
Birth–3 mo/ 6–11 lb/ 2.5–5.4 kg	½ dppr[c] (0.4 mL)					
4–11 mo/ 12–17 lb/ 5.5–7.9 kg	1 dppr[c] (0.8 mL)		½ tsp			
12–23 mo/ 18–23 lb/ 8.0–10.9 kg	1½ dppr[c] (1.2 mL)		¾ tsp			
2–3 y/ 24–35 lb/ 11.0–15.9 kg	2 dppr[c] (1.6 mL)	2 tab	1 tsp			
4–5 y/ 36–47 lb/ 16.0–21.9 kg		3 tab	1½ tsp			

263

TABLE 1 (Continued)

	Suspension Drops and Original Drops 80 mg/0.8 mL Dropperful[c]	Chewable[a] Tablets 80-mg tabs	Suspension[a] Liquid and Original Elixir 160 mg/5 mL	Junior[a] Strength 160-mg Caplets/ Chewables	Regular[b] Strength 325-mg Caplets/ Tablets	Extra Strength[b] 500-mg Caplets/ Gelcaps
6–8 y/48–59 lb/ 22.0–26.9 kg		4 tab	2 tsp	2 cap/tab		
9–10 y/60–71 lb/ 27.0–31.9 kg		5 tab	2½ tsp	2½ cap/ tab		
11 y/72–95 lb/ 32.0–43.9 kg		6 tab	4 tsp	3 cap/tab		
Adults & children ≥ 12 y ≥ 96 lb ≥ 44.0 kg				4 cap/tab	1 or 2 caps/ tabs	2 caps/ gel

[a]Doses should be administered 4 or 5 times daily. Do not exceed 5 doses in 24 h.

[b]No more than 8 dosage units in any 24-h period. Not to be taken for pain for more than 10 days or for fever for more than 3 days unless directed by a physician.

[c]Dropperful.

264

TABLE 2
Common Drug Levels[a]

Drug	When to Sample	Therapeutic Levels	Usual Half-Life	Potentially Toxic Levels
Antibiotics				
Gentamicin	Peak: 30 min after 30-min infusion (peak level not necessary if extended-interval dosing: 6 mg/kg/dose) Trough: <0.5 h before next dose	Peak: 5–8 µg/mL Trough: <2 µg/mL <1.0 µg/mL for extended intervals (6 mg/kg/dose) (peak levels not needed with extended-interval dosing)	2 h	Peak: >12 µg/mL
Tobramycin Amikacin Vancomycin	Same as above Same as above Peak: 1 h after 1-h infusion Trough: <0.5 h before next dose	Same as above Peak: 20–30 µg/mL Peak: 30–40 µg/mL	Same as above 2 h 6–8 h	Same as above Peak: >35 µg/mL Peak: >50 µg/mL Trough: >15 µg/mL

TABLE 2
(Continued)

Drug	When to Sample	Therapeutic Levels	Usual Half-Life	Potentially Toxic Levels
Anticonvulsants				
Carbamazepine	Trough: just before next oral dose	8–12 µg/mL (monotherapy) 4–8 µg/mL (polytherapy)	15–20 h	Trough: >12 µg/mL
Ethosuximide	Trough: just before next oral dose	40–100 µg/mL	30–60 h	Trough: >100 µg/mL
Phenobarbital	Trough: just before next dose	15–40 µg/mL	40–120 h	Trough: >40 µg/mL
Phenytoin	May use free phenytoin to monitor[b] Trough: just before next dose	10–20 µg/mL	Concentration-dependent	>20 µg/mL
Primidone	Trough: just before next dose (primidone is metabolized to phenobarb; order levels separately)	5–12 µg/mL	10–12 h	>12 µg/mL
Valproic acid	Trough: just before next dose	50–100 µg/mL	5–20 h	>100 µg/mL

266

Bronchodilators

Drug	Timing	Therapeutic Range	Half-life	Toxic Level
Caffeine	Trough: just before next dose	Adults 5–15 µg/mL Neonates 6–11 µg/mL	Adults 3–4 h Neonates 30–140 h	20 µg/mL
Theophylline (IV)	IV: 12–24 h after infusion started	5–15 µg/mL	Nonsmoking adults 8 h Children and smoking adults 4 h	>20 µg/mL
Theophylline (PO)	Peak levels: not recommended Trough level: just before next dose	5–15 µg/mL		

Cardiovascular Agents

Drug	Timing	Therapeutic Range	Half-life	Toxic Level
Amiodarone	Trough: just before next dose	1–2.5 µg/mL	30–100 days	>2.5 µg/mL
Digoxin	Trough: just before next dose (levels drawn earlier than 6 h after a dose will be artificially elevated)	0.8–2.0 ng/mL	36 h	>2 ng/mL

**TABLE 2
(Continued)**

Drug	When to Sample	Therapeutic Levels	Usual Half-life	Potentially Toxic Levels
Disopyramide	Trough: just before next dose	2–5 µg/mL	4–10 h	>5 µg/mL
Flecainide	Trough: just before next dose	0.2–1.0 µg/mL	11–14 h	>1.0 µg/mL
Lidocaine	Steady-state levels are usually achieved after 6–12 h	1.2–5.0 µg/mL	1.5 h	>6.0 µg/mL
Procainamide	Trough: just before next oral dose	4–10 µg/mL NAPA + Procaine: 5–30 µg/mL	Procaine: 3–5 h NAPA: 6–10 h	>10 µg/mL >30 µg/mL NAPA + Procaine: 0.5 µg/mL
Quinidine	Trough: just before next oral dose	2–5 µg/mL	6 h	
Other Agents				
Amitriptyline plus nortriptyline	Trough: just before next dose	120–250 ng/mL		
Nortriptyline	Trough: just before next dose	50–140 ng/mL		
Lithium	Trough: just before next dose	0.5–1.5 mEq/mL	18–20 h	>1.5 mEq/mL

Imipramine plus desipramine	Trough: just before next dose	150–300 ng/mL
Desipramine	Trough: just before next dose	50–300 ng/mL
Methotrexate	By protocol	<0.5 μmol/L after 48 h
Cyclosporine	Trough: just before next dose	Highly variable Renal: 150–300 ng/mL (RIA) Hepatic: 150–300 ng/mL	Highly variable
Doxepin	Trough: just before next dose	100–300 ng/mL
Trazodone	Trough: just before next dose	900–2100 ng/mL

[a]Results of therapeutic drug monitoring must be interpreted in light of the complete clinical situation. For information on dosing or interpretation of drug levels contact the pharmacist or an order for a pharmacokinetic consult may be written in the patient's chart. Modified and reproduced with permission from the *Pharmacy and Therapeutics Committee Formulary*, 41st ed., Thomas Jefferson University Hospital, Philadelphia, PA.
[b]More reliable in cases of uremia and hypoalbuminemia.

TABLE 3
Local Anesthetic Comparison Chart for Commonly Used Injectable Agents

Agent	Proprietary Names	Onset	Duration	Maximum Dose mg/kg	Volume in 70-kg Adult[a]
Bupivacaine	Marcaine, Sensoricaine	7–30 min	5–7 h	3	70 mL of 0.25% solution
Lidocaine	Xylocaine, Anestacon	5–30 min	2 h	4	28 mL of 1% solution
Lidocaine with epinephrine (1:200,000)		5–30 min	2–3 h	7	50 mL of 1% solution
Mepivacaine	Carbocaine	5–30 min	2–3 h	7	50 mL of 1% solution
Procaine	Novocaine	Rapid	30 min–1 h	10–15	70–105 mL of 1% solution

[a]To calculate the maximum dose if not a 70-kg adult, use the fact that a 1% solution has 10 mg of drug per milliliter.

270

TABLE 4
Comparison of Systemic Steroids

Drug	Relative Equivalent Dose (mg)	Mineralo-corticoid Activity	Duration (h)	Route
Betamethasone	0.75	0	36–72	PO, IM
Cortisone (Cortone)	25.00	2	8–12	PO, IM
Dexamethasone (Decadron)	0.75	0	36–72	PO, IV
Hydrocortisone (Solu-Cortef, Hydrocortone)	20.00	2	8–12	PO, IM, IV
Methylprednisolone acetate (Depo-Medrol)	4.00	0	36–72	PO, IM, IV
Methylprednisolone succinate (Solu-Medrol)	4.00	0	8–12	PO, IM, IV
Prednisone (Deltasone)	5.00	1	12–36	PO
Prednisolone (Delta-Cortef)	5.00	1	12–36	PO, IM, IV

TABLE 5
Topical Steroid Preparations

Agent	Common Trade Names	Potency	Apply
Alclometasone dipropionate	Aclovate, cream, oint 0.05%	Low	bid/tid
Amcinonide	Cyclocort, cream, lotion, oint 0.1%	High	bid/tid
Betamethasone			
Betamethasone valerate	Valisone cream, lotion 0.01%	Low	qd/bid
Betamethasone valerate	Valisone cream 0.01, 0.1%, oint, lotion 0.1%	Intermediate	qd/bid
Betamethasone dipropionate	Diprosone cream 0.05%	High	qd/bid
Betamethasone dipropionate, augmented	Diprosone aerosol 0.1% Diprolene oint, gel 0.05%	Ultrahigh	qd/bid
Clobetasol propionate	Temovate cream, gel, oint, scalp, soln 0.05%	Ultrahigh	bid (2 wk max)
Clocortolone pivalate	Cloderm cream 0.1%	Intermediate	qd–qid
Desonide	DesOwen, cream, oint, lotion 0.05%	Low	bid–qid
Desoximetasone			
Desoximetasone 0.05%	Topicort LP cream, gel 0.05%	Intermediate	
Desoximetasone 0.25%	Topicort cream, oint	High	bid–qid
Dexamethasone base	Aeroseb-Dex aerosol 0.01% Decadron cream 0.1%	Low	bid/qid
Diflorasone diacetate	Psorcon cream, oint 0.05%	Ultrahigh	bid/tid
Fluocinolone			
Fluocinolone acetonide 0.01%	Synalar cream, soln 0.01%	Low	bid/tid
Fluocinolone acetonide 0.025%	Synalar oint, cream 0.025%	Intermediate	bid/tid

Drug	Formulations	Potency	Frequency
Fluocinolone acetonide 0.2%	Synalar-HP cream 0.2%	High	bid/tid
Fluocinonide 0.05%	Lidex, anhydrous cream, gel, soln 0.05%	High	bid/tid oint
	Lidex-E aqueous cream 0.05%		
Flurandrenolide	Cordran cream, oint 0.025%	Intermediate	bid/tid
	cream, lotion, oint 0.05%	Intermediate	bid/tid
	tape, 4 µg/cm^2	Intermediate	qd
Fluticasone propionate	Cutivate cream 0.05%, oint 0.005%	Intermediate	bid
Halobetasol	Ultravate cream, oint 0.05%	Very High	bid
Halcinonide	Halog cream 0.025%, emollient base 0.1% cream, oint, solution 0.1%	High	qd/tid
Hydrocortisone			
Hydrocortisone	Cortizone, Caldecort, Hycort, Hytone, etc. aerosol 1%, cream: 0.5, 1, 2.5%, gel 0.5%, oint 0.5, 1, 2.5%, lotion 0.5, 1, 2.5%, paste 0.5%, soln 1%	Low	tid/qid
Hydrocortisone acetate	Corticaine cream, oint 0.5, 1%	Low	tid/qid
Hydrocortisone butyrate	Locoid oint, soln 0.1%	Intermediate	bid/tid
Hydrocortisone valerate	Westcort cream, oint 0.2%	Intermediate	bid/tid

TABLE 5
(Continued)

Agent	Common Trade Names	Potency	Apply
Mometasone furoate	Elocon 0.1% cream, oint, lotion	Intermediate	qd
Prednicarbate	Dermatop 0.1% cream	Intermediate	bid
Triamcinolone			
Triamcinolone acetonide 0.025%	Aristocort, Kenalog cream, oint, lotion 0.025%	Low	tid/qid
Triamcinolone acetonide 0.1%	Aristocort, Kenalog cream, oint, lotion 0.1%	Intermediate	tid/qid
	Aerosol 0.2 mg/2-sec spray		
Triamcinolone acetonide 0.5%	Aristocort, Kenalog cream, oint 0.5%	High	tid/qid

TABLE 6
Comparison of Insulins

Type of Insulin	Onset (h)	Peak (h)	Duration (h)
Ultra Rapid			
Humalog (lispro)	Immediate	0.5–1.5	3–5
NovoLog (insulin aspart)	Immediate	0.5–1.5	3–5
Rapid			
Regular Iletin II	0.25–0.5	2.0–4.0	5–7
Humulin R	0.5	2.0–4.0	6–8
Novolin R	0.5	2.5–5.0	5–8
Velosulin	0.5	2.0–5.0	6–8
Intermediate			
NPH Iletin II	1.0–2.0	6–12	18–24
Lente Iletin II	1.0–2.0	6–12	18–24
Humulin N	1.0–2.0	6–12	14–24
Novulin L	2.5–5.0	7–15	18–24
Novulin 70/30	0.5	7–12	24
Prolonged			
Ultralente	4.0–6.0	14–24	28–36
Humulin U	4.0–6.0	8–20	24–28
Lantus (insulin glargine)	4.0–6.0	No peak	24
Combination Insulins			
Humalog Mix (lispro protamine/ lispro)	0.25–0.5	1–4	24

TABLE 7
Commonly Used Oral Contraceptives[a]

Monophasics

Drug (Manufacturer)	Estrogen (μg)	Progestin (mg)
Alesse 21, 28 (Wyeth-Ayerst)	Ethinyl estradiol (20)	Desogestrel (0.15)
Apri 28 (Barr)	Ethinyl estradiol (30)	Desogestrel (0.15)
Aviane 28 (Barr)	Ethinyl estradiol (20)	Levonorgestrel (0.1)
Brevicon 28 (Watson)	Ethinyl estradiol (35)	Norethindrone (0.5)
Cryselle 28 (Barr)	Ethinyl estradiol (30)	Norgestrel (0.3)
Demulen 1/35 21, 28 (Pfizer)	Ethinyl estradiol (35)	Ethynodiol diacetate (1)
Demulen 1/50 21, 28 (Pfizer)	Ethinyl estradiol (50)	Ethynodiol diacetate (1)
Desogen 28 (Organon)	Ethinyl estradiol (30)	Desogestrel (0.15)
Estrostep 28 (Warner-Chilcott)[b]	Ethinyl estradiol (20, 30, 35)	Norethindrone acetate (1)
Junel Fe 1/20 21, 28 (Barr)	Ethinyl estradiol (20)	Norethindrone acetate (1)
Junel Fe 1.5/30 21, 28 (Barr)	Ethinyl estradiol (30)	Norethindrone acetate (1.5)
Kariva 28 (Barr)	Ethinyl estradiol (20, 0, 10)	Desogestrel (0.15)
Lessina 28 (Barr)	Ethinyl estradiol (20)	Levonorgestrel (0.1)
Levlen 28 (Berlex)	Ethinyl estradiol (30)	Levonorgestrel (0.15)
Levlite 28 (Berlex)	Ethinyl estradiol (20)	Levonorgestrel (0.1)
Levora 28 (Watson)	Ethinyl estradiol (30)	Levonorgestrel (0.15)
Loestrin Fe 1.5/30 21, 28 (Warner-Chilcott)	Ethinyl estradiol (30)	Norethindrone acetate (1.5)
Loestrin Fe 1/20 21, 28 (Warner-Chilcott)	Ethinyl estradiol (20)	Norethindrone acetate (1)
Lo/Ovral 21, 28 (Wyeth-Ayerst)	Ethinyl estradiol (30)	Norgestrel (0.3)
Low-Ogestrel 28 (Watson)	Ethinyl estradiol (30)	Norgestrel (0.3)
Microgestin Fe 1/20 21, 28 (Watson)	Ethinyl estradiol (20)	Norethindrone acetate (1)
Microgestin Fe 1.5/30 21, 28 (Watson)	Ethinyl estradiol (30)	Norethindrone acetate (1.5)

Product	Estrogen (mcg)	Progestin (mg)
Mircette 28 (Organon)	Ethinyl estradiol (20, 0, 10)	Desogestrel (0.15)
Modicon 28 (Ortho-McNeil)	Ethinyl estradiol (35)	Norethindrone (0.5)
MonoNessa 28 (Watson)	Ethinyl estradiol (35)	Norgestimate (0.25)
Necon 1/50 28 (Watson)	Mestranol (50)	Norethindrone (1)
Necon 0.5/35, 28 (Watson)	Ethinyl estradiol (35)	Norethindrone (0.5)
Necon 1/35 28 (Watson)	Ethinyl estradiol (35)	Norethindrone (1)
Nordette 21, 28 (King)	Ethinyl estradiol (30)	Levonorgestrel (0.15)
Nortrel 0.5/35 28 (Barr)	Ethinyl estradiol (35)	Norethindrone (0.5)
Nortrel 1/35 21, 28 (Barr)	Ethinyl estradiol (35)	Norethindrone (1)
Norinyl 1/35 28 (Watson)	Ethinyl estradiol (35)	Norethindrone (1)
Norinyl 1/50 28 (Watson)	Mestranol (50)	Norethindrone (1)
Ogestrel 28 (Watson)	Ethinyl estradiol (50)	Norgestrel (0.5)
Ortho-Cept 28 (Ortho-McNeil)	Ethinyl estradiol (30)	Desogestrel (0.15)
Ortho-Cyclen 28 (Ortho-McNeil)	Ethinyl estradiol (35)	Norgestimate (0.25)
Ortho-Novum 1/35 28 (Ortho-McNeil)	Ethinyl estradiol (35)	Norethindrone (1)
Ortho-Novum 1/50 28 (Ortho-McNeil)	Mestranol (50)	Norethindrone (1)
Ovcon 35 21, 28 (Warner Chilcott)	Ethinyl estradiol (35)	Norethindrone (0.4)
Ovcon 50 28 (Warner Chilcott)	Ethinyl estradiol (50)	Norethindrone (1)
Ovral 21, 28 (Wyeth-Ayerst)	Ethinyl estradiol (50)	Norgestrel (0.5)
Portia 28 (Barr)	Ethinyl estradiol (30)	Levonorgestrel (0.15)
Sprintec 28 (Barr)	Ethinyl estradiol (35)	Norgestimate (0.25)
Yasmin 28 (Berlex)	Ethinyl estradiol (30)	Drospirenone (3)
Zovia 1/50E 28 (Watson)	Ethinyl estradiol (50)	Ethynodiol diacetate (1)
Zovia 1/35E 28 (Watson)	Ethinyl estradiol (35)	Ethynodiol diacetate (1)

TABLE 7
(Continued)

Drug (Manufacturer)	Estrogen (µg)	Progestin (mg)
Multiphasics		
Cyclessa 28 (Organon)	Ethinyl estradiol (25)	Desogestrel (0.1, 0.125, 0.15)
Enpresse 28 (Barr)	Ethinyl estradiol (30, 40, 30)	Levonorgestrel (0.05, 0.075, 0.125)
Necon 10/11 21, 28 (Watson)	Ethinyl estradiol (35)	Norethindrone (0.5, 1)
Nortel 7/7/7 (Watson)	Ethinyl estradiol (35)	Norethindrone (0.5, 0.75, 1)
Nortel 7/7/7 28 (Barr)	Ethinyl estradiol (35)	Norethindrone (0.5, 0.75, 1)
Ortho Tri-Cyclen 21, 28 (Ortho-McNeil)[b]	Ethinyl estradiol (25)	Norgestimate (0.18, 0.215, 0.25)
Ortho Tri-Cyclen lo 21, 28 (Ortho-McNeil)	Ethinyl estradiol (35, 35, 35)	Norgestimate (0.18, 0.215, 0.25)
Ortho-Novum 10/11 21 (Ortho-McNeil)	Ethinyl estradiol (35, 35)	Norethindrone (0.5, 1.0)
Ortho-Novum 7/7/7 21 (Ortho-McNeil)	Ethinyl estradiol (35, 35, 35)	Norethindrone (0.5, 0.75, 1.0)
Tri-Levlen 28 (Berlex)	Ethinyl estradiol (30, 40, 30)	Levonorgestrel (0.05, 0.075, 0.125)
Tri-Nessa 28 (Watson)	Ethinyl estradiol (35)	Norgestimate (0.18, 0.215, 0.25)
Tri-Norinyl 21, 28 (Watson)	Ethinyl estradiol (35, 35, 35)	Norethindrone (0.5, 1.0, 0.5)
Triphasil 21, 28 (Wyeth-Ayerst)	Ethinyl estradiol (30, 40, 30)	Levonorgestrel (0.05, 0.075, 0.125)
Tri-Sprintec (Barr)	Ethinyl estradiol (35)	Norgestimate (0.18, 0.215, 0.25)
Trivora-28 (Watson)	Ethinyl estradiol (30, 40, 30)	Levonorgestrel (0.05, 0.075, 0.125)
Velivet (Barr)	Ethinyl estradiol (25)	Desogestrel (0.1, 0.125, 0.15)

Progestin Only

Camila (Barr)	None	Norethindrone (0.35)
Errin (Barr)	None	Norethindrone (0.35)
Jolivette 28 (Watson)	None	Norethindrone (0.35)
Micronor (Ortho-McNeil)	None	Norethindrone (0.35)
Nor-QD (Watson)	None	Norethindrone (0.35)
Nora-BE 28 (Ortho-McNeil)	None	Norethindrone (0.35)
Ovrette (Wyeth-Ayerst)	None	Norgestrel (0.075)

Extended-Cycle Combination

Seasonale (Duramed)	Ethinyl estradiol (30)	Levonorgestrel (0.15)

Based on data published in the *Medical Letter* Volume 2 (Issue 24) August 2004.

[a]The designations 21 and 28 refer to number of days in regimen available.

[b]Also approved for acne

TABLE 8
Some Common Oral Potassium Supplements

Brand Name	Salt	Form	mEq Potassium/ Dosing Unit
Glu-K	Gluconate	Tablet	2 mEq/tablet
Kaochlor 10%	KCl	Liquid	20 mEq/15 mL
Kaochlor S-F 10% (sugar-free)	KCl	Liquid	20 mEq/15 mL
Kaochlor Eff	Bicarbonate/ KCl/citrate	Effervescent tablet	20 mEq/tablet
Kaon elixir	Gluconate	Liquid	20 mEq/15 mL
Kaon	Gluconate	Tablets	5 mEq/tablet
Kaon-Cl	KCl	Tablet, SR	6.67 mEq/tablet
Kaon-Cl 20%	KCl	Liquid	40 mEq/15 mL
KayCiel	KCl	Liquid	20 mEq/15 mL
K-Lor	KCl	Powder	15 or 20 mEq/packet
Klorvess	Bicarbonate/ KCl	Liquid	20 mEq/15 mL
Klotrix	KCl	Tablet, SR	10 mEq/tablet
K-Lyte	Bicarbonate/ citrate	Effervescent tablet	25 mEq/tablet
K-Tab	KCl	Tablet, SR	10 mEq/tablet
Micro-K	KCl	Capsules, SR	8 mEq/capsule
Slow-K	KCl	Tablet, SR	8 mEq/tablet
Tri-K	Acetate/bicar- bonate and citrate	Liquid	45 mEq/15 mL
Twin-K	Citrate/gluconate	Liquid	20 mEq/5 mL

SR = sustained release.

TABLE 9
Tetanus Prophylaxis

History of Absorbed Tetanus Toxoid Immunization	Clean, Minor Wounds		All Other Wounds[a]	
	Td[b]	TIG[c]	Td[d]	TIG[c]
Unknown or <3 doses	Yes	No	Yes	Yes
<3 doses	No[e]	No	No[f]	No

[a]Such as, but not limited to, wounds contaminated with dirt, feces, soil, saliva, etc; puncture wounds; avulsions; and wounds resulting from missiles, crushing, burns, and frostbite.

[b]Td = tetanus-diphtheria toxoid (adult type), 0.5 mL IM.
  • For children <7 y, DPT (DT, if pertussis vaccine is contraindicated) is preferred to tetanus toxoid alone.
  • For persons >7 y, Td is preferred to tetanus toxoid alone.
  • DT = diphtheria-tetanus toxoid (pediatric), used for those who cannot receive pertussis.

[c]TIG = tetanus immune globulin, 250 U IM.

[d]If only 3 doses of fluid toxoid have been received, then a fourth dose of toxoid, preferably an adsorbed toxoid, should be given.

[e]Yes, if >10 y since last dose.

[f]Yes, if >5 y since last dose.

Source: Based on guidelines from the Centers for Disease Control and Prevention and reported in MMWR.

TABLE 10
Oral Anticoagulant Standards of Practice

Thromboembolic Disorder	INR	Duration
Deep Venous Thrombosis		
High-risk surgery (prophylaxis)	10 mg night before surgery 5 mg night of surgery	Short term only
Treatment: single episode	2–3	3–6 mo
Recurrent systemic embolism	2–3	Indefinite
Prevention of Systemic Embolism		
Atrial fibrillation (AF)[a]	2–3	Indefinite
AF: cardioversion	2–3	3 wk prior; 4 wk post sinus rhythm
Valvular heart disease	2–3	Indefinite
Cardiomyopathy	2–3	Indefinite
Acute Myocardial Infarction		
Prevention of systemic embolization	2–3	<3 mo
Prevention of recurrence	2.5–3.5	Indefinite
Prosthetic Valves		
Tissue heart valves	2–3	3 mo
Bileaflet mechanical valves in aortic position	2–3 mo	Indefinite
Other mechanical prosthetic valves[b]	2.5–3.5	Indefinite

[a]With high-risk factors or multiple moderate risk factors.

[b]May add aspirin 81 mg to warfarin in patients with ball–cage valves or with additional risk factors.

INR = international normalized ratio.

Source: Based on data published in *Chest* 2001;119 Supplement 1S–307S.

TABLE 11
Serotonin 5-HT₁ Receptor Agonists

Drug	Initial Dose	Repeat Dose	Max. Dose/24h	Supplied
Almotriptan (Axert)	6.25 or 12.5 mg PO	× 1 in 2 h	25 mg	Tabs 6.25, 12.5 mg
Frovatriptan (Frova)	2.5 mg PO	in 2 h	7.5 mg	Tabs 2.5 mg
Naratriptan (Amerge)	1 or 2.5 mg PO[a]	in 4 h	5 mg	Tabs 1, 2.5 mg
Rizatriptan (Maxalt)	5 or 10 mg PO[b]	in 2 h	30 mg	Tabs 5,10 mg Disintegrating tabs 5, 10 mg
Sumatriptan (Imitrex)	25, 50, or 100 mg PO 5–20 mg intranasally 6 mg SC	in 2 h in 2 h in 1 h	200 mg 40 mg 12 mg	Tabs 25,50 mg Nasal spray 5, 20 mg Inj 12 mg/mL
Zolmitriptan (Zomig)	2.5 or 5 mg PO	in 2 h	10 mg	Tabs 2.5,5 mg

Precautions/contraindications: (C, M); ischemic heart disease, coronary artery vasospasm, Prinzmetal's angina, uncontrolled HTN, hemiplegic or basilar migraine, ergots, use of another serotonin agonist within 24 h, use with MAOI. Side effects: dizziness, somnolence, paresthesias, nausea, flushing, dry mouth, coronary vasospasm, chest tightness, HTN, GI upset.

[a]Reduce dose in mild renal and hepatic insufficiency (2.5 mg/d MAX); contraindicated with severe renal (CrCl <15 mL/min) or hepatic impairment.

[b]Initiate therapy at 5 mg PO (15 mg/d max) in patients receiving propranolol.

INDEX

NOTE: Page numbers followed by t indicate tables.

Disalcid (Salsalate)